ALTERNATIVE APPROACHES TO HUMAN BLOOD RESOURCES IN CLINICAL PRACTICE

DEVELOPMENTS IN HEMATOLOGY AND IMMUNOLOGY

Volume 33

The titles published in this series are listed at the end of this volume.

Alternative Approaches to Human Blood Resources in Clinical Practice

Proceedings of the Twenty-Second International Symposium on Blood Transfusion, Groningen 1997, organized by the Red Cross Blood Bank Noord Nederland

edited by

C. Th. SMIT SIBINGA and P. C. DAS

Red Cross Blood Bank Noord Nederland, The Netherlands

and

J.C. FRATANTONI

C.L. McIntosh & Ass., Rockville, MD, U.S.A.

SPRINGER SCIENCE+BUSINESS MEDIA, B.V.

A C.I.P. Catalogue record for this book is available from the Library of Congress.

ISBN 978-1-4613-7571-5 ISBN 978-1-4615-5619-0 (eBook)
DOI 10.1007/978-1-4615-5619-0

Printed on acid-free paper

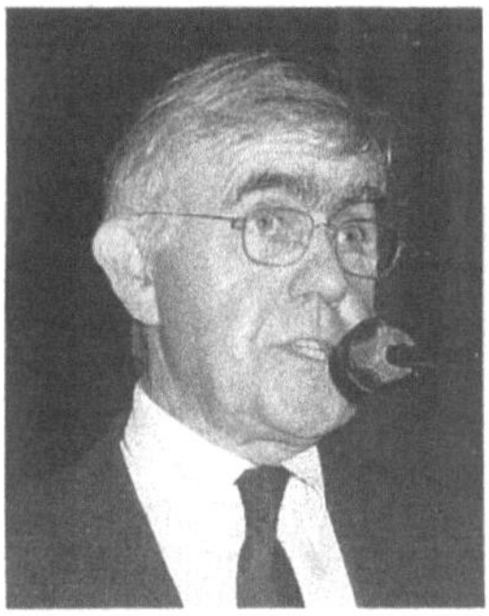

Dr. Cees Th. Smit Sibinga
Initiator and Organizer

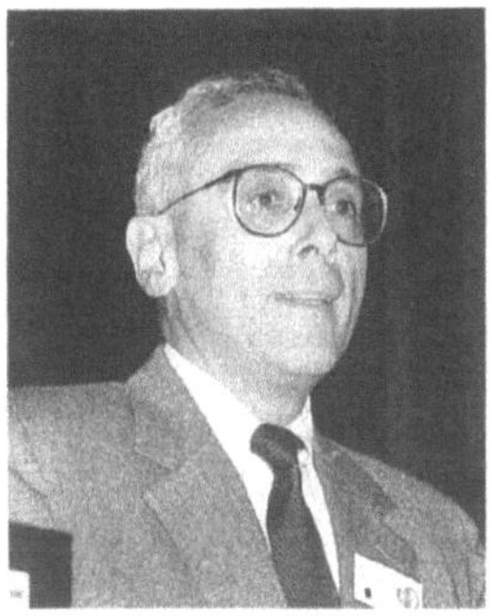

Dr. Joseph C. Fratantoni
Chairman

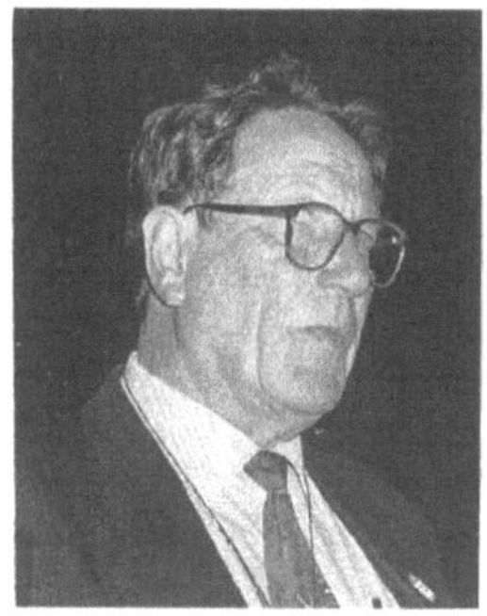

Prof. Dr. Jon J. van Rood
Opening Address

Baxter

Acknowledgement

This publication has been made possible through the support of Baxter, which is gratefully acknowledged.

CONTENTS

MODERATORS AND SPEAKERS

Moderators

J.F. Fratantoni (chairman)	– C.L. McIntosh & Associates Inc., Rockville, MD, USA
P.C. Das	– Red Cross Blood Bank Noord Nederland, Groningen, NL
L.T. Goodnough	– Washington University School of Medicine, St. Louis, MO, USA
C.Th. Smit Sibinga	– Red Cross Blood Bank Noord Nederland, Groningen, NL
C.R. Valeri	– Naval Blood Research Laboratory, Boston, MS, USA
H.J.C. de Wit	– Red Cross Blood Bank Noord Nederland, Groningen, NL
J.Th.M. de Wolf	– Academic Hospital Groningen, Department of Haematology, Groningen, NL

Speakers

W.G. van Aken	– Central Laboratory for the Blood Transfusion of the Dutch Red Cross, Amsterdam, NL
J.P. AuBuchon	– Dartmouth-Hitchcock Medical Center, Lebanon, NH, USA
P.L. Baele	– University Clinic St. Luc, Department of Anaesthesiology, Brussels, B
P.C. Hébert	– Loeb Medical Research Institute, Ottawa, Ontario, C
F. Falkenburg	– Eurocord Foundation Nederland, Leiden, NL
D. Fergusson	– Ottawa Civic Hospital, Clinical Epidemiology Unit, Ottawa, Ontario, C
A.W.M.M. Koopman-van Gemert	– Hospital Gooi-Noord, Blaricum, NL
A. Laupacis	– Ottawa Civic Hospital, Ottawa, Ontario, C
L. de Leij	– Academic Hospital Groningen, Department of Clinical Immunology, Groningen, NL

W.G. Murphy – Blood Transfusion Service Board, Dublin, IRL

D.M. Nicolson – Viragen (Scotland) Ltd., Midlothian, UK

V. Rocha – European Researc Project of Cord Blood Transplantation, Paris, F

R.K. Spence – Staten Island University Hospital, Staten Island, NY, USA

E.G.E. de Vries – Academic Hospital Groningen, Department of Clinical Oncology, Groningen, NL

R.M. Winslow – Veterans Affairs Medical Center, UC San Diego, San Diego, CA, USA

Prepared discussant

S. Middleton – Andaris Ltd., Nottingham, UK

FOREWORD

Approaches to Human Blood Resources in Clinical Practice. This is certainly a timely topic in a world in which it becomes more and more difficult to motivate the public to donate an ever increasing number of units of blood. It is obvious that this confronts us with the need to use the existing supply as efficiently as possible and explore alternative sources, which in part could replace blood. This course will address this issue.

This meeting exemplifies Cees Smit Sibinga's foresight when he started these meetings 22 years ago. These symposia have become quite well known in the transfusion world, and rightly so.

I think it is appropriate to congratulate Cees Smit Sibinga in putting the program of this year together. I am happy that we have in the Netherlands top level professionals in blood transfusion medicine, such as Cees Smit Sibinga and his colleagues. Thanks to their expertise we now have in the Netherlands an officially recognised speciality in blood transfusion medicine of which the curriculum has been approved. It is for that reason most unfortunate that the Netherlands is one of the very, very few countries in which there is no university chair in blood transfusion medicine. I feel that I can say this so strongly, because, at my farewell party as chief of the Department of Immuno–hematology and Blood Bank in Leiden, I expressed the wish that also in the Netherlands we soon would have a chair in transfusion medicine. This was now more than six years ago. As Hegel put it: "If the end of the world is imminent go to the Netherlands: everything happens there 50 years later!"

I can imagine that some of you wonder why I should open this meeting, and I will try to explain that to you. In the first place I have been interested in blood transfusion and blood banking since 1950 when I for the first time entered a blood bank in New York in the Presbyterian Hospital to donate blood. I was living at that time as a clinical clerk on a dollar a day and I wanted to take my girlfriend out. One unit of blood was $10 and that was a lot of money at that time. I can assure you that I have often given blood, but never for money again.

In 1952 I became, as a junior resident of internal medicine, responsible for the blood bank. I have enjoyed being the boss of the blood bank until the early 90's. I have also received blood transfusion both in the context of platelet transfusion experiments (and suffered from a non haemolytic TR) and clinically during an operation. Finally, in the last ten years I had the opportunity to watch the blood transfusion field from a fourth position, as chairman of the Medical Advisory Committee (MAC) of the Dutch Blood Transfusion Board, in which it was our task to scrutinise the whole process of donation of blood by the donor, the processing in the blood bank and the evaluation of the results of the blood transfusion. I have thus been involved in blood transfusion in many different ways. And as I am standing here anyhow I would like to use this opportunity to share with you a few of my thoughts on blood transfusion practice in the years to come.

The point we are of course all interested in is BTY2000 or the state of affairs of blood transfusion in the year 2000. There are at least three issues which need our attention; the issue of logistics, the issue of safety and the issue of effectiveness.

As far as the logistics are concerned the field is doing well. We are set on a course which is clearly heading towards unification, standardisation, and internationalisation. Everything said and done, I would call the way things are developing as far as logistics is concerned, optimal and for that reason will not spend more time on it.

About the second topic, that of safety, I am far less happy. Safety is of course the prime concern of patients who receive the blood, and rightly so. We can truly say that blood transfusion is an extremely safe procedure. I just heard that the likelihood of dying of a blood transfusion is in the same order of magnitude of being killed in a thunder storm. Still it is certain that not everyone is satisfied and it is completely understandable that patients whose life depends on a regular blood transfusion will feel that safe is still not safe enough. This is understandable and of course we should listen and discuss this.

Nevertheless, sometimes this leads to a situation in which we strive to *maximal* safety, but where one can wonder whether the money needed for that is spend *optimally*.

To give you one example, not too long ago the MAC received from the Ministry of Health the question whether or not blood donors should be screened for HTLV-I, a virus which is extremely uncommon in the Netherlands. The MAC of the Dutch Transfusion Board studied the incidence, risk, costs and benefit of HTLV-I screening. And from that we learned that the costs would be about DFl. 8 million a year and the profit would be that in all probability 1 human life could be saved in 10 years. In other words, one human life at the cost of DFl. 80 million.

At the same time that our report on HTLV-I testing had been sent to the minister, the central laboratory of the Red Cross opened its new processing facility. The Minister of Health came over to open it and referred to this report and said: "Of course a human life is worth DFl. 80 million and we will therefore screen for HTLV-I", which was contrary to the advice the Medical Advisory Committee had given. It is of course wonderful that the Ministry of Health thinks the safety of blood can really command such large sums of money, and everybody should be very happy, if there were not a few questions which remain unanswered.

What were the arguments of the Ministry of Health to decide, contrary to the advice of the Medical Advisory Committee, to start the screening for HTLV-I?

Did the fear of liability play a role? Almost certainly it did and for anyone who watched the impact of AIDS HIV on transfusion medicine quite understandably so. But there is also the nagging question whether when such a large sum of money is spent on HTLV-I screening, there would be no other side effects of blood transfusion which need to be taken care of.

Of course such complications exist, bacterial infections which kill more patients than viral infections and immunological complications varying from non-haemolytic transfusion reactions to the deadly Graft-versus-Host disease.

To bring the discussion on this problem in focus, i.e. the contrast between the wish of the patients (but also the public and the politicians) for maximal safety of blood products on the one hand and the obvious need to spend the available funds optimally, which implies that also the other complications should be taken care of, we organised a symposium a year ago on "optimal versus maximal safety of the blood transfusion products"[1]. The meeting was mainly focussed on an inventory of the problems one encounters when trying to make a choice between optimal and maximal blood transfusion policies.

It was soon clear that there should be follow-up meetings, hopefully on an international level. There was already during this first meeting a consensus that in a discussion on the choice between maximal and optimal safety not only the experts, but also the public should take a part.

As far as effectiveness is concerned, here too the situation is heterogeneous: on one side the effectiveness of blood, platelets and blood product transfusion has increased enormously and can be (but unfortunately is not always) monitored. On the other hand many potentially very important clinical effects of blood transfusion are largely ignored if not simply forgotten. Blood transfusions can immunise, tolerate and cure cancer (in the case relapse of chronic myeloid leukaemia after bone marrow transplantation), but no-one knows when and how, and (almost) nobody seems to care.

As a result it is very difficult to study these effects of blood transfusion. We should try to change that. To that end it will be of prime importance that each hospital activates its (legally required) blood transfusion committee (BTC) and that these committees will have sufficient authority. Their task should not be limited to the indication of blood and its products; when to give what and how much, but also should include the follow-up.

There again, not only the effectiveness of the transfusion should be monitored by these BTC's but also the early and even more important the late complications; whether infectious or immunological. We need the BTC's and we need them now. Transfusion medicine is a recognised clinical speciality which should be implemented. It is clear that we have come a long way and it is equally clear

---

1. Poel CL van der, Boer JEG de, Reesink HW, Smit Sibinga CTh. Optimale versus maximale veiligheid van de bloedtransfusieketen in Nederland; resultaten van een conferentie. NTvG 1998;142:285-88.

that many issues remain unresolved and that we need the help and support of the public to achieve that. In this awareness process the symposia organised in Groningen already played and continue to play an important role. I am sure you will enjoy the meeting.

Prof. Dr. J.J. van Rood

I. THE CLINICAL SETTING: HOW TO OPTIMISE SUPPORTIVE HAEMOTHERAPY

PRINCIPLES OF SUPPORTIVE HAEMOTHERAPY

W.G. van Aken

Introduction

The safe and adequate supply of blood, blood components and plasma products is indispensable to a variety of medical disciplines. The term haemotherapy is commonly used to indicate the administration of whole blood, cellular blood components, plasma and plasma products as well as certain synthetic products which may replace blood substances. When used in patients who suffer from hereditary or acquired deficiency of certain blood or plasma components such as factor VIII or immunoglobulins, the aim is to correct the lacking factor or component thereby decreasing the risk of e.g., bleeding, infection, or shock. This correction is, however, temporarily due to the limited life span of the administered blood or plasma component. The adjective curative or definitive can only be used restrictive in the context of haemotherapy although in recent years there is evidence that some plasma components (such as immunoglobulins) may cure certain autoimmune diseases. Supportive haemotherapy is used when other treatment modalities, such as irradiation, cytostatic drugs, surgical procedures, affect the volume and the composition of circulating blood or blood cell precursors to such an extent that the clinical condition deteriorates. In clinical practice the distinction between the different types of haemotherapy, i.e. corrective, curative and supportive, is usually not strict. The term supportive haemotherapy is commonly used for a large variety of situations where transfusion of blood , blood components and plasma derivatives is required.

Developments in haemotherapy

Since the last three decades haemotherapy is changing rapidly. Before the 1970s in most countries transfusion of whole blood was used. When, however, plastic blood bags became available for collection and storage of blood donations, practical difficulties related to centrifugation and sterility were solved and component technology started to be introduced. Components such as red cells, platelets and plasma are now prepared aseptically and stored in concentrated form so that patients may be given only the cellular or plasma component that they need. The use of components instead of whole blood has greatly increased the efficiency of blood donations, and improved both the safety of transfusions and the logistics of blood products. Once the availability of blood components started to change, procedures like bone marrow transplantation and open heart surgery, which could not be adequately supported by transfusions of whole blood, became feasible.

At present a variety of products derived from blood and plasma is available for clinical use. Thus, haemotherapy may be "tailored" to individual patient needs. Besides separation of various types of blood cells, additional steps such as filtration, washing and irradiation may be included in component preparation to prevent immune reactions notably in patients which are at risk of developing transfusion reactions. The preparation of single donor platelet concentrates through apheresis is another illustration of the optimal provision of blood components for patients who have become refractory following previous platelet transfusions.

In the area of plasma derivatives the number of concentrates of clotting factors, protease inhibitors and immunoglobulins for clinical application has grown significantly. The purity and safety of these products has been improved, which led to less allergic reactions respectively to a substantial decrease of the risk of viral transmission. Products such as immunoglobulins which formerly could only be safely administered through the intramuscular route, are now also available for intravenous injection which allows the administration of much higher dosages than before. This is not only beneficial to patients with agammaglobulinemia, who formerly experienced painful intramuscular injections, but also for patients with autoimmune diseases such as idiopathic thrombocytopenia which require large dosages of polyvalent immunoglobulins. Another example of improved plasma component therapy is the availability of highly purified clotting factor concentrates which allows patients with severe haemophilia to start home treatment and most important to institute prophylactic substitution of clotting factor concentrates.

It is a matter of definition whether or not haemotherapy, apart from cellular components and plasma derivatives derived from human blood, also includes animal blood products, synthetic substances and DNA-recombinant products. Some of these alternatives are currently considered competitive with products derived from human blood and plasma in terms of safety and cost. It is expected that in the coming years the number of recombinant plasma proteins for clinical usage will grow and gradually - partly or completely – will replace some conventional plasma products. Furthermore haemoglobin solutions will start to compete with red cell concentrates. The availability of recombinant haematopoietic growth factors such as erythropoietin and in the very near future thrombopoietin will affect haemotherapy of a number of diseases.

Table 1. Principles of haemotherapy

– Estimate risks vs. benefits using best evidence
– Identify cause(s) of deficiency
– Administer only component(s) which is (are) deficient
– Products(s) should be as safe as possible
– Monitor (side) effects of blood transfusions

Thus, it is clear that the field of haemotherapy is broad and complex both in terms of products and indications. Acceptance of certain criteria or principles (Table 1) may assist in promoting the optimal and safe usage of these products.

Principles of haemotherapy

Like all other medical treatments, blood transfusions should be prescribed only after weighing the risks and assessment of the benefits of the therapy. In general the potential risks associated with blood transfusions are well known and the application of methods to reduce hazards such as blood group incompatibility, transmission of blood borne diseases, and alloimmunization to blood cell antigens is now routine in blood banks. As a result the blood supply is safer as has ever been. However, as it is not realistic to expect a "zero risk" situation it is important that transfusion practices are not liberalized and that the decision to transfuse is not taken lightly.

Most transfusions are given to prevent adverse events like bleedings, decreased oxygen delivery and drop of blood pressure which are anticipated or occur as part of certain diseases or situations (e.g. surgery). The evidence that blood transfusions have improved mortality and morbidity in defined patient groups is however mostly not substantiated by the results of well designed clinical studies. Whereas the rationale for haemotherapy in patients with clotting factor deficiencies (e.g. haemophilia) has been demonstrated by studies in which outcome was measured, the benefits of red cell transfusion in many indications have not been established in a scientifically satisfactory way.

Secondly, before haemotherapy is started the cause of the deficiency. which is the reason for the transfusion of blood or blood components, should in principle be identified. This seems self evident but very often transfusions are given without sufficient information about the nature and the severity of the disease or the condition for which the patient is admitted. It is evident that there are conditions, notably emergency situations, when the clinical diagnosis is not yet established or the outcome of laboratory measurements is not available whereas the severity of the disease does not allow further delay until blood transfusion is started. However, frequently perioperative red cell transfusions are given without sufficient evidence that oxygen delivery is likely to be increased. The so-called transfusion trigger, i.e. the lower limit of normovolemic anaemia at which transfusion of red cells is indicated, is not well established. Recent studies suggest that the practice of starting transfusion only when the haemoglobin level is less than 10 g/dL is no longer uniformly accepted [1]. Even in elderly patients red cell transfusions may not be necessary with haemoglobin levels equal or higher than 8 g/dL. However, it is questionable if it is allowed to decide purely on the basis of this parameter, as it is necessary to carefully consider clinical parameters (e.g. mental status, cardiac condition) and the risk of additional blood loss.

Since component therapy is currently available in most hospitals it is logical to advocate that only the component for which the patient is deficient should be administered. The usage of whole blood for transfusion has dropped significantly in recent years and the need for such transfusion is considered non existent. Similarly, there is consensus that fresh frozen plasma should only be transfused in a limited number of disorders such as thrombotic thrombocytopenic purpura, bleeding episodes in severe liver disease, and rare clotting factor deficiencies (e.g. factor V deficiency) for which no concentrates are available. However, there continue to be variations in the consumption of blood products, not only between hospitals but also between countries. Consensus development conferences as well as recommendations of a number of national and international organizations have contributed to defining standards regarding the indications for treatment but much work needs still to be done to harmonize the proper usage [2].

There are several other important issues of the practice of component therapy which are not yet settled. Firstly, the degree of deficiency which necessitates treatment with blood components or plasma derivatives. As was already briefly discussed for red cell transfusions, it is important to determine the risk benefit ratio notably for patients receiving fewer than 4 to 5 units of red cell concentrates. For the assessment of the need for platelet transfusions the distinction is whether or not the vascular system is intact and next if risk factors (such as sepsis, and concurrent use of drugs) are present. The number and function of platelets required to prevent oozing from, intact blood vessels is much less compared to the number needed to control blood loss when vascular damage is present. Platelet transfusions are indicated in patients with active bleeding as a result of a documented severe deficiency in either platelet number or function. In situations accompanied by massive bleeding where there is consensus to transfuse platelets if the platelet count is less than 50×10^9/l, other clinical criteria need to be taken into account [3].

Another question relates to the extent at which the deficiency should be corrected. Is it necessary to continue haemotherapy until the level of blood cells or plasma factors has been normalised or is it sufficiently safe and efficient to transfuse, to suboptimal levels? Obviously the answer will depend on the nature and circumstances of the clinical situation of individual patients but once again scientific evidence is required.

The dosage schedule for various blood products varies considerable among different hospitals and clinical departments for reasons which are not clear.

The next principle, i.e. the blood product should be as safe as possible, is pertinent to the responsibilities of blood banks and fractionation centers as manufacturers of blood and plasma products. Donor selection, screening of all donations with licensed reagents using validated methods, virus inactivation techniques where possible and fulfilling current Good Manufacturing Practice (cGMP) are among the most important measures to guarantee optimal safety. However, safety is also dependent on the transfusion policy and practice in hospitals. Compatibility testing, storage and delivery of blood components and surveillance of the optimal usage of blood and blood products are among the tasks of the hospital transfusion service. The hospital transfusion committee should develop and monitor the transfusion policy which is then executed by various clinicians. In addition other bodies such as the hospital infection committee should be involved when it is uncertain if infections in recipients are due to blood transfusions or nosocomial (i.e. HCV).

Finally, systematic monitoring of the effects and adverse reactions of transfusions is necessary to control the quality and the safety of blood and plasma products. Post marketing surveillance is already performed for pharmaceuticals and more recently has also been introduced for plasma products. As for blood cell concentrates and plasma initiatives such as haemovigilance (France) and SHOT (UK), have been taken to optimize the complete chain from donor to recipient instead of only the production of these products.

Conclusion

The field of haemotherapy is rapidly moving towards a large range of products derived from human blood and plasma as well as from alternative sources. Most likely, competition between several products derived from different sources will stimulate clinical studies to provide more evidence about their risks and benefits. Good Transfusion Practice requires adherence to certain principles such as outlined. At the same time newly emerging transmissible agents will require constant surveillance of blood donor populations.

Reference

1. Carson JL, Duff A, Berlin JA. Perioperative transfusion and postoperative mortality. JAMA 1998;279:199-205.
2. Task Force on Blood Component Therapy. Practice guidelines for blood component therapy: a report by the American Society of Anaesthesiologists Task Force on Blood Component Therapy. Anaesthesiology 1996;84:732-47.
3. Consensus Conference on Platelet Transfusion. Proc R Coll Physicians. Edinb. 1998; 28:43-5.

WHAT SHOULD TRIGGER A TRANSFUSION?

W.G. Murphy

Introduction

Transfusion rates vary widely between [1-4], and probably also within [5,6] clinical centres, for procedures that might reasonably be expected to have similar transfusion demands or transfusion rates. The local practice may be defined by a number of factors, such as the local consensus on the postoperative haemoglobin level or platelet transfusion level, the preferences of opinion leaders in the local clinical community [7], the availability of a transfusion committee with an authoritative surveillance system, variations in supply or in local or regional risks or public perceptions of those risks.

While the above factors may influence what *does* trigger a transfusion, they do not necessarily define what *should* trigger a transfusion. The fact that variations do exist from clinician to clinician and from place to place indicates that the state of knowledge necessary to define best practice beyond reasonable doubt has not yet been reached for transfusion. This is probably more true for red cells than for platelets, and for both cellular components than for plasma; a large variation in plasma consumption suggests that in the presence of a reasonable consensus on indications [8,9] that poor penetration of current standards contributes in some part to transfusion practice and would indicate that clinician education is an important component of what should trigger a transfusion.

The situation is further complicated by the variation in risk from transfusion over time as well as from place to place. For some considerable time into the future it may not be possible to apply a general trigger for transfusion of cellular or non-cellular components.

However it should be possible to define certain broad principles as to what should trigger a transfusion, which will not differ from the principles applied to any therapeutic intervention planned in any patient. A transfusion should be triggered by a clear knowledge of the ability of the product transfused to achieve the desired therapeutic effect, a clear understanding of the risk involved in the transfusion of the product to be used for the patient being transfused, and even more ideally, a consent of the patient to the transfusion based on a clear understanding of the risks involved both in receiving and in not receiving the transfusion.

Red blood cell transfusion triggers

A transfusion of red cells is indicated when oxygen capacity is critically impaired or can be expected to become so in spite of other measures available and applicable. While this is reasonably self evident, the risk to the patient of an adverse outcome if no transfusion is received (i.e. the real indication for the transfusion) will depend on tissue oxygen delivery and requirement, on the rate of blood loss and on the presence of pre-existing and perhaps occult cardiovascular or other systems' disease. The risk of a contributory effect of pre-existing cardiorespiratory disease will vary with the patient's age, sex, and lifestyle, and will not be accurately predictable for the individual at the time the decision needs to be made about transfusion.

The area for debate on what should trigger a transfusion is mainly limited at present to haemoglobin or haematocrit levels [10-12]; this is an inappropriate limitation for several reasons. Haemoglobin level is limited as a surrogate for tissue oxygen delivery, which will vary according to several additional factors, including cardiac output and the red cell oxygen dissociation curve. Tissue oxygen requirements also vary independently of the red cell mass or the oxygen delivery capability of the blood and circulatory system, further limiting the usefulness of haemoglobin level as a trigger for red cell transfusion [11,12].

The point at which a transfusion is triggered also depends on the availability of alternatives for transfusion. Emerging haemoglobin solutions may dramatically alter transfusion triggers [13,14]; their place in the management of patients requiring support of oxygen delivery capacity will need to be carefully established by clinical trials.

The risk from blood transfusions is low; the risk of a serious misadventure in current practice is probably in the order of 1 in 100,000 though an accurate overall figure is not at present available [15]. It will be very difficult to demonstrate that withholding transfusion in a given setting will entail a lesser risk than transfusion for adverse outcome. Very few trials have addressed this question, and no published studies have had the power to resolve the issue in elective settings [4]. Blair et al randomised patients following gastrointestinal haemorrhage and with a haemoglobin level between 8 and 10 gm/dl to transfusion or to withholding transfusion; rebleeding and overall mortality were significantly higher in the transfused group [16]. The reason for this finding is unclear but may be related to the findings of the later studies of Marik & Sibbald whose data suggested that transfusions of older red blood cells can induce intestinal mucosal anoxia [17], which may have impaired local natural haemostasis.

This illustrates a major problem that exists in interpreting the results of trials of red cell transfusions. Red cells for transfusions are stored for up to 42 days, and are generally considered to be of therapeutic equivalence throughout their storage life. There are no data to support this universally held belief; if anything the reported data suggest the contrary to be true [17-19], and point to the need for careful clinical trials of red cells of different ages in different clinical settings, particularly in critically ill patients.

General availability of direct tissue oxygen delivery measurement would contribute to the improvement of the clinical ability to define the transfusion needs in individual patients, but would still not substitute for the results of good clinical trials.

Various studies have indicated that tissue perfusion is optimal at haemoglobin levels of 10 gms of haemoglobin [20,21] (which is not to say that patients *transfused to this level have optimal tissue oxygen delivery*). While conclusive evidence that this level correlates with optimal clinical outcome in various patient groups is unavailable the existing data do support the general consensus that there is little or no requirement to transfuse patients to a higher haemoglobin level [4,10-12]. Studies on the lower level necessitating transfusion are confined mainly to observational studies on patients refusing transfusions for religious reasons [22], or not receiving transfusions because of the unavailability of blood for transfusion [23]. These studies, though informative in general terms cannot provide a basis for defining risk free or minimal risk transfusion triggers in a broad range of clinical settings, mainly because of the current understanding of the low risk of transfusion in many countries. However we cannot be sure that new pathogens have not already entered the blood supply, so that our confidence in the level of risk for transfusion is uncertain. This makes the necessity for addressing the unresolved issues in red cell transfusion triggers all the more important.

What is needed to answer the question *what should trigger a red blood cell transfusion?* is the ability to determine the individual patient's oxygen delivery needs, the ability of available therapeutic modalities to meet those needs and up to date knowledge of the risks involved in meeting those needs along with the risks to the patient of leaving the needs unaddressed.

A comprehensive approach to a transfusion trigger will also require consideration of the dose required. Almost all transfusions are given in units, which contain 50 gms or more of red cell haemoglobin. This is probably a useful unit of formulation; certainly a lower one would result in some patients getting exposed to increased numbers of donors per therapeutic dose, which is almost certainly undesirable; conversely a higher unit volume may improve the risk benefit profile of red cell transfusions. In the meantime it is probably reasonable to state that in stable settings the necessity for transfusion needs to be reassessed on a unit by unit basis in an adult patient.

Transfusion triggers for platelet transfusions

Consensus as to what constitutes a trigger for platelet transfusion is generally possible [24-26], and can be based to some degree at least on useful studies comparing transfusion with no transfusion, so that the risks of not transfusing platelets in several settings can be estimated with some degree of confidence. As always, the applicability of the findings in one clinical study and in one clinical unit is not universal, and the general unwillingness to apply Gmür's strategy of withholding prophylactic platelet transfusion when the morning platelet count is above 5×10^9/L [27] reflects this; however it is generally accepted that the benefits of transfusing above a level of 10×10^9/L are unlikely to outweigh the current risks in patients receiving prophylactic platelet transfusions for bone marrow failure and who do not have any other significant haemostatic impairment [3,26]. Whether this position would change if there were a significant change in the risks of platelet transfusion, such as the routine introduction of virus inactivation of platelets [28], remains to be seen.

While prophylaxis in thrombocytopenic non-bleeding patients probably represents the single most common reason for platelet transfusion at present, a very large proportion of transfusions are given for haemostasis in bleeding thrombocytopenic patients and for surgical patients.

For bleeding thrombocytopenic patients the diagnosis constitutes the trigger; what is far from clear however is what product the patient should be transfused with, and in what dose so as to maximise the likelihood of benefit and to minimise the risk of transfusion. A similar situation exists for platelet transfusions in surgical patients: all platelet transfusions are treated as being of equal value in spite of the lack of substantive evidence to support this position. As is also the case for prophylactic transfusions it is not clear whether one type of platelet preparation is superior to another, or whether length of storage influences outcome in this indication, or whether a dose response curve can be derived.

Further problems exist in defining transfusion triggers for platelet transfusions in surgical patients. Recommendations vary as to whether in the massive transfusion setting transfusion of haemostatic agents including platelets should await the results of blood counts and clotting tests or whether it is reasonable to transfuse on the basis of clinical signs and history in the presence of microvascular bleeding [29-33]. Similar difficulties will exist in patients following cardiopulmonary bypass or during liver transplantation. At present sufficient grounds do not exist for the dogmatic setting of triggers in these settings; clinical conditions will often vary considerably from any ideal standard, the rate of change in the patient may be such as to render the use of time consuming measurements of very questionable benefit [29], and the risk of withholding platelets in any particular setting is impossible to compute at present. Probably the best that can be achieved in the current situation is to conclude that where the clinical conditions exist to provide a possibility for haemostatic failure due to thrombocytopenia or platelet function failure (such as rapid large volume transfusion with associated hypotension or cardiopulmonary bypass, especially redo surgery) along with the presence of microvascular bleeding then platelet transfusion is likely to be indicated. It should not generally be an absolute requirement that platelet counts be available before treatment is to commence [11], but equally it should not be assumed that thrombocytopenia is the only or main cause of the clinical haemostatic failure and coagulation testing should be ordered to support the clinical diagnosis.

The trigger for repeat or continued platelet transfusions in continuing haemorrhage in patients with bleeding due to thrombocytopenia or platelet function disorders is usually the observed therapeutic response. In patients with established bleeding an incrementing platelet transfusion is more likely to result in haemostatis than a non incrementing one [34,35]. In bleeding patients for whom an incrementing platelet transfusion cannot be given, either because compatible platelets are not available for a patient who is refractory because of an immunological cause, or because the patient is refractory because of a non-immunological reason, it is common practice to give multiple doses of platelets, often as fresh as possible. Published evidence that confirms the benefit of this approach is currently lacking, although recent studies suggest a rationale for transfusing unmatched platelets in this setting [36]: it is possible that platelets that do not survive to circulate in vivo can provide useful haemostatic activity by increasing fibrin deposition at the site of vascular injury.

Transfusion triggers for plasma transfusions

The use of plasma transfusion varies widely from country to country and from centre to centre, although it is probably the simplest blood component of all for which to define clinical indications and non-indications, and for which to apply audit standards [1,7,8,11]. It is also, by the same token the component for which a risk benefit ratio may be most easily determined, and favourably manipulated. The situation with regard to plasma is further simplified by the fact there are few grounds for dissent over variability of efficacy over the shelf life of the product (unlike red cells and platelets) or depending on the techniques of collection. This makes large variation in the use of the component particularly difficult to comprehend or justify.

The indications for plasma transfusion are treatment of thrombotic thrombocytopenic purpura, treatment of complex coagulopathies and treatment of plasma protein deficiencies where an alternative is not available. The indications for plasma transfusion are so few that it is difficult to see where any problem might lie in deciding whether an indication exists. Thus (other than for TTP) for a patient justifiably to receive a plasma transfusion the existence of an appropriate deficiency state must be established; for the most part this means that the presence of a clinical significant coagulopathy must be diagnosed. Difficulties may arise in determining at what point in a developing coagulopathy it becomes useful to transfuse a patient with plasma. While it may not always be necessary to have confirmation of a deficiency state by coagulation testing before treatment is instituted, a guess based on the number of transfusions the patient has already had is generally not considered sufficient justification for the risks of transfusion; clinical evidence of abnormal coagulation should be present [7,8,11].

For reversal of coumarin effect plasma may be indicated in certain settings, particularly where factor concentrate is unavailable or undesirable in a patient with established haemorrhage [37]; however transfusion will need to be approached cautiously in many of these patients because of the additional risks of volume overload in the presence of valvular heart disease.

In TTP all that remains to be established in terms of the transfusion trigger once the diagnosis is made is how much to give, at what interval, and for how long. In general most patients will require infusions of approximately one plasma volume per day for an average of seven or eight days [38]; considerably more may be necessary and many weeks of therapy are sometimes required. The therapeutic response may be guided by the plasma LDH and the platelet count, and the necessity to re-introduce therapy after remission is guided by careful monitoring of the platelet count. Plasmapheresis should be used in association with plasma therapy based on the available evidence [38]. Why plasma therapy works so predictably in TTP is a complete mystery [39], so that it could be maintained that in this condition, which is one of the firmest indications for blood component therapy, one of the principal triggers for transfusion is our inability to identify the need for it.

References

1. Sirchia G, Giovanetti AM, McClelland DBL, Fracchia GN. Safe and good use of blood in surgery (SANGUIS). Luxembourg: European Commission, 1994.
2. Murphy WG, Phillips P, Gray A, et al. Blood use for surgical patients: A study of Scottish hospital transfusion practices. JR Coll Surg Edinb 1995;40:10-13.
3. Murphy MF, Murphy W, Wheatley K, Goldstone AH. Survey of use of platelet transfusions in centres participating in MRC leukaemia trials. Brit J Haematol 1997;97,1(Abstract):59
4. Carson JL, Duff A, Berlin JA, et al. Perioperative blood transfusion and postoperative mortality. JAMA 1998;279;199-205.
5. McCullough J, Steeper TA, Connelly DP, et al. Platelet utilization in a univerity hospital. JAMA 1988;259:2414-18.
6. Milne AA, Murphy WG. Current blood transfusion practice in aortic aneurysm surgery in Scotland. JR Coll Surg Edinb 1995;40:104-8.
7. Nichols MD, White G. Red cell, plasma and albumin transfusion decision triggers. Anaesth Intensive Care 1993;21:156-62.
8. British Committee for Standards in Haematology. Guidelines for the use of fresh frozen plasma. Transf Med 1992;2:57-63.
9. NIH Consensus Conference. Fresh frozen plasma: indications and risks. JAMA 1985; 253:551-53.
10. Consensus statement on red cell transfusion. Transf Med 1994;4:177-78.
11. American Society of Anaesthesiologists Task Force on Blood Component Therapy. Practice Guidelines for Blood Component Therapy. Anesthesiology 1996;84:732-47.
12. Lundsgaard-Hansen P, Djoran JE, Blauhut B. Is there a generally valid, minimum acceptable hemoglobin level? Infusionstherapie 1989;16:167-275.
13. Winslow RM, Vandegriff KD, Intaglietta M Eds. Blood Substitutes, New Challenges. Boston: Birkhauser, 1996.
14. Gould SA, Moore EE, Moore FA, et al. Clinical utility of human polymerized hemoglobin as a blood substitute after acute trauma and urgent surgery. J. Trauma; 1997: 43:325.
15. Williamson LM, Love EM. Reporting serious hazards of transfusion. The SHOT Program. Trans Med Rev 1998;12:28-35.
16. Blair SD, Janvrin SB, McCollum CN, Greenhalgh RM. Effect of early blood transfusion on gastrointestinal haemorrhage. Brit J Surg 1986;73:783-85.
17. Marik PE, Sibbald WJ. Concepts in emergency and critical care. JAMA 1995;273: 1439-44.
18. Purdy FR, Tweeddale MG, Merrick PM. Association of mortality with age of blood transfused in septic ICU patients. Can J Anaesthiol 1997;44,12:1256-61.
19. Martin CM, Sibbald WJ, Herbert P, Schweisser I. Age of transfused red blood cells is associated with ICU length of stay (Abstract). Clin Invest Med 1994;17:B21,123.
20. Messmer K. Hemodilution. Surg Clin North Am 1975;55:569.
21. Messmer KFW. Acceptable hematocrit levels in surgical patients. World J Surg 1987;11:41-46.

22. Carson JL, Spence RK, Poses RM, Bonavita G. Severity of anaemia and operative mortality and morbidity. Lancet 1988;727-29.
23. Lackritz EM, Campbell CC, Trenton K, et al. Effect of blood transfusion on survival among children in a Kenyan hospital. Lancet 1992;340:524-28.
24. British Committee for Standards in Haematology. Guidelines for platelet transfusions. Transf Med 1992;2:311-18.
25. Consensus Conference. Platelet transfusion therapy. JAMA 1987;257:1777-80.
26. Consensus Conference on Platelet Transfusion. Royal College of Physicians of Edinburgh, November 1997.
27. Gmür J, Burger J, Schanz U, Fehr J, Schaffner A. Safety of stringent prophylactic platelet transfusion policy for patients with acute leukaemia. Lancet 1991;338;1223-26.
28. Corash L. Inactivation of viruses in human cellular blood components. Vox Sang 1994;67:211-16.
29. Horsey PJ. Multiple trauma and massive transfusion. (Editorial) Anaesthesia 1997; 52:1027-29.
30. Mollison PL, Engelfriet CP, Contreras M. Blood Transfusion in Clinical Medicine. 10th Ed. Oxford: Blackwell Science, 1997.
31. McClelland DBL (ed). Handbook of Transfusion Medicine 2nd Ed. London: HMSO, 1996.
32. Murphy WG, Davies MJ, Eduardo A. The haemostatic response to surgery and trauma. Brit J Anaesth 1993;70:205-13.
33. Ciavarella D, Reed RL, Counts RB, et al. Clotting factor levels and the risk of diffuse microvascular bleeding in the massively transfused patient. Brit J Haematol 1987; 67:365-68.
34. Becker GA, Tuccelli M, Kunicki T, et al. Studies of platelet concentrates stored at 22C and 4C. Transfusion 1973;13:61-68.
35. Murphy WG, Palmer JP, Green RHA. The management of haemorrhage in the refractory non-alloimmunized thrombocytopenic patient. Vox Sang 1994; 67(Suppl 3): 99-103.
36. Mazzara R, Escolar G, Garrido M, et al. Procoagulant effect of incompatible platelet transfusions in alloimmunized refractory patients. Vox Sang 1996;71:84-89.
37. British Committee for Standards in Haematology. Guidelines on oral anticoagulation: second edition. J Clin Pathol 1990;43:177-83.
38. Rock GA, Kenneth MD, Shumak KH, et al. Comparison of plasma exchange with plasma infusion in the treatment of thrombotic thrombocytopenic purpura. N Engl J Med 1991;325:393-97.
39. Murphy WG, Moore JC, Warkentin TE, Hayward CPM, Kelton JG. Thrombotic thrombocytopenic purpura. Blood Coagulation and Fibrinolysis 1992,3:655-59.

THE EFFICACY OF TECHNOLOGIES TO MINIMISE PERI-OPERATIVE ALLOGENEIC TRANSFUSION

A. Laupacis, D. Fergusson[1]

Introduction

Concern about the side-effects of allogeneic blood transfusion, especially the transmission of viral infections, has led to the development of a variety of methods intended to minimise peri-operative transfusion. These include pharmacological agents (aprotinin, desmopressin (DDAVP), tranexamic acid (TXA), epsilon aminocaproic acid (EACA) and erythropoietin (EPO)), pre-operative autologous donation (PAD), acute normovolemic haemodilution (ANH), and intra- and post-operative cell salvage. We have performed meta-analyses of randomised trials of all of the technologies except cell salvage, using exposure to peri-operative allogeneic blood transfusion as the primary outcome [1-4]. The results are summarised here.

Methods and materials

Literature search and study selection

A Medline search was performed with no restrictions for the dates 1966 to 1996 (March 1997 for aprotinin, DDAVP, TXA and EACA), to identify all articles with any of the following terms as a text word: aprotinin; DDAVP; desmopressin acetate; l-desamino-8-D-arginine vasopressin; tranexamic acid; epsilon-aminocaproic acid; 6-aminocaproic acid; erythropoietin; blood transfusion, autologous; or haemodilution. An extensive EMBASE search was done as well. All the titles and abstracts were examined for studies evaluating the efficacy of the technologies for minimising peri-operative blood use. The manufacturers of the drugs were asked to identify any articles or reports on this subject. The references of all relevant randomised trials, reports, review articles, and previous meta-analyses [5,6] were searched for other potentially useful trials.

Only randomised trials in which the technologies were compared with a concurrent control, and which described the proportion of patients receiving at least

---

1. The International Study of Peri-operative Transfusion (ISPOT) Investigators. (Complete list of investigators and affiliations at the back of the paper). This work was carried out at the Clinical Epidemiology Unit, Loeb Research Institute, University of Ottawa, Ottawa, Canada.

one unit of allogeneic red blood cells were included. Studies were included irrespective of whether they were full publications, abstracts or letters to the editor; used placebo or open-label controls; or were published in English or non-English journals. Because they have been shown to lead to biased estimates of treatment effect [7,8], we excluded articles that were described as randomised, but in which clinicians could have been aware of which treatment the patient would receive (e.g. allocation by chart number, birth date, etc.). Duplicate publications, studies of children, non-elective surgery, and trials in which patients were randomised post-operatively were excluded.

Data collection

Data from the studies were independently abstracted onto study data forms by two individuals. Disagreements were resolved by consensus. Except for the meta-analysis of acute normovolemic haemodilution, no attempt was made to conceal the identity of the author or the medium of publication. When necessary, authors were contacted for clarification (e.g. to ensure that the same

Tabel 1. Efficacy of drugs: overall and subgroup analyses*

	Aprotinin		**Desmopressin**		**Tranexamic acid**	
	Odds ratio (95% CI)	**Trials**	**Odds ratio (95% CI)**	**Trials**	**Odds ratio (95% CI)**	**Trials**
Overall	0.31 (.25-0.39)	45	0.98 (0.64-1.50)	12	0.50 (0.34-0.76)	12
Control:						
Placebo	0.33 (0.24-0.45)	28	0.95 (0.62-1.46)	11	0.63 (0.33-1.23)	5
Open label	0.28 (00.21-0.39)	17	4.81 (0.22-105.18)	1	0.37 (0.23-0.59)	7
ASA use:						
No pts on ASA	0.26 (0.16-0.43)	17	0.75 (0.29-1.97)	2	0.42 (0.17-1.01)	2
Some pts on ASA	0.34 (0.27-0.44)	16	1.26 (0.81-1.94)	5	0.87 (0.46-1.64)	6
All pts on ASA	0.26 (0.11-0.61)	3	0.21 (0.07-0.62)	3	–	–
Type of surgery:						
Primary	0.29 (0.19-0.44)	26	0.63 (0.36-1.11)	7	0.50 (0.26-0.96)	5
Primary and repair	0.33 (0.27-0.40)	7	1.65 (1.01-2.68)	5	0.71 (0.38-1.34)	4
Repair	0.27 (0.14-0.51)	4	–	–	0.12 (0.01-1.14)	1
Transfusion threshold:						
>100 gm/L	0.16 (0.07-0.35)	10	0.70 (0.34-1.42)	2	0.41 (0.16-1.02)	3
80-100 gm/L	0.23 (0.12-0.45)	10	–	–	0.31 (0.11-0.82)	2
<80 gm/L	0.43 (0.31-0.60)	15	1.54 (0.85-2.81)	2	0.64 (0.32-1.27)	4
Jadad quality score:						
>3	0.36 (0.25-0.52)	26	0.95 (062-1.46)	11	0.63 (0.33-1.23)	5
<3	0.29 (0.22-0.39)	19	4.81 (0.22-105.18)	1	0.37 (0.23-0.59)	7

* Number of trials in subgroups do not always equal the overall number because data is not reported in all trials.

Aprotinin		PROPORTION TRANSFUSED Treatment	Control
Overall:		1599/3355	1769/2453
Type of Control:	Placebo	800/1888	730/1140
	Open-Label	799/1467	1039/1313
Dose:	High	1148/2286	1629/2233
	Medium	170/499	270/498
	Low	281/570	281/509
ASA Use:	No Pts. on ASA	282/629	349/494
	Some Pts. on ASA	557/1316	485/731
	All Pts. on ASA	40/73	47/57
Type of Surgery:	Primary	615/1554	628/992
	Repeat	175/336	127/164
	Both Primary & Repeat	681/1121	885/1083
Transfusion Threshold:	>100 Hgb	722/1186	889/1076
	80-100 Hgb	160/425	206/338
	<80 Hgb	478/1346	424/733

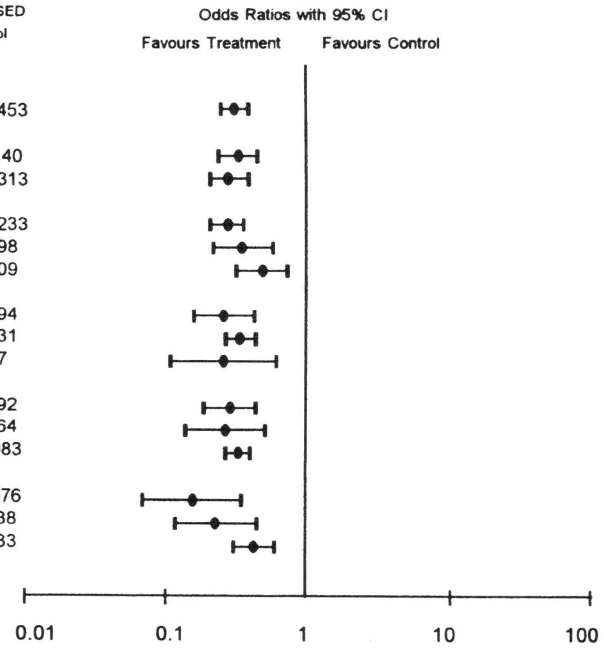

Figure 1. Summary of the overall odds ratios associated with aprotinin, and the results of important secondary analyses, expressed as odds ratios with 5% confidence intervals.

patients were not included in more than one report from the same author), and the author of one large study of aprotinin was contacted to determine the proportion of patients transfused with allogeneic red blood cells [9] (the paper reported the proportion transfused with any allogeneic blood product). The primary outcome measure was the proportion of patients receiving at least one unit of allogeneic packed red blood cells. Other data abstracted from the studies were the dose of medication used for pharmaceutical agents; the volume of blood withdrawn for ANH; the type of surgery (primary or re-operation), perioperative myocardial infarction, re-operation because of bleeding and preoperative use of aspirin for cardiac surgery; the route of administration (intravenous or subcutaneous) and the total dose [low (<1800 units/kg) or high (>1800 units/kg)] of erythropoietin; the intra and post-operative transfusion thresholds reported (haemoglobin >100 g/l, 80-100 g/l or <80 g/l; haematocrit was converted to haemoglobin by multiplying by 3.3); and the methodological quality of the study report using the Jadad scale [10]. The Jadad scale contains questions about three items: the process of randomisation, double blinding, and the description of withdrawals. Possible scores vary from 0 (worst score) to 5 (best score). If blood transfusion was only reported in millilitres, this value was divided by 300 ml to determine the mean number of units transfused. If patients were taking aspirin within 7 days of the operation, they were considered to be on the drug. A total dose of aprotinin was calculated, assuming that an intravenous transfusion lasted four hours (e.g. if 2 million units were given intravenously and added to the prime, and 0.5 million units were infused intravenously, the total dose was 6 million units).

Analysis

Data were analysed using Meta-Analyst [11] (random effects model). Results are presented as odds ratios with 95% confidence intervals (CI) and p values. An odds ratio of 1.0 suggests that there was no difference between treatment and control, an odds ratio less than one suggests that fewer patients in the treatment group received at least one allogeneic transfusion, and an odds ratio of greater than one suggests that more patients in the treatment group received at least one allogeneic transfusion. A p value <0.05 was considered statistically significant. Tests for heterogeneity were performed for each meta-analysis, and if positive, the studies that appeared to be the major contributors to the heterogeneity were evaluated in an attempt to discover the reasons.

Results

Aprotinin

There were 45 trials of aprotinin for cardiac surgery [9,12-54] which studied a total of 5808 patients. The largest trial randomised 1784 patients, and the median size of the trials was 63 patients. The overall odds ratio, when all trials were included was 0.31 (95%CI 0.25 to 0.39; p<0.0001). In order to determine whether aprotinin was more effective in some patients than others, we evaluated its efficacy in a number of subgroups including the dose of aprotinin, type of surgery, aspirin use, the transfusion threshold, the type of control used and the Jadad score (Table 1, Figure 1). The efficacy of aprotinin was similar in all subgroups of patients, except for statistically non-significant trends towards a greater effect of aprotinin in studies using a higher dose, and in the studies in which the transfusion threshold was >100 g/l of haemoglobin compared with those in which the transfusion threshold was <80 g/l . The test for heterogeneity was statistically significant among the high dose aprotinin trials (p=0.001), but we were unable to identify any clinical or methodological reason for this.

Patients receiving aprotinin required fewer re-operations because of bleeding after surgery than patients in the control group [mean 1.8% versus 5.2%; OR 0.46 (95%CI 0.29 to 0.73; p=0.001)]. There was no statistically significant difference in the frequency of peri-operative myocardial infarction [8.0% in aprotinin treated patients and 5.6% in patients in the control groups: OR 1.12 (95%CI 0.82 to 1.53; p=0.48)].

Desmopressin

There were 12 studies of desmopressin for cardiac surgery [34,35,55-64] involving a total of 793 patients, all but one of them placebo-controlled. The largest study enrolled a total of 99 patients, and the median size was 65 patients. Most studies used a dose of 0.3 μg/kg intravenously at the end of cardiopulmonary bypass. Desmopressin had no statistically significant effect upon the proportion of patients receiving transfusion [odds ratio 0.98 (95%CI 0.64 to 1.50; p=0.92)] (Figure 2). However, on subgroup analyses, the efficacy of desmopressin appeared to vary depending upon the use of aspirin (Table 1, Figure 2). In studies in which no patients received aspirin the odds ratio was 0.75 (95%CI 0.29 to 1.97; p=0.56), compared with an odds ratio of 1.26 (95%CI 0.81 to 1.94; p=0.30) if some patients received aspirin, and an odds ratio of 0.21 (95%CI 0.07 to 0.62; p= 0.005) if all patients were taking aspirin.

In the six trials that reported re-operations for bleeding, 2.0% of patients receiving desmopressin underwent surgery compared with 2.8% in the control groups [odds ratio 0.87 (95%CI 0.23 to 3.27; p=0.83)]. The frequency of peri-operative myocardial infarction was 4.4% in patients treated with desmopressin and 1.6% in patients in the control group [OR 1.85 (95%CI 0.74 to 4.62; p=0.19)].

Tranexamic acid

There were twelve eligible studies of TXA for cardiac surgery [36,37,43,45, 49,50,54,57,65-68] with a total of 882 patients (median sample size 47). The majority of studies used a 10 mg/kg bolus followed by a 1 mg/kg infusion for 10 to 12 hours. TXA decreased the proportion of patients receiving at least one unit of allogeneic blood [OR 0.50 (95%CI 0.34 to 0.76; p=0.0009)] (Figure 2). The efficacy of tranexamic acid appeared similar in all subgroups studied (Table 1, Figure 2).

There was no statistically significant effect of TXA on peri-operative myocardial infarction [0.4% in the TXA groups versus 1.8% in the control - OR 0.50 (95%CI 0.13 to 1.93; p=0.30)] or re-operations because of bleeding [2.4% in

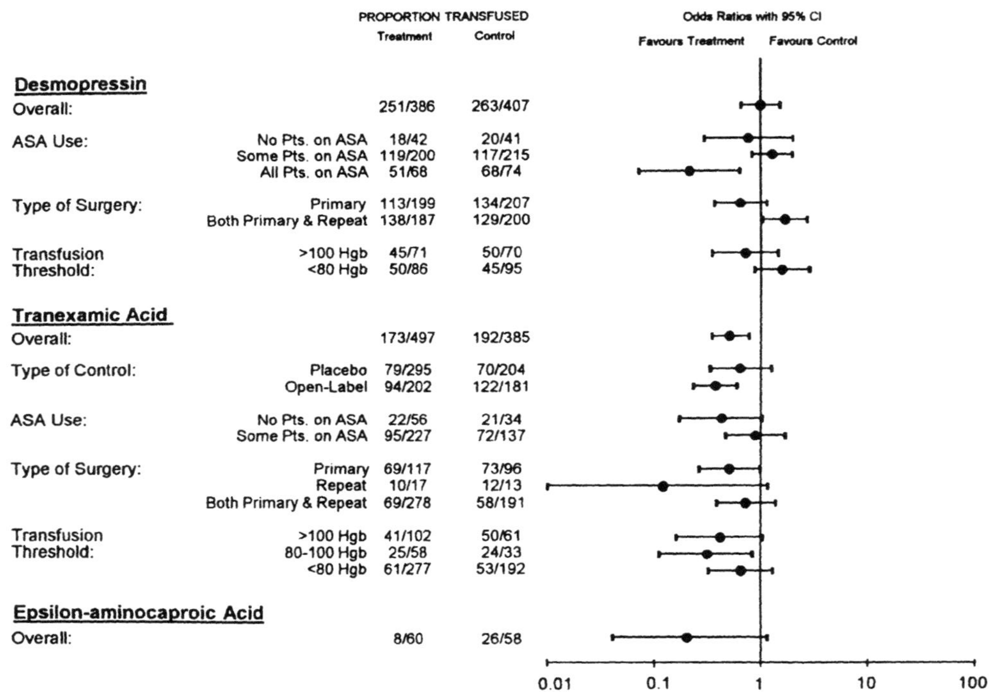

Figure 2. Summary of the overall odds ratios associated with desmopression, tranexamic acid and aminocaproic acid, and the results of important secondary analyses, expressed as odds ratios with 95% confidence intervals.

patients receiving TXA and 2.9% in patients in the control group: OR 0.93 (95%CI 0.35 to 2.46; p=0.88)].

Epsilon aminocaproic acid

There were only three eligible studies of EACA for cardiac surgery [36,54, 69], with a total of 118 patients. There was no statistically significant effect of EACA on the proportion of patients transfused with allogeneic blood, although the odds ratio was considerably less than 1.0 [OR 0.20 (95%CI 0.04 to 1.12; p=0.07)] (Figure 2).

Erythropoietin to augment autologous donation

Most studies evaluating erythropoietin to augment autologous donation were done in orthopaedic patients. There were 11 studies including a total of 825 patients [70-80], with a median sample size of 62. Erythropoietin therapy was associated with a statistically significant decrease in the proportion of patients transfused with allogeneic blood [odds ratio 0.42 (95%CI 0.28 to 0.62; p<0.0001)] (Figure 3). There was no difference between the efficacy of high and low doses of erythropoietin [odds ratio 0.41 (95%CI 0.26 to 0.65;p=0.0002)] versus 0.48 [odds ratio 95%CI 0.24 to 0.96; p=0.04)] (Figure 3). The odds ratio associated with subcutaneous erythropoietin [odds ratio 0.32 (95%CI 0.18 to 0.57;p=0.0001)] was less than that for intravenous use [odds ratio 0.52 (95%CI 0.31 to 0.89;p=0.016)], but this difference was not statistically significant. There were five trials of erythropoietin to augment autologous donation in patients undergoing cardiac surgery [81-85] with a total of 224 patients, and the odds ratio was 0.25 (95%CI 0.08 to 0.82;p=0.02). The odds ratio in placebo-controlled studies of erythropoietin (orthopaedic and cardiac) was 0.45 (95%CI 0.14 to 1.44;p=0.18) compared with 0.04 (95%CI 0.01 to 0.29;p=0.001) in studies with open-label controls. Study reports with a Jadad score ≥3 had a similar odds ratio compared to studies with a score <3.

Erythropoietin alone

There were three randomized trials of erythropoietin alone in orthopaedic surgery [86-88] with a total of 684 patients, and two studies in cardiac surgery [89, 90] with a total of 108 patients (Figure 3). There was no statistically significant heterogeneity in these analyses. The odds ratio for the studies in orthopaedic patients was 0.36 (95%CI 0.24 to 0.56;p=0.0001) and the odds ratio for the studies in cardiac patients was 0.09 (95%CI 0.03 to 0.28;p<0.0001).

Pre-operative autologous donation

There were 6 randomized trials comparing PAD with a control group [91-96] in colorectal surgery for bowel cancer (3 studies), hip arthroplasty (2 studies) and liver resection (1 study). The sample sizes of the studies varied from 31 to 423 with a total of 933 patients. All six trials demonstrated a statistically significant decrease in exposure to allogeneic blood in patients who predeposited autologous blood compared with those who did not. The odds ratio when all of these studies were combined was 0.17 (95%CI, 0.08 to 0.32) (Figure 4). The odds

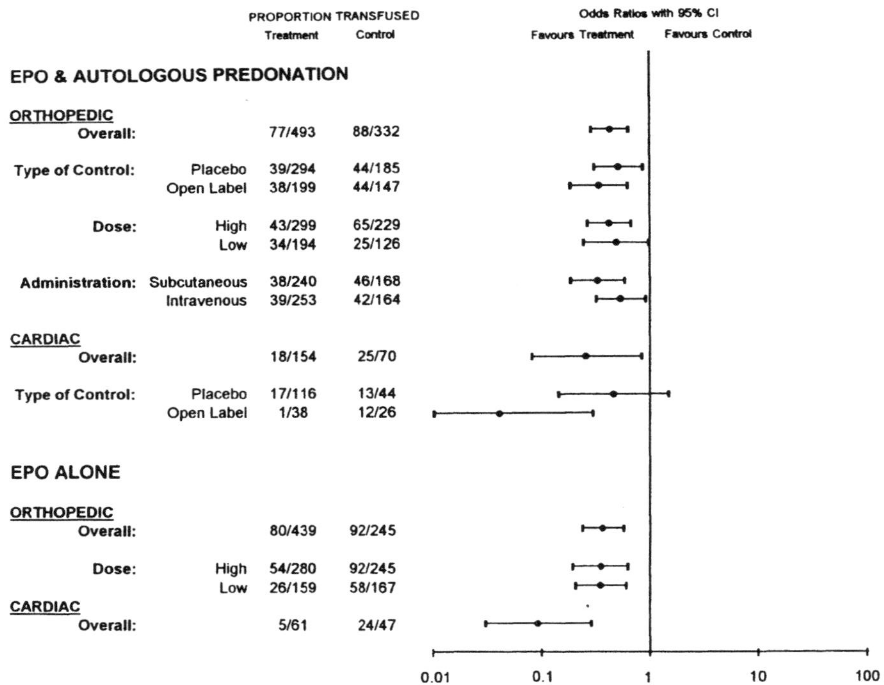

Figure 3. Proportion of patients transfused, and in subgroups of patients treated with erythropoietin, expressed as odds ratios with 95% confidence intervals.

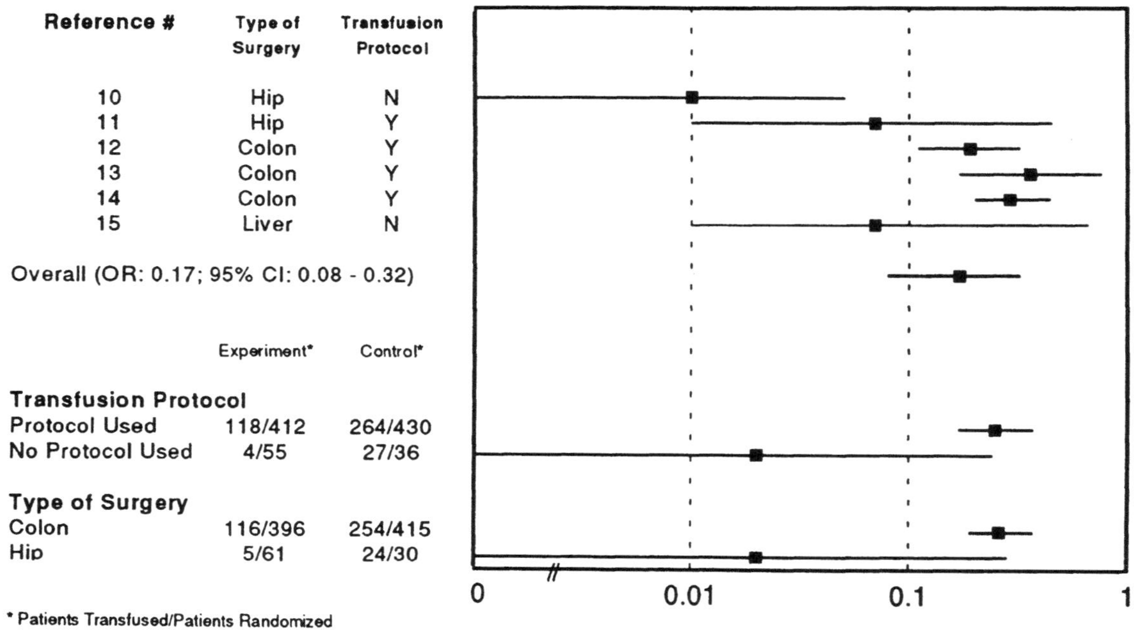

Figure 4. Proportion of patients transfused with allogeneic blood in the randomised trials of pre-operative autologous donation, expressed as odds ratios with 95% confidence intervals.

ratio for colorectal surgery was 0.26 (95% CI, 0.19 to 0.37), compared with 0.20 (95% CI, 0.00 to 0.28) in patients who underwent hip arthroplasty. The odds ratio in studies in which a transfusion protocol was reported was 0.25 (95% CI, 0.17 to 0.37) compared with 0.02 (95% CI, 0.00 to 0.24) in those that did not report a transfusion protocol (Figure 4). Five randomized studies reported the total number of units transfused (allogeneic and autologous). Autologous donors were more likely to receive any transfusion (allogeneic and/or autologous red blood cells), with an odds ratio of 3.03 (95% CI, 1.70 to 5.39). These results were minimally affected when the analysis was restricted to the four studies that reported a transfusion protocol (OR 3.29, 95% CI 1.59 to 6.82).The test for heterogeneity was significant when all trials were combined. However, when the trials were analysed separately according to the type of surgery, and the use of a transfusion protocol, the heterogeneity was no longer statistically significant (Figure 4).

Acute Normovolemic Haemodilution

Sixteen randomized trials of acute normovolemic haemodilution (ANH), reported in 15 publications [97-111], described the proportion of patients exposed to at least one unit of allogeneic blood. A total of 615 patients were enrolled, and the median sample size of the trials was 30 (range 20-103]. When all eligible trials were considered, ANH significantly reduced the likelihood of exposure to at least one unit of allogeneic blood (OR 0.31; 95% CI 0.15,0.62). When surgical procedures were considered individually, ANH was effective in reducing the likelihood of exposure to at least one unit of allogeneic blood in cardiac and miscellaneous procedures but not in orthopaedic surgery (Figure 5). Marked heterogeneity of results was found in both the overall and individual procedure analyses mentioned above.

In trials in which the volume of blood withdrawn during haemodilution was less than 1000 mL the reduction in the likelihood of transfusion failed to reach statistical significance (OR 0.43; 95% CI 0.18, 1.02). On the other hand, studies in which 1000 mL of autologous blood or more was withdrawn prior to surgery showed large and statistically significant reductions in the likelihood of transfusion (OR 0.16; 95% CI 0.04, 0.65). Trials without transfusion protocols showed marked reductions in the likelihood of exposure to allogeneic blood (OR 0.12; 95% CI 0.04, 0.37), while studies with a transfusion protocol failed to show statistically significant reductions in the likelihood of receiving an allogeneic transfusion (OR 0.64; 95% CI 0.31, 1.31).

Discussion

The main findings of these meta-analyses were that aprotinin, TXA, erythropoietin (both to augment autologous predonation and on its own) and PAD all decrease exposure to peri-operative allogeneic blood transfusion. Desmopressin is not efficacious, and there are too few trials of EACA to establish its efficacy.

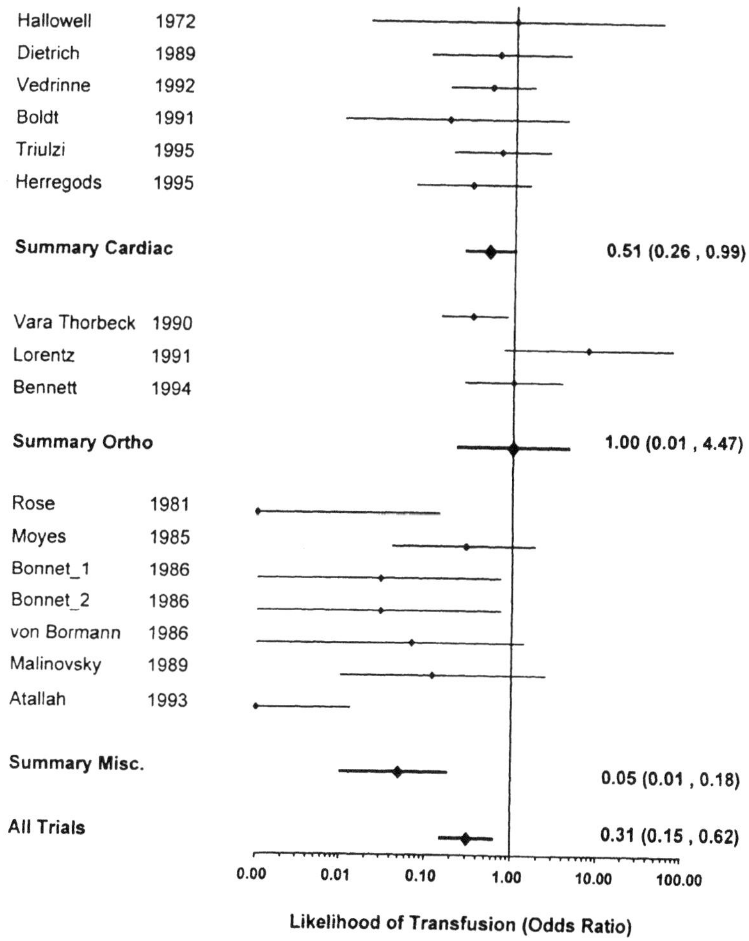

Figure 5. Proportion of patients transfused with allogeneic blood in the randomized trials of acute normovolemic haemodilution, expressed as odds ratios with 95% confidence intervals.

There was so much heterogeneity in the meta-analysis of ANH, and most of the trials were of such poor methodological quality, that it is presently difficult to determine whether ANH is efficacious or not.

The reporting of side-effects in the randomized trials was frequently incomplete. However, there were too few patients enrolled in the studies of pharmaceutical agents to reliably exclude the possibility of a small but clinically important increase in thrombotic side-effects such as myocardial infarction or graft thrombosis. This is particularly true of erythropoietin in cardiac surgery, where one study found a higher rate of death in patients receiving erythropoietin than in control patients [112]. Although this was not statistically significant and may have occurred by chance, only 332 cardiac surgery patients were studied in all of the randomized trials included in this meta-analysis.

It is also concerning that patients who predonated autologous blood were considerably more likely to receive any blood transfusion (autologous and/or allogeneic) than those who did not, a finding that has been reported by others [113]. Since the chance of a fatal haemolytic transfusion reaction is in the same order of magnitude as the chance of receiving HIV from an allogeneic transfusion [114,115], it is possible that autologous donors, if they are more likely to receive transfusion of any kind, are ultimately placed at higher risk than non donors.

The limitations of these meta-analyses should be acknowledged. Firstly, the sample sizes of most of the studies included in these meta-analyses were small. Except for the meta-analysis of aprotinin in cardiac patients, which included 5808 patients, all of the other meta-analyses included less than 1000 patients. Meta-analyses of other interventions, containing more patients than were included in most of the meta-analyses in this study, have still reached false conclusions about efficacy when their results were compared with subsequent "definitive" large trials [116]. Thus, the results of this meta-analysis must be interpreted with caution, especially the subgroup analyses, such as the efficacy of desmopressin in patients receiving aspirin. Secondly, there was unexplained heterogeneity in the meta-analysis of ANH which makes the results difficult to interpret. Thirdly, the frequency of post-operative myocardial infarction, the need for re-operation because of bleeding, and side-effects were not reported in all studies. This supports the belief of others that uniform and comprehensive standards are needed when reporting the results of these studies [117].

The results of these meta-analyses suggest that further large randomized trials using clear transfusion guidelines need to be done. Questions of particular interest include comparison of high and low doses of aprotinin, determining whether ANH is efficacious, establishing whether desmopressin truly is efficacious in cardiac patients on aspirin, and direct comparison of these technologies with each other and with "optimal clinical management". Economic evaluations should be incorporated into the design of these studies to determine the cost-effectiveness of the various options, and side-effects should be carefully evaluated.

Acknowledgements

We thank Drs. O. Benavente, J. Cooper, J. Pagliarello, O. Rosaeg, and B. Schmidt, and Ms. B. Malanka for translating some of the articles, Dr. Malcolm Hing for help with abstracting data from studies, Ms. Jesse McGowan, Ms. Shin and Ms. June MacLeod for assistance with the literature searches, and Mrs. Karen Weeks for her secretarial assistance.

References

1. Laupacis A, Fergusson D, for the International Study of Peri-operative Transfusion (ISPOT) Investigators. Drugs to minimize peri-operative blood loss in cacrdiac surgery - Meta-analyses using peri-operative blood transfusion as the outcome. Anesth Analgesia 1997;85:1258-67.
2. Forgie M, Wells P, Laupacis A, Fergusson D, for the International Study of Peri-operative Transfusion (ISPOT) Investigators. Pre-operative autologous donation decreases allogeneic transfusion but increases exposure to all red cell transfusion. Arch Intern Med 1998;158:610-16.
3. Bryson GL, Laupacis A, Wells GA, for the International Study of Peri-operative Transfusion. Does acute normovolemic haemodilution reduce perioperative allogeneic transfusion? A meta-analysis. Anesth Analgesia 1998;86:9-15.
4. Laupacis A, Fergusson D, for the International Study of Peri-operative Transfusion (ISPOT) Investigators. Erythropoietin to minimize peri-operative blood transfusion. Four meta-analyses of randomized trials. Transfus Med (under review).
5. Fremes SE, Wong BI, Lee E, et al. Meta-analysis of prophylactic drug treatment in the prevention of postoperative bleeding. Ann Thorac Surg 1995;58:1580-88.
6. Cattaneo M, Harris AS, Stroberg U, Mannucci PM. The effect of desmopressin on reducing blood loss in cardiac surgery - A meta-analysis of double-blind, placebo-controlled trials. Thromb Haem 1995;74:1064-70.
7. Chalmers TC, Celano P, Sacks HS, Smith H. Bias in treatment assignment in controlled clinical trials. N Engl J Med 1983;309:1358-61.
8. Schultz KF, Chalmers I, Hayes RJ, Altman DG. Empirical evidence of bias: dimensions of methodological quality associated with estimates of treatment effect in controlled trials. JAMA 1995;273:408-12.
9. Lemmer JH, Dilling EW, Morton JR, et al. Aprotinin for primary coronary artery bypass grafting: A multicenter trial of three dose regimens. Ann Thorac Surg 1996;62:1659-68.
10. Jadad AR, Moore A, Carroll D, et al. Assessing the quality of reports of randomized clinical trials: Is blinding necessary? Contr Clinical Trials 1996;17:1-12.
11. Meta-Analyst.977. Lau J, Chalmers TC. 1990.
12. Kalangos A, Tayyareci G, Pretre R, Di Dio P, Sezerman O: Influence of aprotinin on early graft thrombosis in patients undergoing myocardial revascularization. Eur J Cardio-Thorac Surg 1994;8:651-56.
13. Lemmer JH, Jr., Stanford W, Bonney SL, et al. Aprotinin for coronary bypass operations: efficacy, safety, and influence on early saphenous vein graft patency. A multicenter, randomized, double-blind, placebo-controlled study. J Thorac Cardiovasc Surg 1994;107:543-51.
14. Bidstrup BP, Underwood SR, Sapsford RN, Streets EM. Effect of aprotinin (Trasylol) on aorta-coronary bypass graft patency. J Thorac Cardiovasc Surg 1993;105:147-52.

15. Rodrigus IE, Vermeyen KM, De Hert SG, Amsel BJ, Walter PJ. Efficacy and safety of aprotinin in aortocoronary bypass and valve replacement operations: a placebo-controlled randomized double-blind study. Perfusion 1996;11;313-18.
16. Royston D, Bidstrup BP, Taylor KM, Sapsford RN. Effect of aprotinin on need for blood transfusion after repeat open-heart surgery. Lancet 1987;ii:1289-91.
17. Bidstrup BP, Royston D, Sapsford RN, Taylor KM. Reduction in blood loss and blood use after cardiopulmonary bypass with high dose aprotinin (Trasylol). J Thorac Cardiovasc Surg 1989;97:364-72.
18. Fraedrich G, Weber C, Bernard C, Hettwer A, Schlosser V. Reduction of blood transfusion requirement in open heart surgery by administration of high doses of aprotinin – preliminary results. Thorac Cardiovasc Surg 1989;37:89-91.
19. Locatelli A, Bertollo D, Bianchi T, et al. Aprotinin in cardiosurgery: a randomized prospective study with different protocols for use. Minerva Anestesiologica 1990; 56:973-975.
20. Dietrich W, Spannagl M, Jochum M, et al. Influence of high-dose aprotinin treatment on blood loss and coagulation patterns in patients undergoing myocardial revascularization. Anesthesiology 1990;73:1119-26.
21. Boldt J, Zickmann B, Czeke A, Herold C, Dapper F, Hempelmann G. Blood conservation techniques and platelet function in cardiac surgery. Anesthesiology 1991; 75:426-32.
22. Gherli T, Porcu A, Padua G, et al. Reducing bleeding during extracorporeal circulation interventions by high doses of aprotinin. Minerva Cardioangiol 1992;40: 121-26.
23. Deleuze P, Loisance DY, Feliz A, et al. Reduction of pre- and postoperative blood loss with aprotinin (Trasylol) during extracorporeal circulation. Arch Mal Coeur Vaiss 1991;84:1797-1802.
24. Vedrinne C, Girard C, Jegaden O, et al. Reduction in blood loss and blood use after cardiopulmonary bypass with high-dose aprotinin versus autologous fresh whole blood transfusion. J Cardiothorac Vasc Anesth 1992;6:319-23.
25. Dietrich W, Barankay A, Hahnel C, Richter JA. High-dose aprotinin in cardiac surgery: three years' experience in 1,784 patients. J Cardiothorac Vasc Anesth 1992; 6:324-27.
26. Mohr R, Goor DA, Lusky A, Lavee J. Aprotinin prevents cardiopulmonary bypass-induced platelet dysfunction. A scanning electron microscope study. Circulation 1992;86(suppl II):II405-9.
27. Cosgrove DM, Heric B, Lytle BW, et al. Aprotinin therapy for reoperative myocardial revascularization: a placebo-controlled study. Ann Thorac Surg 1992;54:1031-36.
28. Baele PL, Ruiz-Gomez J, Londot C, Sauvage M, Van Dyck MJ, Robert A. Systematic use of aprotinin in cardiac surgery: influence on total homologous exposure and hospital cost. Acta Anaesthesiologica Belgica 1992;43:103-12.
29. Bailey CR, Kelleher AA, Wielogorski AK. Randomized placebo-controlled double-blind study of three aprotinin regimens in primary cardiac surgery. Br J Surg 1994; 81:969-73.
30. Carrera A, Martinez MV, Garcia-Guiral M, Herrero E, Peral A, Planas A. Use of high doses of aprotinin in cardiac surgery. Rev Esp Anestesiol Reanim 1994;41:13-19.
31. Maccario M, Fumagalli C, Deangelis R, et al. Comparison between low and high doses of aprotinin in heart surgery. Minerva Anestesiologica 1994;60:315-20.
32. Murkin JM, Lux J, Shannon NA, et al. Aprotinin significantly decreases bleeding and transfusion requirements in patients receiving aspirin and undergoing cardiac operations. J Thorac Cardiovasc Surg 1994;107:554-61.

33. Swart MJ, Gordon PC, Hayse-Gregson PB, et al. High-dose aprotinin in cardiac surgery – a prospective, randomized study. Anaesth Intensive Care 1994; 22:529-33.
34. Rocha E, Hidalgo F, Llorens R, Melero JM, Arroyo JL, Paramo JA. Randomized study of aprotinin and DDAVP to reduce postoperative bleeding after cardiopulmonary bypass surgery. Circulation 1994;90:921-27.
35. Casas JI, Zuazu-Jausoro I, Mateo J, et al. Aprotinin versus desmopressin for patients undergoing operations with cardiopulmonary bypass. J Thorac Cardiovasc Surg 1995;110:1107-17.
36. Penta de Peppo A, Danilo Pierri M, Scafuri A, et al. Intraoperative antifibrinolysis and blood-saving techniques in cardiac surgery. Tex Heart Inst J 1995; 22:231-36.
37. Corbeau JJ, Monrigal JP, Jacob JP, et al. Comparaison des effet de l'aprotinine et de l'acide tranexamique sur le saignement en chirurgie cardiaque. Ann Fr Anesth Reanim 1995;14:154-61.
38. Levy JH, Pifarre R, Schaff HV, et al. A multicenter, double-blind, placebo-controlled trial of aprotinin for reducing blood loss and the requirement for donor-blood transfusion in patients undergoing repeat coronary artery bypass grafting. Circulation 1995; 92:2236-44.
39. Lab M, Welz A, Kochs M, Mayer G, Schwandt M, Hannekum A. Aprotinin in elective primary bypass surgery: Graft patency and clinical efficacy. Eur J Cardio-thorac Surg 1995;9:206-10.
40. Dietrich W, Dilthey G, Spannagl M, Jochum M, Braun SL, Richter JA. Influence of high-dose aprotinin on anticoagulation, heparin requirement, and celite- and kaolin-activated clotting time in heparin-pretreated patients undergoing open-heart surgery. Anesthesiology 1995;83:679-89.
41. D'Ambra MN, Akins CW, Blackstone E, et al. Aprotinin in primary valve replacement and reconstruction: A multicenter, double- blind, placebo-controlled trial. J Thorac Cardiovasc Surg 1996;112:1081-89.
42. Harder MP, Eijsman L, Roozendaal KJ, van Oeveren W, Wildevuur CRH. Aprotinin reduces intraoperative and postoperative blood loss in membrane oxygenator cardiopulmonary bypass. Ann Thorac Surg 1991;51:936-41(abstract).
43. Isetta C, Gunness TK, Samat C, et al. Antifibrinolytic treatment and homologous transfusion in cardiac surgery. Eur Heart J 1993;14:424.
44. Liu B, Belboul A, Radberg G, et al. Effect of reduced aprotinin dosage on blood loss and use of blood products in patients undergoing cardiopulmonary bypass. Scand J Thorac Cardiovasc Surg 1993;27:149-55.
45. Blauhut B, Harringer W, Bettelheim P, Doran JE, Spath P, Lundsgaard-Hansen P. Comparison of the effects of aprotinin and tranexamic acid on blood loss and related variables after cardiopulmonary bypass. J Thorac Cardiovasc Surg 1994;108:1083-91.
46. Hardy JF, Desroches J, Belisle S, Perrault J, Carrier M, Robitaille D. Low-dose aprotinin infusion is not clinically useful to reduce bleeding and transfusion of homologous blood products in high-risk cardiac surgical patients. Can J Anaesth 1993;40:625-31.
47. Bailey CR, Wielogorski AK. Randomised placebo controlled double blind study of two low dose aprotinin regimens in cardiac surgery. Br Heart J 1994; 71:349-53.
48. Tabuchi N, Huet RC, Sturk A, Eijsman L, Wildevuur CR. Aprotinin preserves haemostasis in aspirin-treated patients undergoing cardiopulmonary bypass. Ann Thorac Surg 1994;58:1036-39
49. Pugh SC, Wielogorski AK. A comparison of the effects of tranexamic acid and low-dose aprotinin on blood loss and homologous blood usage in patients undergoing cardiac surgery. J Cardiothorac Vasc Anesth 1995;9:240-44.

50. Speekenbrink RG, Vonk AB, Wildevuur CR, Eijsman L. Hemostatic efficacy of dipyridamole, tranexamic acid, and aprotinin in coronary bypass grafting. Ann Thorac Surg 1995;59:438-42.
51. Alvarez JM, Quiney NF, McMillan D, et al. The use of ultra-low-dose aprotinin to reduce blood loss in cardiac surgery. J Cardiothorac Vasc Anesth 1995;9:29-33.
52. Wendel HP, Heller W, Michel J, et al. Lower cardiac troponin T levels in patients undergoing cardiopulmonary bypass and receiving high-dose aprotinin therapy indicate reduction of perioperative myocardial damage. J Thorac Cardiovasc Surg 1995; 109:1164-72.
53. Bidstrup BP, Royston D, McGuinness C, Sapsford RN. Aprotinin in aspirin-pretreated patients. Perfusion 1990;5(suppl):77-81.
54. Menichetti A, Tritapepe L, Ruvolo G, et al. Changes in coagulation patterns, blood loss and blood use after cardiopulmonary bypass: aprotinin vs tranexamic acid vs epsilon aminocaproic acid. J Cardiovasc Surg 1996;37:401-7.
55. Salzman EW, Weinstein MJ, Weintraub RM, et al. Treatment with desmopressin acetate to reduce blood loss after cardiac surgery. A double-blind randomized trial. N Engl J Med 1986;314:1402-6.
56. Frankville DD, Harper GB, Lake CL, Johns RA. Hemodynamic consequences of desmopressin administration after cardiopulmonary bypass. Anesthesiology 1991; 74:988-96.
57. Horrow JC, Van Riper DF, Strong MD, Brodsky I, Parmet JL. Hemostatic effects of tranexamic acid and desmopressin during cardiac surgery. Circulation 1991;84: 2063-70.
58. Marquez J, Koehler S, Strelec SR, et al. Repeated dose administration of desmopressin acetate in uncomplicated cardiac surgery: a prospective, blinded, randomized study. J Cardiothorac Vasc Anesth 1992;6:674-76.
59. Ansell J, Klassen V, Lew R, et al. Does desmopressin acetate prophylaxis reduce blood loss after valvular heart operations? A randomized, double-blind study. J Thorac Cardiovasc Surg 1992;104:117-23.
60. Gratz I, Koehler J, Olsen D, et al. The effect of desmopressin acetate on postoperative hemorrhage in patients receiving aspirin therapy before coronary artery bypass operations. J Thorac Cardiovasc Surg 1992;104:1417-22.
61. Dilthey G, Dietrich W, Spannagl M, Richter JA. Influence of desmopressin acetate on homologous blood requirements in cardiac surgical patients pretreated with aspirin. J Cardiothorac Vasc Anesth 1993;7:425-30.
62. Sheridan DP, Card RT, Pinilla JC, et al. Use of desmopressin acetate to reduce blood transfusion requirements during cardiac surgery in patients with acetylsalicylic-acid-induced platelet dysfunction. Can J Surg 1994;37:33-36.
63. Temeck BK, Bachenheimer LC, Katz NM, Coughlin SS, Wallace RB. Desmopressin acetate in cardiac surgery: a double-blind, randomized study. South Med J 1994; 87:611-15.
64. Spyt TJ, Weerasena NA, Bain WH, Lowe GDO, Rumley A. The effects of desmopressin acetate (DDAVP) on haemostasis and blood loss in routine coronary artery bypass surgery: a randomized, double-blind trial. Perfusion 1990;(suppl):57-61.
65. Horrow JC, Van Riper DF, Strong MD, Grunewald KE, Parmet JL. The dose-response relationship of tranexamic acid. Anesthesiology 1995;82:383-92.
66. Coffey A, Pittmam J, Halbrook H, Fehrenbacher J, Beckman D, Hormuth D. The use of tranexamic acid to reduce postoperative bleeding following cardiac surgery: a double-blind randomized trial. Am Surg 1995;61:566-68.
67. Katsaros D, Petricevic M, Snow NJ, Woodhall DD, Van Bergen R. Tranexamic acid reduces postbypass blood use: A double-blind, prospective, randomized study of 210 patients. Ann Thorac Surg 1996;61:1131-35.

68. Shore-Lesserson L, Reich DL, Vela-Cantos F, Ammar T, Ergin MA. Tranexamic acid reduces transfusions and mediastinal drainage in repeat cardiac surgery. Anesth Analgesia 1996;83:18-26.
69. Daily PO, Lamphere JA, Dembitsky WP, Adamson RM, Dans NF. Effect of prophylactic epsilon-aminocaproic acid on blood loss and transfusion requirements in patients undergoing first-time coronary artery bypass grafting. A randomized, prospective, double-blind study. J Thorac Cardiovasc Surg 1994;108:99-106.
70. Goodnough LT, Rudnick S, Price TH, et al. Increased preoperative collection of autologous blood with recombinant human erythropoietin therapy. N Engl J Med 1989;321:1163-68
71. Bormann B von, Weidler B, Friedrich M, von Andrian-Werburg H. Recombinant erythropoietin in autologous blood donation. Anaesthesist 1991;40:386-90
72. Mercuriali F, Zanella A, Barosi G, et al. Use of erythropoietin to increase the volume of autologous blood donated by orthopedic patients. Transfusion; 1993;33:55-60
73. Biesma DH, Kraaijenhagen RJ, Marx JJ, van de Wiel A. The efficacy of subcutaneous recombinant human erythropoietin in the correction of phlebotomy-induced anemia in autologous blood donors. Transfusion 1993;33:825-29
74. Beris P, Mermillod B, Levy G, et al. Recombinant human erythropoietin as adjuvant treatment for autologous blood donation. A prospective study. Vox Sang 1993;65: 212-18
75. Goodnough LT, Price TH, Friedman KD, et al. A phase III trial of recombinant human erythropoietin therapy in nonanemic orthopedic patients subjected to aggressive removal of blood for autologous use: dose, response, toxicity, and efficacy. Transfusion 1994;34:66-71
76. Biesma DH, Marx JJM, Kraaijenhagen RJ, Franle W, Messinger D, van de Wiel A. Lower homologous blood requirement in autologous blood donors after treatment with recombinant human erythropoietin. Lancet 1994;344:367-70
77. Schlaeppi B, Gunter P, Nydegger UE. Enhancing the efficacy of preoperative autologous blood donation by erythropoietin. Transf Sci 1994;15:171-77
78. Yuen K, Matthews JP. Recombinant human erythropoietin (R-HuEPO) and autologous donation. Document from Janssen Cilag Limited 1995.
79. Price TH, Goodnough LT, Vogler WR, et al. The effect of recombinant human erythropoietin on the efficacy of autologous blood donation in patients with low hematocrits – a multicenter, randomized, double-blind, controlled trial. Transfusion 1996; 36:29-36
80. Tryba M, Kindler D, Schulte-Tamburen A. Preoperative use of low dose human erythropoietin in combination with parenteral iron substitution for the stimulation of autologous blood donation in patients before elective orthopaedic surgical interventions. The role of epoetin alpha in surgery. Forging the link in blood conservation. Published by Adelphi Communications, UK 1995; 6-7.
81. Watanabe Y, Fuse K, Naruse Y, et al. Subcutaneous use of erythropoietin in heart surgery. Ann Thorac Surg 1992;54:479-83
82. Kulier AH, Gombotz H, Fuchs G, Vuckovic U, Metzler H. Subcutaneous recombinant human erythropoietin and autologous blood donation before coronary artery bypass surgery. Anesth Analg 1993;76:102-6
83. Schmoeckel M, Nollert G, Mempel M, Mempel W, Reichart B. Effects of recombinant human erythropoietin on autologous blood donation before open heart surgery. Thorac Cardiovasc Surg. 1993;41:364-68
84. Hayashi J, Kumon K, Takanashi S, et al. Subcutaneous administration of recombinant human erythropoietin before cardiac surgery: a double-blind, multicenter trial in Japan. Transfusion 1994;34:142-46

85. Walpoth BH, Galliker B, Spirig P, Haeberli A, Rosenmund A, Althaus U, Nydegger UE. Use of epoetin alpha in autologous blood donation programs for patients scheduled for elective cardiac surgery. Sem Hematol1996;22(suppl 2);75-76.
86. Canadian Orthopedic Perioperative Erythropoietin Study Group. Effectiveness of perioperative recombinant human erythropoietin in elective hip replacement. Lancet 1993;341:1227-32
87. De Andrade JR, Jove M, Landon G, Frei D, Guitfoyle M, Young D. Baseline hemoglobin as a predictor of risk of transfusion and response to epoetin alfa in orthopedic surgery patients. J Bone Joint Surg Am 1966;78-A:62-72.
88. Faris PM, Ritter MA, Abels RI, American Erythropoietin Study Group. The effects of recombinant human erythropoietin on perioperative transfusion requirements in patients having a major orthopaedic operation. J Bone Joint Surg 1996;78-A:62-72
89. D'Ambra MN, Lynch KE, Boccagno MS, Vlahakes GJ. The effect of perioperative administration of recombinant human erythropoietin (r-HuEPO) in CABG patients: a double blind, placebo-controlled study. Anesthesiology 1992;77:A159
90. Sowade O, Warnke H, Scigalla P, et al. Avoidance of allogeneic blood transfusions by treatment with Epoetin Beta (Recombinant Human Erythropoietin) in patients undergoing open-heart surgery. Blood. 1997;89:411-18
91. Elawad AR, Jonsson S, Laurell M, Fredin HO. Predonation autologous blood in hip arthroplasty. Acta Orthop Scand 1991; 62:218-22.
92. Lorentz A, Osswald PM, Schilling M, Jani L. A comparison of autologous transfusion procedures in hip surgery. Anaesthesist 1991;40:205-13.
93. Hoynck van Papendrecht MA, Hop W, Langenhorst BL, Kothe FC, Marquet RL, Jeekel J. Feasibility of a predeposit autologous blood donation program in colorectal cancer patients: results from a randomized clinical study. Vox Sang 1992;62:102-7.
94. Heiss MM, Mempel W, Jauch KW, et al. Beneficial effect of autologous blood transfusion on infectious complications after colorectal cancer surgery. Lancet 1993; 342: 1328-33.
95. Busch OR, Hop WC, Hoynck van Papendrecht MA, Marquet RL, Jeekel J. Blood transfusions and prognosis in colorectal cancer. N Engl J Med 1993; 328:1372-76.
96. Kajikawa M, Nonami T, Kurokawa T, et al. Autologous blood transfusion for hepatectomy in patients with cirrhosis and hepatocellular carcinoma: use of recombinant human erythropoietin. Surgery 1994; 115:727-34.
97. Hallowell P. Transfusion of fresh autologous blood in open-heart surgery. A method for reducing blood bank requirements. J Thorac Cardiovasc Surg 1972;64:941-48.
98. Dietrich W, Barankay A, Dilthey G, et al. Reduction of blood utilization during myocardial revascularization. J Thorac Cardiovasc Surg 1989;97:213-19.
99. Boldt J, Kling D, Weidler B, et al. Acute preoperative hemodilution in cardiac surgery: volume replacement with a hypertonic saline-hydroxyethyl starch solution. J Cardiothorac Vasc Anesth 1991;5:23-28.
100. Vedrinne C, Girard C, Jegaden O, et al. Reduction in blood loss and blood use after cardiopulmonary bypaass with high-dose aprotinin versus autologous fresh whole blood transfusion. J Cardiothorac Vasc Anesth 1992;6:319-23.
101. Herregods L, Foubert L, Moerman A, et al. Comparative study of limited normovolaemic haemodilution in patients with left main coronary artery stenosis. Anaesthesia 1995;50:950-53.
102. Triulzi DJ, Gilmor GD, Ness PM, et al. Efficacy of autologous fresh whole blood or platelet-rich plasma in adult cardiac surgery. Transfusion 1995;35:627-34.
103. Lorentz A, Osswald PM, Schilling M, Jani L. A comparison of autologous transfusion procedures in hip surgery. Anaesthesist 1991;40:205-13.

104. Vara Thorbeck R, Rosell Pradas J, Mekinassi KL, et al. Prevention of thromboembolic disease and post-transfusional complications using normovolemic hemodilution in arthroplasty surgery of the hip. Rev Chir Orthop Reparatrice Appar Mot 1990;76:267-71.
105. Bennett SR. Perioperative autologous blood transfusion in elective total hip prosthesis operations. Ann R Coll Surg Eng 1994;76:95-98.
106. Rose D, Coutsoftides T. Intraoperative normovolemic hemodilution. J Surg Res 1981;31:375-81.
107. Moyes DG, Mistry BD, Conlan AA. Normovolaemic haemodilution using dextran 70 in thoracic surgery. S Afr Med J 1985;67:762-64.
108. von Bormann B, Weidler B, Boldt J, et al. Acute normovolemic hemodilution in extensive surgical interventions. Chirurg 1986;57:457-64.
109. Bonnet MC, Julia JM, Mathieu-Daude JC, du Cailar J. Value of hemodilution in maxillofacial surgery for postoperative traumatic edema and graft viability. Ann Fr Anesth Reanim 1986;5:243-84.
110. Malinovsky JM, Bouyer L, Rusterholtz T, et al. Saving of blood products by normovolemic hemodilution in prostate resection. Ann Fr Anesth Reanim 1989;8(suppl): R120.
111. Atallah MM, Abdelbaky SM, Saied MM. Does timing of hemodilution influence the stress response and overall outcome? Anesth Analg 1993;76:113-17.
112. EPREX (epoetin alpha) product monograph, Janssen-Ortho Inc, Canada, 1996
113. Kanter MH, van Maanen D, Anders KH et al. Preoperative autologous blood donations before elective hysterectomy. JAMA 1996; 276:798-801.
114. Linden JV, Kaplan HS. Transfusion errors: causes and effects. Transf Med Rev 1994;8:169-83.
115. Linden JV, Paul B, Dressler KP. A report of 104 transfusion errors in New York State. Transfusion 1992;32:601-6.
116. LeLorier J, Gregoire G, Benhaddad A, Lapierre J, Derderian F. Discrepancies between meta-analyses and subsequent large randomized, controlled trials. N Engl J Med 1997;337:536-42.
117. Lemmer JH Jr. Reporting the results of blood conservation studies: The need for uniform and comprehensive methods. Ann Thorac Surg 1994;58:1305-6.

* The International Study of Peri-operative Transfusion (ISPOT) Investigators are the following:

Coordinating Centre and Canadian Investigators -

Phil Wells, MD; George Wells, PhD; Fraser Rubens, MD; Annette O'Connor, PhD; Laura McAuley BSc; Andreas Laupacis, MD (Chair); Jack Kitts, MD; Paul Hebert, MD; Ian Graham, PhD; Dean Fergusson, MHA (Coordinator); Greg Bryson, MD. Clinical Epidemiology Unit, Loeb Research Institute, Ottawa Civic Hospital, University of Ottawa, Ottawa, Ontario, Canada.

Investigators

UNITED STATES: Chris Hillyer, MD; Jeff Etchason, MD; Angela Blair. Emory University School of Medicine, Atlanta, Georgia and the Kerr L. White Institute for Health Services Research, Decatur, Georgia

UNITED KINGDOM: Brian McClelland, MD; Patricia Phillips. Scottish Health Service. Edinburgh, Scotland.

SPAIN: Jordi Gol-Freixa, MD; Antonio Garcia. Agencia de evaluacion de Tecnologias Sanitarias, Madrid

NETHERLANDS: Ankie Koopman-van Gemert, MD, PhD. Laren (NH).

JAPAN: Akinori Hisashige, MD, PhD. University of Tokushima, Tokushima.
ISRAEL: Nachum Egoz MD, MPH; Luis Gaitini MD; Somri Mustafa MD. Bnai Zion Medical Center, Haifa.
FRANCE: Luc Noel, MD; Centre Hospitalier de Versailles, Versailles. Rachid Salmi, PhD; Charlotte Huet, MD; Université Victor Segalen Bordeaux II, Bordeaux.
DENMARK: Helga Sigmund, MSc. Danish Hospital Institute, Copenhagen
AUSTRALIA: Katherine McGrath, MD; Kim Henderson. Hunter Area Pathology Service, Newcastle. David Henry, MD. Newcastle.
Funding:
Dr. Laupacis received the First Fellowship from the International Society of Technology Assessment in Health Care, funded by the PPP Medical Trust, United Kingdom in order to do this study. The Ottawa Coordinating Centre has received funding from Janssen Ortho Inc, Canada, the Australian Group from the National Health and Medical Research Council and the Hunter Area Pathology Services, the Scottish Group from the Scottish National Blood Transfusion Service and the Clinical Resources & Audit Group of the Scottish Health Service, the French Group from Haemonetics France, Ortho Diagnostics France and University Segalen Bordeaux 2, and the group from the United States from the Baxter Healthcare Corporation Biotech Group and the Emory Center for Clinical Evaluation Sciences.

EVIDENCE-BASED TRANSFUSION MEDICINE OR THE NEED TO EVALUATE CLINICAL OUTCOME

J.Th.M. de Wolf

Evidence based medicine

Evidence based medicine (EBM) is the process of systematically finding, appraising, and subsequently using research findings as the basis for clinical decisions. In practice it means an integration of individual clinical expertise with the best available external clinical evidence from systemic research. EBM will never replace clinical skills, clinical judgement and clinical experience. In the concept of EBM a clinical problem will be turned into a clear clinical question and then relevant clinical articles will be searched for, critically appraised (evaluated) for validity and usefulness and the results are finally implemented in clinical practice [1-4].

Posing the question

The questions that initiate the process of EBM can relate to diagnosis, treatment, prognosis, quality of care, or economics of care. For instance concerning the case of white blood cell reduction of blood products for all transfusion recipients, the following questions can be formulated: how large is the incidence of febrile non-haemolytic transfusion reactions in patients receiving RBC or platelet concentrates; to what extend can this be prevented by the use of leukocyte-depleting filters, and finally what is de clinical relevance for patients in general and for selected groups of patients in particular [5].

Finding the evidence

The second step is the search for the best available external evidence. Two types of electronic databases are available. First, bibliographic sources like Medline or Pubmed in which can be searched on bibliographic terms as authors, keywords, or titles. Access into these databases might be gained by the medical library in the hospital or by the world wide web site: http://www.nlm.nih.gov/. Second, publication-based databases like the Cochrane Database of Systemic reviews, journals like ACP Journal Club (a bimonthly supplement of the Annals of Internal Medicine, from the American College of Physicians) and Evidence-based Medicine or the two journals combined on a single CD-ROM as Best Evidence (American College of Physicians, 1997).

Evaluating the evidence

The third step is to evaluate, or appraise, the evidence for its validity and clinical usefulness. A set of evaluating questions are developed for different sorts of clinical research articles on diagnosis, therapy, prevention, harm, prognosis, screening, guidelines, quality and economics of care [6,7]. Critical appraisal questions for treatment prevention could concern: randomisation, inclusion criteria or follow-up. Treatment or prevention results can further be evaluated by determining the absolute and relative risk reduction (ARR, RRR), and the 95% confidence interval of these parameters. The question whether the benefits of a prevention or treatment are worth the harm and costs can be evaluated by the calculation of the number needed to treat or number needed to harm. (NNT/NNH: 1/ARR) [8].

Acting on the evidence

The final step is to act upon the identified, valid and relevant evidence. One of the most difficult aspects of EBM is the implementation of the presented evidence, especially because it concerns a change in medical behaviour.

Besides an integration of the best available external clinical evidence of systemic research in clinical practice, EBM has several other advantage [9-11]: it is probably one of the best methods for a life-long self directed learning to maintain a high level of clinical competence of the physician and an excellent quality of patient care, it improves reading habits and clinician's understanding of research methods and makes them more critical in using data. Further, EBM might provide a better communication with patients about the rationale behind management decisions, and by that, it might help patients and doctors in making decisions.

Evidence-based medicine and blood transfusion

The wish to come to a more rationalised use of blood products might be dictated by motives of potential adverse effects such as the transmission of infections, immunological risks like haemolytic reactions and graft versus host disease. Other considerations to come to a more rationalised use of blood products concern the great variability in transfusion practice, publications reporting inappropriate/unnecessary use of blood components, the wish of physicians to quantify the quality of the treatment, and finally the growing pressure from patients and society to come to a more explicit medical behaviour. Patients want to know more about the rationale behind the decision to transfuse: why is a transfusion necessary, what are the expected benefits, what are the risks of transfusion in one's own country besides in other parts of the world, are there alternatives, what are the benefits and risks of the alternatives and what determines the preferences? The great variability in the use of blood products in Europe has become clear from the SANGUIS (Safe ANd Good Use of blood In Surgery) study. Ten Duis described more in detail the results of total hip replacement for osteoarthritis in 1647 patients in 10 European countries [12]. The percentage of patients that received blood ranged from 29 to 100 per hospital, the number of units RBC per transfused patient ranged between 1 and 4, and the haematocrit at discharge for the transfused patients ranged between 27 and 36. In only 23% of the cases the reason for the transfusion of RBC was documented. The wide variation in the use of RBC might be an indication for ill-defined criteria for transfusion or differences in application of the criteria. On the other hand in many hospitals it seemed possible to perform a total hip replacement in more then 50% of the patients without the use of RBC, suggesting that in the hospitals in which nearly 100% of the patients were transfused part of the patients received blood unnecessary. These practices could partly be explained by a lack of effective methods to translate scientific knowledge into clinical practice. From the problems around the implementation guidelines we know that changing the medical behaviour of physicians is a very complicated process.

Petra Denig from the Department of Clinical Pharmacology and Health Sciences from the University of Groningen, investigated the drug choice behaviour of physicians [13]. This research gives insight in possibilities and impossibilities to influence these prescribing choices. Two main interventional strategies can be distinguished: restrictive strategies in which prescribing is limited, by for instance requiring a special request form or to limit treatment options to certain physicians. This strategy can be effective in limiting the use of certain drugs but does not influence inappropriate use. Voluntary strategies have an educational or guiding nature. Three forms can be identified.

- Communication and dissemination of information is directed at improving knowledge.
- Guidelines, protocols and algorithms can help the physician to implement new medical behaviour in clinical practice.
- Presenting feedback data shows the physicians what they actually do, and where clinical practice can be further improved. It can make the physician aware of certain behaviour and a motivation to change.

In her thesis Denig described the effects of different intervention strategies. The most unsuccessful strategy is reported from printed material. Developing a guideline and sending this to physicians may improve knowledge but seldom changes behaviour. The same is true for feedback data. Just sending them to the individual physician will not be very effective. The combination of printed material, feedback, discussion of the results in the group of physicians and recommendations for specific situations is the most successful strategy, probably because of the impact of the groups' process.

As a consequence of these considerations we developed the following strategy to improve some transfusion practices. The transfusion committee of the hospital developed a guideline for the transfusion of RBC: the 4-5-6 rule. With separate departments the transfusion practice of the department and the guideline were discussed. Thereupon the prospectively collected data concerning the transfusion practice were discussed with the department in order to further improve the quality of the transfusion policy. As we all know the trigger to start a transfusion is difficult to define. Traditional is the 100/30 trigger: a haemoglobin level of 100 g/l or 6 mmol/l and a haematocrit of 30% often leads to the transfusion of RBC. We know that the need for extra oxygen transporting capacity in bleeding or otherwise anaemic patients will not only be determined by the haemoglobin level, but also by age, type of anaemia, velocity of its development, cardiopulmonary function and especially the possibilities to compensate for anaemia and haemodilution. In order to make the implementation of all these factors in the decision to transfuse RBC easier, we introduced the physical status classification of the American Society of Anaesthesiologists (Table 1). Altogether we came to the 4-5-6 rule (Table 2). Most important in this 4-5-6 rule is that physicians are guided along other parameters then the haemoglobin level before the decision is made to transfuse a patient. Furthermore, this guideline has the approval of all specialists transfusing blood in our hospital: anaesthesiologists, surgeons and internists.

Table 1. Physical status classification of American Society of Anesthesiologists (ASA)

I	Healthy patient
II	Mild systemic disease, no functional limitations
III	Severe systemic disease, definite functional limitations
IV	Severe systemic disease that is a constant threat to life
V	Moribund, not expected to live 24 hours irrespective of operation

Table 2. The 4-5-6 rule

Consider a transfusion if there is a Hb < 4 mmol/l (Ht 18%) and:

- Acute blood loss in an otherwise healthy person (ASA I) < 60 years, normovolemic and blood loss in one locus

Consider a transfusion if there is Hb < 5 mmol/l (Ht 23%) and:

- Acute blood loss in otherwise healthy persons (ASA I) > 60 years, normovolemic and blood loss in one locus
- Acute blood loss in otherwise healthy persons < 60 years, normovolemic and blood loss in more then one locus (polytrauma patients)
- A pre-operative patient < 60 years and an expected blood loss > 500 ml
- Fever
- Post-operative period after uncomplicated open heart surgery
- ASA II/III patients with uncomplicated operation

Consider a transfusion if there is a Hb < 6 mmol/l (Ht 28%) and:

- An ASA IV patient
- A patient not able to increase cardiac output to compensate for haemodilution
- A septic/toxic patient
- A patient with serious lung disease
- A patient with symptomatic cerebrovascular disease

A few examples

First we looked at the transfusion practice in patients operated for a total hip replacement (no re-operations). After the introduction of the 4-5-6 rule the % of patients who did not receive blood during hospital stay increased from 53 to 72, especially because less patients received 1 or 2 units of blood. During our retrospective analysis of 598 patients with total hip replacement, we noticed that for unknown reasons women received significantly more and more frequently blood transfusions. After the introduction of the 4-5-6 rule these differences disappeared. Although we only studied officially the transfusion practice in patients with hip operations we looked at the same time into the transfusion practice in patients who underwent total knee replacement in the same department. Although the number of patients is still small, the results were remarkable: the number of patients who needed blood during hospital stay decreased from 52% (106/204) to 15% (9/60). Another example concerns the patients operated for a coronary artery bypass graft. After the introduction of the 4-5-6 rule the number of patients transfused in the operating room decreased from 26% (72/278) to 9% (26/300), in the intensive care from 53% to 41%, in the ward from 9% to 8% and in total the number of patients receiving allogeneic blood during their hospital stay decreased from 64% to 49%.

Evidence-based guidelines

The Canadian Medical Association published in 1997 the first evidence-based guidelines for red blood cell and plasma transfusion for adults and children [14] in which each recommendation was rated, based on the strength of the supporting evidence. Three levels of evidence were distinguished:

- Level-I: evidence obtained from at least one properly randomized controlled trial;
- Level-II: evidence obtained from well-designed controlled trials without randomisation, cohort or case-control analytic studies;
- Level-III: opinions of respected authorities, based on clinical experience, descriptive studies or reports of expert committees.

The observation that hardly any recommendation could be supported by level-I evidence should be considered a challenge for workers in the field of clinical transfusion medicine to provide the necessary scientific evidence for the value of not only blood products but also for its alternatives.

References

1. Sackett DL, Richardson WS, Rosenberg W, Haynes RB. Evidence-based Medicine. How to practice & teach EBM. Churchill Livingstone 1997.
2. Lockett T. Evidence-based and Cost-effective Medicine. Radcliffe Medical Press, Oxford and New York, 1997.
3. http://hiru.mcmaster.ca/.
4. http://cebmjr2.ox.ac.uk/.
5. Sirchia G, Rebulla P. Evidence-based medicine: the case for white cell reduction. Transfusion 1997;37:543-49.
6. Users' Guide To The Medical Literature. JAMA 1996-1997 or http://hiru.mcmaster.ca/ebm/userguide/default.htm.
7. Sackett DL, Haynes RB, Guyatt GH, Tugwell P. Clinical epidemiology. A basic science for clinical medicine. Little, Brown and Company, second ed. 1991.

8. Guyatt GH, Sackett DL, Cook DJ. Users' Guide To The Medical Literature. II How to use an article about therapy or prevention. A. Are the results of the study valid? B. What are the results and will they help me in caring for my patients? JAMA 1993; 270:2598-601 and 271:59-63.
9. Rosenberg W, Donald A. Evidence based medicine: an approach to clinical problem solving. BMJ 1995;310:1122-26.
10. Bordley DR, Fagan M, Theige D. Evidence-based Medicine: a powerful educational tool for clerkship education. Am J Med 1997;102:427-32.
11. Sackett DL, Rosenberg WMC. Evidence-based medicine. Tijdschr voor Praktijk Evaluatie 1996;16:63-70.
12. Ten Duis HJ, Dalen KC van, Giovanetti AM, Smit Sibinga CTh, Sirchia G. Het gebruik van bloed en bloedproducten bij totale heupartroplastieken in 31 Europese ziekenhuizen, 1990/'91. Ned Tijdschr Geneesk 1996;140:1307-12.
13. Denig P. Drug choice in medical practice. Rationales, routines, and remedies. Thesis. Groningen 1994, The Netherlands.
14. Expert Working Group. Guidelines for red blood cell and plasma transfusion for adults and children. Can Med Assoc J 1997:156:11(suppl).

DISCUSSION

J.C. Fratantoni, C.Th. Smit Sibinga

R.K. Spence, New Jersey, NY, USA: Let me ask a prerogative question. Since the title of this discussion was to optimise haemotherapy let me ask you to make an assumption that the optimal approach to transfusion would be to eliminate all risk. Since we know that we can never completely eliminate all risk from allogeneic transfusion does it make sense then that all our efforts should be focused on eliminating allogeneic transfusion completely because that is where mostly the risk lies. I wonder what the panel's comments might be on that. If we will look at evidence based medicine there is no level 1 evidence based medicine that allogeneic transfusion is a benefit and I doubt if I will ever see a randomised controlled trial of allogeneic transfusion. So, if we are going to optimise transfusion therapy should not we get rid of blood completely?

W. Murphy, Dublin, IRL: What we are trying to do is not optimise transfusion practice. What we are trying to do is optimise patient care. There is no point in designing trials that go out of their way to look at one particular aspect without having a meaningful end-point of optimised patient care. So, yes you should get rid of allogeneic transfusion, but only when shown in a series of proper prospective controlled trials that it is a better therapy.

W.G. van Aken, Amsterdam, NL: I am a bit surprised by this question, because it looks as if autologous transfusion is an alternative without risks and it is not.

R.K. Spence: Well, further to the discussion there is some pretty good evidence from people who have been working with Jehovah's witness patients and using alternatives such as cell-salvage, erythropoietin drug therapy, that you can do in the majority of all surgical procedures, 95% of them, without ever relying on allogeneic blood. So, there is that kind of evidence. Of course, you are not going to find a randomised controlled trial of transfusion versus these alternatives in the Jehovah's witness, because they simply will not tolerate it, but the evidence we have from thousands of witnesses shows us that that is the case. We know for example at cardiac surgery, that we find it harder and harder to find patients that are going to be transfused because of cardiac surgeons are doing much better jobs not giving blood. If we look at all the trials, it shows that some people are doing the surgery with very little blood, others are doing it with a lot. So if we look at that as an alternative goal, to do 95% of all our surgical patients without need for allogeneic blood, that might be the alternative we should be looking at. I am not saying that there are no risks to autologous blood, but clearly they are defined risks that don't exist for autologous blood.

C.Th. Smit Sibinga, Groningen, NL: Would you then discriminate between the immediate pre- and perioperative autologous and the predonation, predeposit autologous. I think if your surgical procedures follow good standard practice that you could do with much less than what usually is being consumed. In a number of surgical procedures much could be salvaged and used, or in the acute normovolemic haemodilution setting be used which is autologous. In the fact the effects have been shown by Laupacis in his survey. That makes it different to the practice of predonation.

R.K. Spence: I think we should look at innovative ways to redefine what we do to optimise patient care and one of those may be to have the people in the blood bank business helping the surgeons with the alternatives in developing them. Better haemodilution products, better autologous predonation programmes etc. So, I think that if we can make the autologous predonation process simpler and safer by moving haemodilution showing that it is a very cost effective alternative to predonation for the urologic patient. Then, we can differentiate in that set, but again a lot of the work has to be done. Should not we be focusing on doing those kind of things, following up on those areas that dr. Laupacis has identified and that other people have identified as well. If we are going to talk about dollars spent, how much money do we spend doing p24 antigen tests when we know it is not cost effective in the long run; how much money do we spend waiting for the prion to show up and not being able to identify it. How much money do we spend for the HIV variant that we cannot identify. I do not know and I think those are serious questions we need to ask. But this is meant more to be fun to take a look at the issues and maybe approach it from a different side.

J.C. Fratantoni, Rockville, MD, USA: The statement was made by dr. Murphy that we have to look for concurrence from the patients, get them to understand the risk. I would like to suggest that the patient may not be the most important person. The patient in the bed is already fairly compromised and that is one opinion. But the opinion that seemed to be weighing in more heavily with regard to public reaction, that is of the general public. It is often the relatives of patients who may have had some harm done. Certainly patients with haemophilia in the eighties have been an extremely influential group. So, I wonder if you would like to react to that, have some comments on how we deal with that group.

W. Murphy: Not particularly is the answer. I would see patient consent really to be a tool to allow us to critically examine what we do rather than putting it forward as a necessity. Certainly, people have completed the conclusion yes it should be done, but it is just one tool in necessing how to do it. Another tool might be how you would explain this to a particularly offensive or aggressive group of newspaper reporters, health correspondents. How would they agree with your position; they are just tools really.

A. Laupacis, Ottawa, C: I think it is clear that patients are concerned about allogeneic blood. I am not so sure that it is clear they are particularly well informed about the risks of allogeneic blood as well as the risks and benefits of the alternatives. I think we as physicians often say "a patient is demanding this and therefore there is nothing we can do. We know that this is not being driven by a lot of evidence but is being driven by politics". I am not sure that this is entirely true. We just recently completed a survey of patients in our institution undergoing cardiac and orthopaedic surgery. We asked them what they thought their likelihood of receiving allogeneic blood was. Their answers were wildly unrealistic. The average patient thought that they had a 100% chance of getting someone else's blood if they did not predonate and they had a 0% chance of getting someone else's blood if they did predonate. Therefore, it seems to me that there is a potential for engaging in some sort of dialogue in terms of education to make sure that the kind of expectations out there in the public terms of the pros and cons of transfusion are realistic.

J.Th.M. de Wolf, Groningen, NL: Personally, I do not think that the whole discussion about the lowest risk is in the patient's interest. I think that the patient has a fear and I do not think that the right answer is to rationalise it and to look at 1 in 100,000, 500,000 or 600,000. For me the most important thing is how can I treat my patients best. We can treat patients with chemotherapy and we can prevent infections by using growth factors. But at the same time you can treat patients with antibiotics. For me it is interesting to know and I think in the interest of the patient, what strategy is the best. So I like to know and I like to come to the evidence what transfusion practice is the most important. What is the role of predonation, what is the role of aprotinin or something else. But in the whole if you talk about the aprotinin it reduces blood loss but on the other hand if you use aprotinin, in what way does it enhance thrombosis for instance. The balance that will eventually lead to a practice. Not for me to figure a risk of 1 in 500,000 or 1 in a million.

J.P. AuBuchon, Lebanon, NH, USA: I like to continue the discussion about patient education and what is driving our system of choice in transfusion medicine. I agree with dr. Laupacis that in a one and one type of situation whether you are in a cab or whether you are standing at the patient's bedside, you can often make the patient understand the real risks and options of the different alternatives. Usually, at least in the hospital in my experience the patient in that situation after having been explained all the alternatives, even in America usually says well whatever you think is best doc I go along with that. They are not in the situation at that point to demand other alternatives beyond what you can explain to them rationally is the best for them, because they do not have the experience and if you have indeed laid out the options truthfully they will probably agree with you. It seems at least in the US at the moment what is really driving blood banks in a particular direction in terms of more donor questions or more testing, is the public perception of risk or the risk as portrayed by various political leaders often for purposes that are not necessarily directed toward improved health. They may have other motives behind that disguise of improved health for patients. So, the educational tasks that I think we face at least in my country is now not a one in one situation per million, but one or a small group anyway speaking of 250,000,000 trying to make them understand.

A. Lust, Aalst, B: Isn't it a pity that most of the influencing and education comes from that 15 billion dollar company money and not from all those competent doctors who are in transfusion medicine. It is the 15 billion dollar market that influences people and influences our governments.

H.J.C. de Wit, Leeuwarden, NL: That might be, but there is another example that makes us think and make things difficult: evidence based medicine versus public awareness and what people see as a risk, risk perception. The example is silicon breast prosthesis. Although there is no medical evidence that it causes immunological failure or problems in patients, the billion dollar industry recently had to pay billions of dollars to patients having immunological problems without real scientific proof for that. That makes the question much more difficult, that makes that evidence based medicine has its limits, because the best thing as a doctor to do is to see in a patient what is outcome regarding all things to benefit the patient. But you cannot always see everything and a perception of the public is another. For example in terms of production of a blood product you cannot make it pure, there are contaminants that cause side-effects. Why don't you remove contaminants to avoid side-effects although it is not proven that those side-effects are serious or relevant. Perhaps a comment on this.

J.Th.M. de Wolf: We should not remove for instance cell fragments because of assumed side-effects. I think really that if you change your product you must give the evidence that the patient will be better of. If you have adverse effects which occur rarely but if they occur, are very serious there is another problem. Concerning the risks, there is a difference between evidence based medicine and politics that is mentioned earlier, but that does not mean evidence based medicine should not be practised. If our minister tells us that without any reason products from cows should not be used in medicine, well let it be so, but it does not mean that evidence based medicine should not be practised.

A. Laupacis: I am not an expert on this but my understanding from my colleagues is that one of the things that really drives patients is whether they have any control over that risk. Patients know that if they predonate their own blood they will be able to decrease that risk, while they have no control whatsoever over the risk of cardiac surgery or orthopaedic surgery itself. So, I think that is one of the things that makes risk in transfusion so much more emotional, and why those very small risks seem to drive patients more than the much larger risks such as there is the 5% risk of dying at the time of bypass surgery.

J.C. Fratantoni: We are told that people are particularly concerned about risks they cannot control, from things they do not understand and transfusion wins on both counts which helps to explain why people who ride a motorcycle without a helmet are concerned about the safety of transfusion.

H.R. Tahhan, Norfolk, VA, USA: Dr. Laupacis, you presented evidence about DDAVP in open heart surgery. You did not talk about DDAVP in uraemic patients who are undergoing procedures; did you look into this?

A. Laupacis: We only confined ourselves to the use of desmopressin in patients who were healthy aside from their coronary artery or valvular disease. Therefore we did not evaluate desmopressin in uraemic patients.

H.R. Tahhan: This may not be proper, but why don't you combine the tranexamic acid and the aminocaproic acid studies together because they act almost similarly and you might have a better meta-analysis.

A. Laupacis: We did not do this, because in my view, there is enough trouble with pooling all of these studies within one drug, let alone between two drugs.

H.R. Tahhan: I have a final comment about evidence based medicine. Clearly, level one evidence is not available yet and I can tell you from experience that level three evidence does not help when you discuss transfusion medicine issues with surgeons, orthopaedists and others. So, I would say that level two is the best we can rely on now, but we clearly need level one evidence; level three evidence, which is opinion from authoritative, sources, is not satisfactory.

R.K. Spence: I just wanted to comment on what I think we need to avoid when we all leave here and that is how we use evidence and how we careful should not use evidence in the Johny Cocoran fashion. For those of you who do not remember Johny Cocoran, he was O.J. Simpson's attorney and what I consider the Johny Cocoran effect is that although O.J. was guilty, he used the evidence to get him of. What I heard dr. Laupacis say to us was that if I have my patient predonate blood that my patient now has two-thirds less chance of getting someone else's blood and that is what meta-analysis at the best showed. Now what dr. Laupacis also said, and remember he said this was his bias, is that this study showed the patient that predonate is more likely to be transfused. But the evidence shows that he is transfused with his own blood more than he is with somebody else's blood and until such time as the evidence shows that the risk from mismatch etcetera for autologous blood is greater than it is for allogeneic blood then you have to take a look at the risk balance. I would say that when I would talk to a patient about autologous pre-donation I would say to him that the best evidence I have is that you are going to avoid allogeneic blood two/thirds more than if you do not pre-donate. I do not know if that is the case, correct me if I am wrong, but I think that that is what I heard. I want to be careful about how I use data and we have all to be careful. We use these data so that evidence based medicine is good, but when we translate it into actual clinical practice with our patients we got to be very careful about how we present it because that is where the risk is defined for the patient.

A. Laupacis: You have the interpretation generally right. We do have to balance the risk of allogeneic blood versus autologous transfusion. Expressing these rare risks is incredibly difficult. We are mostly used to talking to patients about a 20% chance of something happening rather than a one in a million chance. Our group is actually in the process of developing a decision aid that we hope to give to patients that summarises the results of these trials as best we can. We have been struggling with how to present this information and the best we have come up with so far is to compare the risks of these small events with risks that people are familiar with, such as the chance of dying in a car crash, being hit by lightning.

L.H. Siegenbeek van Heukelom, Alkmaar, NL: The best transfusion is the transfusion not given. There is a special patient group, the Jehovah's witnesses and they are going to the extremes to this axioma. Can we learn something of this group of Jehovah's witnesses to have the transfusion rate going down. To what extremes are we accepting these patients. How far do they want to go. I think as an internist you have to learn and to listen and to see if you can change your treatment scheme. Is there something of evidence of transfusion medicine in this group?

A. Laupacis: I would like to take exception with your comment that the best transfusion is always the transfusion not given. As dr. Murphy and others have said, we really do not know what the optimal perioperative transfusion level is. I think that there is no question that a lot of patients can be operated on without major disasters and tolerate a very low haematocrit. However, the question is "is that optimal practice?"

R.K. Spence: I agree with you completely. I just comment briefly about 2000 Jehovah's witness patients across the board a variety of surgical procedures eliminating cardiac[1]. The focus was developed from what Carson and I did earlier[2], a smaller number of Jehovah's witnesses where we identified variables that effected outcome aside from haemoglobin level. We were able to show that you can do reasonably well with a Jehovah's witness but when haemoglobin drops mortality rises. The question Carson posed was what is the relationship to cardiopulmonary disease. I think it is the first real evidence we have about cardio-

1. Carson JL, Spence RK, Poses RM, Bonavita G. Severity of anaemia and operative mortality and morbidity. Lancet 1988;i:727-29.
2. Carson JL, Duff A, Poses RM et al. Effect of anaemia and cardiovascular disease on surgical mortality and morbidity. Lancet 1996;348:1055-60.

pulmonary function and activity in a patient as an indication of mortality and associated with transfusion. When you get below 8 there is a statistically significant difference in outcome and the patient is not transfused if he has cardiopulmonary disease and that is by history. It shows that very good evidence. So, clearly you need to define that population. Maybe that patient needs a haemoglobin of 10 as a better way to go and finally the best evidence I got from that meeting in Paris was that the good way to get your red cells up is 'paté de foie gras' and red wine. I took that home as a good part of the meeting. Clearly there is good evidence now in that group of Jehovah's witnesses that you can do surgery without transfusion, but you get into risk when you get into lower haemoglobin levels and it may also be related to clinical aspects.

W.G. van Aken: It would be interesting to see whether evidence was published about the wine and 'paté de foie gras', a factor related to my remark. I think transfusion medicine requires more evidence to know what we are actually doing. I would like to ask also the opinion of dr. de Wolf about this- because he apparently is a proponent of evidence based medicine and he has a large group of clinicians and physicians who share him. However, there is also a group which takes a more critical view on evidence based medicine and notices disadvantages and limitations. I also treat patients and I also read my journals and if evidence based medicine does indeed something to the medial profession then it is to promote reading, to promote to go back to where did it come from. But very often I must say when you try to put your individual patient into the study to find the evidence you find so many exclusion factors and so many conditions which your patient does not fulfil that the evidence based medicine approach falls short. That is a limitation which I have not heard today but which together with some other limitations mentioned should be taken into account before we introduce evidence based medicine as a sort of panacea for everything.

J.Th.M. de Wolf: I began my talk by saying that evidence based medicine never will replace clinical skills or clinical judgement, but on the other hand doctors are ordinary people, they are not borne with a lot of knowledge. If you treat patients your knowledge must come from somewhere and I think that with all the remarks on trials there is no better evidence. You have your clinical practice and you must integrate and that is I think the most important thing of evidence based medicine. When there is evidence, you have to integrate it into your clinical practice. It is not so that for all your problems evidence based medicine is the solution.

J.C. Fratantoni: Dr. Laupacis, clinical trials are experiments and experiments are situations where variables are manipulated to make it easier to understand the evidence. Clinical trials are always to some extent artificial, and in interpreting them and bringing them back to clinical practice takes a lot of judgement. The question I would like to ask regards the meta-analysis, which is certainly an experiment because you are taking already analysed data and reanalyse them. Those conclusions that you drew in your study were largely based on decisions to transfuse. In those experiments how well was that controlled? How strict were the criteria for transfusion, or were the decision makers blinded, because you have already proven by the evidence regarding autologous pre-donation that the decision makers were biased which is something to be expected.

A. Laupacis: I hear two questions: one is how do people in the studies deal with the decision to transfuse? The answer is: "it varied". Some studies seem to do an extremely good job, and others did not. However, the main issue was whether the same transfusion trigger was used in the two groups within a randomised trial. We hope to determine whether double blind studies and studies that reported a transfusion trigger appear to come up with a different estimate of the odds ratio than those who did not. In general, we found no difference between studies that were double blind and had a transfusion trigger, and those that did not. There was a nice editorial[3] in one of the surgical journals a while ago calling for a standardised methodology in these trials and I would certainly agree with that editorial. The second issue is a more difficult one, which is really the generalisibility of clinical trials and meta-analyses. Two of the major knocks against clinical trials are they tend to be done in expert centres with patients who are most likely to respond, and by expert physicians. Therefore, one is more likely to see an effective therapy than one would in the real world. So if anything, the bias is in favour of finding a benefit. The other knock against clinical trials is that the inclusion criteria for patients may be a lot different from that in the real world. In the final analysis, you have 45 trials of aprotinin and one has a choice between picking one or two that either show that the drug works or does not work, (or what I would prefer to do) to attempt to combine them in a meta analysis and come up with the best estimate of their efficacy.

C.R. Valeri, Boston, MA, USA: In the meta-analysis, was the temperature of the patients and the amount of heparin administered controlled?

A. Laupacis: No.

C.R. Valeri: Both temperature and heparin affect blood loss and the requirements for transfusion of blood products.

A. Laupacis: It seems to me that the important question is whether, within the same trial, the temperature control was the same within the two groups (the aprotinin and placebo group). To the best of my knowledge, this was the case. We were unfortunately unable to look at temperature in these patients.

C.R. Valeri: Yes, heparin produces a platelet dysfunction and induces fibrinolysis and aprotinin will inhibit the fibrinolytic activity. The dose of aprotinin to

3. Lemmer SH Sr. Reporting the results of blood concentration studies: the need for uniform and comprehensive methods. Ann Thorac Surg 1994;58:1305-6.

reduce the bleeding diathesis and to prevent procoagulant activity is an important consideration.

A. Laupacis: We certainly did look at the dose of aprotinin and arbitrarily divided it into low, high and medium doses. We found no evidence that the dose of aprotinin made a large difference.

L. Noel, Versailles, F: We have seen very interesting data from dr. de Wolf concerning the improvement and usage of red cells that are linked to the four, five, six rules. My question is how can you describe the progress to these rules, what is the time span in which these changes were observed and technically do you have a review process of all transfusions during this period with the technician involved which may well be the major incentive, the major code of the change in practice. If I can put the question to our American colleagues I understood that several years ago the joint committee on accreditation stopped demanding that all transfusions should be reviewed which I believe from our European standpoint was a very interesting self-criticising improvement mechanism. So, my question is how close to the clinicians and the users of blood will the regulation system be.

J.Th.M. de Wolf: I think that one of the major points is that you must make a choice between three points; you have to consider more parameters to see if a patient will fall in the group of four, five or six. It is not only a question of the haemoglobin level decreases to 10 or to 6 mmol, so he needs a transfusion. You must consider more parameters and you must think more before you make a decision. Another point is that when we introduced it in the departments at the same time there was a study. So first of all the clinicians were demonstrated what their transfusion practice was in the past. We introduced a new protocol and then came back with the prospective data. I think that those two points make that blood use diminishes. Another point is that the haemoglobin level at discharge decreased in these departments from around 6.5, 7.0 to around 6.0.

C.Th. Smit Sibinga: Dr. van Aken, one of the three principles you put up is: a product as safe as possible. WHO in its recommendation[4] gives four major principles that should be adhered to as close as possible. It is the safety, the purity, the potency and the efficacy of whatever you do in transfusion medicine, specifically relating to the procurement, the supply. I have the impression that at this point in time there is a mixing up of the first two principles the safety and purity, with a tendency to put purity in the place of safety. I do not think that is very appropriate; it may contribute, but should stand as a separate entity; what is your opinion.

W.G. van Aken: Well, I think they are two different items and they should be discussed completely separately. Also there is of course a relation between the

4. Requirements for the collection, processing and quality control of human blood and blood products. WHO Technical Reports Series 626, Geneva 1978.

two but there are some good examples where it was demonstrated that further attempts to purify for instance FVIII, did not lead to improved safety. So, that is why I believe that there is no evidence to keep them separate and discuss them in that way without losing the contact between the two. So, for me safety stands out as first and purity follows.

II. CHEMICAL AND BIOLOGICAL ALTERNATIVES

THE ROLE OF O_2 TRANSPORT IN THE DEVELOPMENT OF THE TRANSFUSION TRIGGER

R.M. Winslow

Introduction

The "transfusion trigger" is that event or set of events which result in a patient receiving a red cell transfusion. Excellent recent discussions have been published regarding the transfusion trigger [1-4], and numerous conferences have been held to specify guidelines or algorithms whereby clinicians can make objective decisions about the use of red cells [5,6]. For many years an empirical transfusion trigger was a haemoglobin concentration of 10 g/dl. If the value was less, the patient received at least 2 units of packed red cells or whole blood, in spite of the well known fact that many patients tolerate modest anaemia quite well [7]. The rationale for such transfusions was that an O_2 reserve needed to be maintained so that if unexpected (or expected) blood loss occurred during surgery, the patient would be in less danger of suffering deficient O_2 delivery to tissue. Guidelines for the transfusion of blood or packed red cells in the face of severe blood loss have been less well defined.

Historically, the risks of red cell transfusion were considered negligible. However, the HIV epidemic served to focus for the public, as well as for physicians, the risks of infectious disease transmission. The goal of "zero risk" blood is now very close at hand [8], but the HIV experience has demonstrated the potential for further problems, and transfusion practices have changed permanently, with the implementation of effective measures for reducing patients' exposure to allogeneic blood.

Now that potential risks of blood products are focused more clearly, indications for all transfusions are carefully examined and transfusions must be justified in patients' records. Traditional transfusion triggers were based on haemoglobin concentration alone (Table 1). However the modern standard of care now dictates a more thorough evaluation of the need for transfusion, and the old "10 g/dl" rule is no longer adequate. Most physicians would agree that transfusion of males and females, young and old, and patients with ischaemic coronary disease, for example, would not have the same triggers, but standards have not been available to sharply define individual differences. There are, in general, two types of indication for transfusion of red blood cells: inadequate O_2 delivery (anaemia), and acute blood loss (volume deple tion). They are different, and there is no reason, *a priori*, to assume the triggers should be the same in the

Table 1. Classical transfusion triggers*

Haemoglobin (g/dl)	Risk	Strategy
> 10	Very low	Avoid
8-10	Low	Avoid; transfuse if improved after trial
6-8	Moderate	Try to avoid Decrease VO_2 Clinical evaluation Volume status Pulmonary status Cardiac status Cerebrovascular status Duration of anaemia Estimated blood loss during surgery Extent of surgery Risk of rebleed
< 6	High	Usually requires transfusion

* Modified from [9].

two instances. This review will focus primarily on the use of red blood cells to restore O_2 transport rather than volume expansion.

The transfusion trigger – current practice

It is almost impossible to summarise the state of current transfusion practice, because data are very difficult to obtain. Probably the best compilation comes from the European SANGUIS study [10] which found tremendous variation from hospital to hospital in regard to the use of blood and blood products.

Current experience suggests that otherwise healthy patients with haemoglobin values of 10 g/dl or greater rarely require pre-operative transfusion, where those with haemoglobin values of less than 7 g/dl will frequently require transfusion [6]. Further distinction between the needs of individual patients is not sharp. In the US, Goodnough [2] examined the haematocrits in respect to blood loss in a group of surgical patients and found 26% of women but 13% of men were transfused in excess of their estimated blood loss. In another study, Friedman [11] found that the same "trigger" was used in both men and women, even though the normal haematocrit ranges for the two sexes is well known to be different, and questioned whether this is appropriate.

In our enthusiasm to spare patients the risks of blood transfusions, there is a risk of undertransfusion. While the NIH consensus conference [6] recommended that the lower safe limit of haemoglobin concentration could be below 10 g/dl, no definite lower limit guideline was provided. Experimental studies by Wilkerson et al. [12] in haemodiluted baboons suggested that a haematocrit of 10% could be reached before the oxygen extraction ratio rose or mortality increased. Cain showed that O_2 delivery was not critical until the haematocrit was less than 10% in dogs [13]. Levine et al. [3] found adaptive physiologic changes during progressive haemodilution down to 15% haematocrit, and a number of studies in progressive haemodilution down to 15% haematocrit, and a number of studies in Jehovah's Witness patients who refuse blood transfusion show that extremely low haemoglobins and haematocrits can be tolerated [14].

Animal studies underscore the risks of undertransfusion. Spahn et al. [15] haemodiluted dogs in whom experimental stenoses had been placed on the left anterior descending coronary artery. They then measured regional function of the myocardium by sonomicrometry,, and found that the lowest haemoglobin concentration tolerated without compromised function was 7.5 g/dl and an increase of as little as 1.9 g/dl by transfusion restored function and O_2 consumption in the affected region. Other investigators have also found that coronary stenosis in dogs limits coronary O_2 supply reserve in progressive haemodilution [16]. In patients, a haematocrit lower than about 28% is associated with significant cardiac ischaemia [17-19]. These animal and clinical studies suggest that the current practice of tolerating haemoglobin concentrations as low as 8 g/dl or haematocrits of 28%, is probably as liberal as is reasonable, and that further lowering the haemoglobin "transfusion trigger", especially in patients at risk for coronary ischaemia, could be very dangerous. In patients in whom the haematocrit must fall below 28%, the astute clinician must assess the patient's ability to compensate for the reduced O_2 capacity and, if there is evidence of ischaemia, careful monitoring of ECG, blood pressure, oxygen saturation and ST segment analysis is indispensable [20].

In order to further define how the transfusion trigger can be sharpened and standards adapted to individual cases, it is necessary to understand the indications for transfusion and the physiology of O_2 transport, and thus to consider some possible physiologic transfusion triggers.

Indications for blood transfusion

Acute blood loss (shock)

In considering the physiology of blood transfusion, it is useful to consider the changes that accompany blood loss (Table 2). Acute blood loss can be considered at 3 levels: mild (up to 20% blood volume), moderate (20-40% blood volume) and severe (over 40% blood volume). Most patients do not survive haemorrhage of greater than 50-60% blood volume [21]. Compensatory mechanisms come into play in all three, but the degree of compensation varies with the severity of blood loss.

Apparently, chemoreceptors play little or no role in the acute response to blood loss at sea level. In environmental hypoxia, arterial PO_2 falls in spite of hyperventilation and alkalosis, and O_2 uptake in the lung is diffusion-limited. When cardiac output rises in this case, an increase in pulmonary red cell transit time will limit full oxygenation of red cells. Thus, the normal sea level response to blood loss is mediated by baroreceptor (pressure) reflexes, including increased heart rate and ventilation. Both increase cardiac output; the former by increasing heart rate and the latter by increasing right heart filling. Hyperventilation causes a fall in PCO_2 and rise in arterial pH, both of which increase arterial haemoglobin saturation via the alkaline Bohr effect. The second response to

Table 2. Physiological responses to blood loss

Blood loss, %				
0	**10 20**	**30 40**	**50 60**	**70 80 90 100**
	Mild	**Moderate**	**Severe**	**Lethal**
	↑albumin synthesis			
	fluid shifts			
	↓ viscosity	—	—	—
	↓ haematocrit	—	—	—
	↑C.O.	—	—	↓ C.O.
	↑ ventilation	—	—	—
	↓PCO_2	—	—	—
		thirst	—	
		↓ blood pressure	—	—
		↓ pH	—	—
		↓ BE	—	—
		↓ lactic acid	—	—
				Infarction
				Death

acute haemorrhage, restoration of blood pressure, is mediated by the almost immediate secretion of vasoactive hormones, catecholamines and angiotensin II. The degree of hormone response is proportional to the degree of blood loss [22]. Both mechanisms, baroreflex and hormone secretion, increase blood pressure and peripheral vascular resistance selectively: that is, blood flow is redistributed in a predictable way, decreasing sharply to muscle, skin, gut and kidney, while being preserved to heart and brain.

A third response to blood loss is a redistribution of water, from the extravascular to the intravascular space. This redistribution is responsible for the falling haemoglobin concentration observed after haemorrhage, and occurs with impressive rapidity. Meyers et al. found in the fetal lamb that haemoglobin concentration was significantly lower after as little as 2 minutes following a 40% controlled haemorrhage [22].

Several mechanisms account for this rapid refilling of the vascular space. First, falling hydrostatic pressure results in a net flux of water from the interstitial to the intravascular space. Second, albumin is mobilised from the interstitial matrix and increases the oncotic pressure of the plasma. Third, albumin synthesis is increased in the liver, as is production of glucose and amino acids which further increase the plasma oncotic pressure. This increase in oncotic pressure contributes to further refilling of the vascular space. Acute reduction of circulating blood volume can impair liver function [23].

As the vascular volume refills, haematocrit falls and consequently, blood viscosity is lowered. Lowered blood viscosity reduces resistance to blood flow, increases venous return to the heart, and maintains or increases cardiac output [24].

If these compensatory mechanisms are inadequate to preserve tissue oxygen requirements, lactic acid may be produced in ischaemic tissues, dropping arterial pH. Acidosis presents a further stimulus to hyperventilation and reduces haemoglobin oxygen affinity *via* the alkaline Bohr effect. This may actually augment tissue oxygen delivery, especially in regions of the circulation in which O_2 requirements are high, such as in cardiac muscle or brain [25].

Finally, erythropoiesis is stimulated. The precise mechanism of this stimulation is not yet completely understood, because, as mentioned above, arterial PO_2 is preserved or increased in haemorrhage. Thus, the renal sensors which signal increased erythropoietin secretion must be sensitive to O_2 flux rather than O_2 concentration (PO_2). In any case, erythropoietin concentration can be seen to rise within 2-3 days of haemorrhage, a reticulocyte response is present between 2-7 days, and, in humans, the haemoglobin concentration can be seen to rise at about 7 days post haemorrhage. Of course, in many surgical patients, this sequence of events may be delayed or prevented if there are other limitations to erythropoiesis such as chronic inflammation, iron deficiency, renal failure or other concomitant problems.

Although most healthy patients can tolerate loss of up to 40% of their blood volume, many surgical patients who are not healthy may be much less tolerant of blood loss. For example, elderly patients with ischaemic heart disease may suffer tissue infarction as a result of decreased organ blood flow. Patients with borderline or inadequate pulmonary function may not be able to maintain arterial oxygenation when red cell capillary transit time decreases with increased cardiac output. Patients with liver disease may not be able to increase albumin synthesis to increase plasma oncotic pressure. And so on. These factors must be kept firmly in mind when considering the clinical indications for transfusion in an individual patient.

To some extent, restitution of blood volume by crystalloid and/or colloid resuscitation can in itself restore cardiac output. Thus, Mitzner et al. [26] found that administration of epinephrine increased cardiac output by 55% due partly to lowered right atrial pressure (caused by improved cardiac function) and increased pressure (caused by the volume shift to the systemic circulation). The choice of plasma expanders in the treatment of shock is still debated, but some workers believe that colloids such as urea-linked succinylated gelatin (Gelofusine) and 6% hetastarch (Hespan) or Pentastarch are more effective than crystalloids in restoring myocardial blood flow and O_2 after acute haemorrhage.

It should be emphasised that blood and red blood cells are not recommended as the first plasma expanders administered to shock patients because of their high viscosity. If the plasma space needs to be expanded in order to restore haemodynamic stability, colloid or crystalloid should be given first, with blood or red blood cells being given after haemodynamic stability is achieved.

Chronic anaemia

Transfusion practices in chronic anaemia are not well documented in the literature, but clinicians tend to use the same haemoglobin and haematocrit "triggers" as in other types of anaemia. This may not be appropriate since chronically anaemic patients develop significant adaptation to their anaemia, including increased cardiac output, expanded plasma volume and hyperventilation.

Transfusion in chronic anaemia may be part of a disturbing indifference in physicians' attitudes and practices. Saxena et al. [27] studied transfusions in 265 iron-deficient patients in a large metropolitan medical centre and found that in the majority of cases, transfusions were given to raise the haematocrit or haemoglobin to arbitrary values, rather than using clinical signs or symptoms as a guide. Furthermore, iron was not prescribed for almost 1/3 of the patients, including those in whom blood was not given when it was clearly indicated.

Haemodilution

Much of the literature concerned with the transfusion trigger does not distinguish between acute blood loss and the more controlled condition, surgical haemodilution. The important difference is that in the latter instance, blood volume is controlled. Thus, strategies for conservation of allogeneic blood in the surgical setting involve removal of blood prior to surgery and replacement with crystalloid or colloid (or both) so that during surgery loss of the patient's red cells can be minimised [28]. These techniques can be very effective in blood-sparing and reducing a patient's transfusion exposure.

A separate but similar situation, however, is the patient who presents with (relatively) long-standing anaemia which is well-compensated. One example of such patients is Jehovah's Witnesses who refuse transfusions on religious grounds [29-31]. Haemoglobins as low as 5 g/dl have been reported not to be associated with increased mortality. Similarly, the recommendation has been made that otherwise healthy African children with haemoglobins of 5 g/dl or higher not be transfused unless congestive heart failure is detected [32]. Some of these children can tolerate haemoglobin concentrations as low as 3 or 3.5 g/dl.

These examples from clinical practice illustrate the importance of understanding that if blood volume is restored, either in the hospital (haemodilution) or by physiologic refilling of the intravascular space (long-standing anaemia) rather low haemoglobin concentrations can be managed successfully in many patients. This concept is in agreement with the above argument that chemoreceptors are relatively less significant in adjusting to haemorrhage than are baroreceptors.

Summary: Clinical transfusion triggers (Table 1)

An enormous amount has been written about the transfusion trigger since the NIH clinical conference in 1988 [6]. In some ways, focusing attention on this issue has resulted in physicians' attitudes drifting away from using "clinical judgement" toward the search for hard, quantitative triggers which relieve the clinician from the responsibility for making a decision [33]. In reality, a decision to transfuse (or not to transfuse) is a clinical judgement, and the careful clinician distills many different data, objective and subjective, in coming to a final decision.

How then should the physician consider the decision to transfuse? Table 1 summarises the classical approach. It is difficult to imagine a situation in which a haemoglobin over 10 g/dl would be desired. The issue of the optimal haematocrit has been explored extensively in the literature, and it appears that there is little justification for maintaining a haematocrit over 35% either at sea level or in high altitude natives [34]. The reason for this is that as haematocrit rises, viscosity rises exponentially with increased resistance to flow and reduced cardiac output [24].

When the haemoglobin is between 8 and 10 g/dl, the risk to most patients is very low. Some patients, especially elderly ones, will report subjective improvement in symptoms of shortness of breath or dyspnea on exertion when their haemoglobins are maintained over 8 g/dl. Transfusion in these patients would appear to be justified, but elevation to values over 10 g/dl would seem unnecessary.

A haemoglobin concentration between 6 and 8 g/dl requires a thoughtful approach to the clinical evaluation of the patient. One should try to avoid transfusion, and a number of alternatives are available such as lowering O_2 (e.g. rest, pharmacologic agents, hypothermia) or treatments to modify the cause of anaemia (e.g. stop bleeding, treat underlying disease). But if neither of these can be done, then a number of specific factors should be evaluated.

When the haemoglobin is less than 6 g/dl few would argue with the decision to transfuse except when the anaemia is of very long standing. Such cases would include, for example, some patients with pernicious anaemia who are well-adapted to a very low haematocrit. But the adaptation is due, in part, to chronically increased cardiac output and expanded blood volume, and too vigorous transfusion can push the patient into overt congestive heart failure.

Physiology of oxygen transport

The "optimal" haematocrit

Because it is easily measured, haematocrit is too frequently equated with O_2 transport capability. What is the "optimal" haematocrit? Obviously, there is no simple answer to this question and certainly none that would apply to all patients. The bulk viscosity of blood increases exponentially with haematocrit, and increased viscosity raises resistance to blood flow, limiting cardiac output in the absence of compensatory mechanisms. As the O_2 capacity of the blood (haemoglobin or haematocrit) increases, cardiac output decreases, and over a wide range of haematocrit there exists an optimum, defined as the point of maximal O_2 delivery. These principles have been studied theoretically [35], in animals [24] and in humans with extensions to high altitude polycythemia [34] and the general conclusion is that 35% haematocrit represents be best combination of cardiac output and haematocrit in healthy animals and humans. If all patients were in perfect health a transfusion trigger could be simply defined as 35%, therefore.

The problem, of course, is that patients, by definition, are not in perfect health, and the ability to compensate for loss of haemoglobin by raising cardiac output, for example, may be quite variable. In addition, it is not always simple to determine which patients can utilise compensatory mechanisms and which cannot, or which ones are in greater danger of localised tissue ischaemia because of restrictions such as coronary stenosis. In order to move beyond the type of formulas provided in Table 1, it is necessary to understand the basic principles of O_2 transport to tissue.

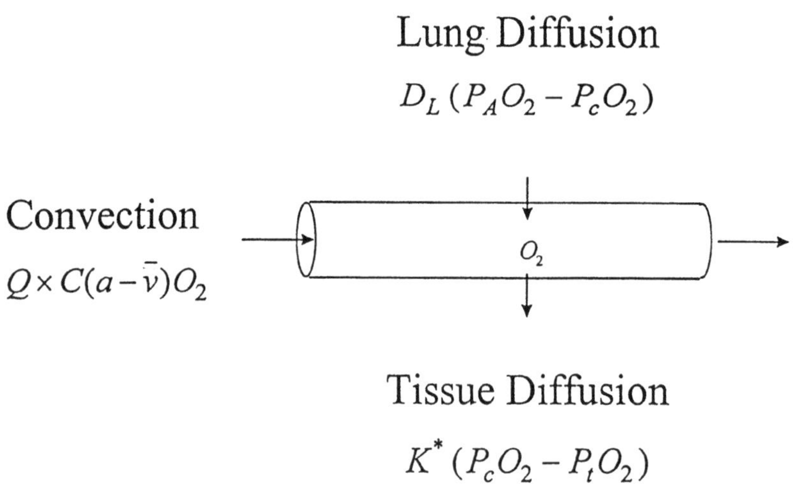

Figure 1. Convective and diffusive O_2 transport. Diffusion refers to the O_2 gradient driven transfer of O_2 from red blood cells to tissue. Convection is the bulk delivery of O_2 to the microcirculation.

Definition of terms

Oxygen transport has 2 components: convection and diffusion (Figure 1).

Convective O_2 transport is the product of the blood flow (cardiac output) and the difference between arterial and mixed venous blood O_2 content. This relationship is simply a statement of the well-known Fick equation:

$$(1)\quad V_{O2} = Q \times (CaO_2 - C\bar{v}O_2)$$

where VO_2 is the O_2 utilised by the body, Q is the cardiac output, and CaO_2 and $C\bar{v}O_2$ are the arterial and mixed venous O_2 contents, respectively.

Diffusive O_2 transport in the lung is described by the diffusion equation:

$$(2)\quad \frac{d(O_2)}{dt} = \frac{100}{V_c} \cdot \frac{D_L}{60} \cdot \left(P_{AO_2} - P_{cO_2}\right)$$

where $d(O_2)/dt$ is the rate of O_2 diffusion into the capillary, PAO_2 is the alveolar PO_2, PcO_2 is the pulmonary capillary PO_2, D_L is the diffusion coefficient for O_2 in the lung and is regarded as a resistance to diffusion. V_c is the volume of capillary blood. Roughton and Forster [36] described the components of this resistance as the in-series sum of a membrane component and the "reactivity" of haemoglobin with O_2:

$$(3)\quad \frac{1}{D_L} = \frac{1}{D_m} + \frac{1}{\theta_{O_2} \times V_c}$$

In this equation, D_M is the diffusion coefficient for the alveolar/capillary membrane interface and is proportional to the thickness of the membrane. (θ_{O_2} is the reaction rate constant of O_2 with haemoglobin.

Diffusion of oxygen from capillaries to tissues is much more difficult to quantitate, because of the inaccessibility of capillary beds to direct measurements. The equations describing tissue diffusion are similar to the description in the lung:

$$(4)\quad \frac{dO_2}{dt} = K^*(P_cO_2 - P_tO_2)$$

where P_tO_2 is the tissue PO_2. The diffusion constant, K^*, can be further defined as:

$$(5)\quad K^* = \frac{D_{O_2}}{r} \times \alpha$$

where D_{O2} is the diffusivity of O_2 in plasma, α is its solubility, and r is the vessel diameter. Hellums [37] concluded, based on mathematical modelling, that about half the total resistance to O_2 diffusion to tissues is intracapillary.

These relationships are conceptually simple, but their exact quantitation is complex. For example, O_2 is dependent on haemoglobin saturation, which, in turn is dependent on the position of the O_2-haemoglobin saturation curve (P50), itself dependent on 2,3-DPG, pH, and PCO_2. pH and PCO_2 are further interdependent, and both are affected by the buffering of haemoglobin. Each of the terms in equations 1-5 has a number of determinants which can vary in different physiological conditions and in disease or pathological states (Figure 2). While complex, all of these variables can be accounted for using mathematical models [38]. The situation in the tissues is slightly more complicated than in the lung but in general represents the mirror image and the principles governing the exchange of gases are the same.

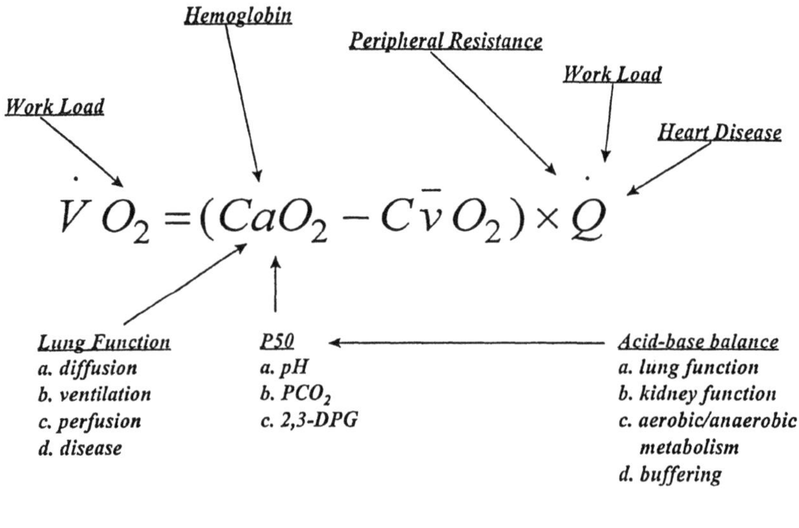

Figure 2. Interactions of the determinants of oxygen transport in health and disease [34].

Autoregulation

Autoregulation is the process whereby the delivery of O_2 to tissues is matched to demand by various combinations of the variables in equations 1-5 and Figure 2. *It is the ability to autoregulate O_2 delivery that determines the individual's need for a red cell transfusion and his/her reaction to it.* Autoregulation can be considered to be a balance between blood flow and O_2 extraction. The mechanisms which ensure autoregulation involve both central nervous and peripheral components. The central nervous mechanisms are comprised of the control of ventilation, hypoxic ventilatory responses, and carotid body reflexes, for example. Peripheral mechanisms are the result of local metabolic controls and have been studied extensively in denervated animals. In such preparations when blood pressure is decreased, oxygen extraction increases.

The oxygen extraction ratio (OER) is the fraction of O_2 that is removed from blood on a passage from the arterial to the venous circulation and is defined:

$$(6)\quad OER = \frac{C(a-\bar{v})O_2}{CaO_2}$$

Arterial O_2 content (CaO_2), venous O_2 content (CvO_2) and their difference ($C(a\text{-}v)O_2$) are determined predominantly by the product of the haemoglobin concentration and fractional saturation, because normally approximately 97% of blood O_2 is carried bound to haemoglobin, the remaining O_2 being physically dissolved in plasma.

As an example of an autoregulation experiment, Shepherd et al. [39] studied decapitated dogs, in whom blood pressure was maintained by infusion of epinephrine. When the blood pressure was lowered by either decreasing the epinephrine infusion or reducing the level of venous blood return to the heart, cardiac output fell precipitously to about 60% of its control value. At the same time, the extraction of O_2 in the circulation increased by a comparable amount, so that tissue oxygen consumption (VO_2) was preserved. Thus the end result of autoregulation was maintenance of tissue homeostasis over a range of different conditions. In other words, the variables in equations 1-6 and Figure 2 can be adjusted in almost infinitely different combinations to keep overall O_2 supply to tissues at a "normal" level. This is a very important concept for the transfusion trigger, because it suggests that need for a 1 to 1 replacement of lost red cells is not necessary because of the body's capacity to compensate through a variety of mechanisms. The problem comes in determining when the compensatory mechanisms are stretched to their limit in a given patient.

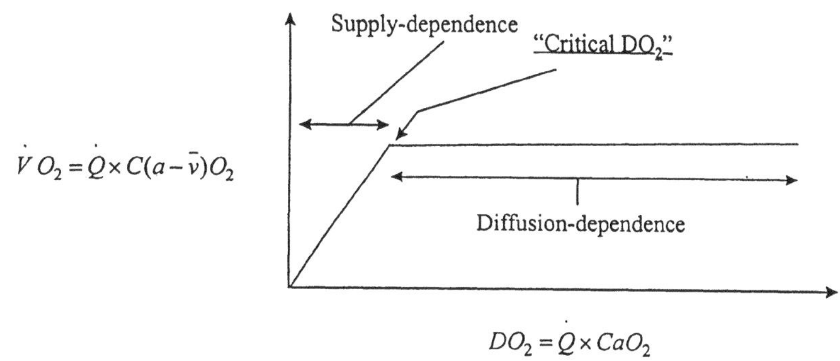

Figure 3. The critical DO_2 ($Q \times CaO_2$). As the haematocrit is reduced, VO_2 is maintained by a combination of rising cardiac output and dropping PO_2. When these compensations no longer suffice, VO_2 falls, and tissue ischaemia occurs. The goal of transfusion therapy is to maintain the O_2 reserve such that this point is not reached.

Oxygen utilisation: DO_2, O_2, and the "critical O_2"

A useful way to consider the limits of compensation was introduced by Cain et al. [13]. They compared the delivery of O_2 (DO_2, cardiac output × arterial O_2 content) with O_2 utilisation (VO_2). This analysis led to the demonstration that as haematocrit is decreased (decreasing DO_2), there is no change in O_2 uptake (O_2) until a "critical" DO_2 is reached, at which point O_2 can no longer be sustained (Figure 3). Thus, DO_2 has two components, called diffusion-limited (above the critical DO_2) and supply-limited (below the critical DO_2) O_2 delivery.

As will be discussed below, patients are in serious danger of organ failure if DO_2 is allowed to drop below the critical value, and the goal of transfusion (and other) therapy, is to maintain DO_2 well above that value so that an appropriate reserve of O_2 is maintained should the patient require it because of blood loss or elevated O_2 requirement.

Physiological transfusion triggers

Using the quantitative framework developed above, it should be possible to identify physiological markers which can be used as a transfusion trigger which might be more useful than haemoglobin or haematocrit (Table 3). While no single trigger provides a clear-cut transfusion indication, the thoughtful clinician observes all possible signs of tissue ischaemia and, based on experience, attempts to transfuse before the critical DO_2 is reached.

Table 3. Potential transfusion triggers

– Blood loss (real, estimated or anticipated)
– Haemoglobin, haematocrit
– Symptoms (ischaemia, e.g. angina)
– Haemodynamics (BP, HR, postural effects)
– O_2 transport (VO_2, OER, PvO_2)
– Metabolic status (lactic acid, pH, base excess)
– Cardiac output
– Ventilation (PCO_2)

Haematocrit/haemoglobin concentration

The most commonly used parameter, the haematocrit (or haemoglobin concentration) is useful in some clinical situations, but not in others, and it is important to be aware of its limitations. For example, in chronic anaemia, an expanded plasma volume gives the impression that the red cell mass is smaller than it really is. In acute blood loss, some time is required for the fluid spaces to re-equilibrate and the haematocrit to once again reflect the red cell mass.

In one study of surgical patients, Cordts et al. [40] found that while haematocrit significantly correlated with red cell mass both intra- and postoperatively, the ability of the haematocrit to predict red cell mass in individual patients was poor. In their study, haemodynamic parameters did not contribute to prediction of the red cell mass, plasma volume, or total blood volume at any time, and the authors believe that some patients, particularly those at risk for coronary ischaemia, may be undertransfused if traditional haematocrit "triggers" are used. Similarly, Kim et al. [41] found that the number of inpatient days did not correlate with the level of haemoglobin at discharge, preoperative haemoglobin, or drop in haemoglobin during hospitalisation. They concluded that use of blood transfusion as a means to shorten hospitalisation is probably not justified. However, in another study of patients with postoperative myocardial ischaemia [18], a postoperative haematocrit less than 28% was found to be associated with significantly more ischaemic events than a haematocrit over 28%.

The haemoglobin concentration in Jehovah's Witness patients who undergo surgery with severe anaemia is only a predictor of overall outcome when less than 3 g/dl. Multiple independent factors influence outcome of these severely anaemic surgical patients, the strongest being sepsis and active bleeding [42].

Mixed venous PO_2

Mixed venous PO_2 (PVO_2) would seem an obviously important parameter to assess adequacy of tissue oxygenation since, in theory, the mixed venous blood should be in equilibrium with tissue. Some clinical studies have shown that PVO_2 decreases when O_2 is supply-dependent (see Figure 3) [22]. However, as is now known, the tissue PO_2 is much lower than mixed venous values [43,44] and PVO_2 can be normal even in severe anaemia [45]. Nevertheless, a decreasing PVO_2 has been used as a classic indicator of reduced tissue oxygenation, and perhaps a dropping value should be more meaningful to clinical evaluation of a given patient than an absolute value. Traditional textbooks of critical care medicine indicate that transfusions may be helpful when the PVO_2 drops.

Mixed venous O_2 saturation (SVO_2) may be a more useful indicator of severe O_2 extraction. Because of the steepness of the haemoglobin-O_2 dissociation curve, when mixed venous PO_2 falls below approximately 30 torr, the haemoglobin saturation falls rapidly. As the haemoglobin reserve depletes, small drops in PO_2 will drop the SO_2 more rapidly. SO_2 falls dramatically at haematocrits less than approximately 20%. In one clinical study, Spiess et al. [46] showed that SvO_2 is a sensitive indicator of overall VO_2 in liver transplant patients. In those patients, removal of the liver with attendant reduction in VO_2 produced a measurable rise in SO_2. When the new liver became functional, SvO_2 fell back to normal values.

O_2 consumption (VO_2)

Haemoglobin concentration may limit maximal O_2 in some circumstances. However, the potential advantages of "blood doping" have not been fully realised and, in general, the increased O_2 associated with transfusion has been marginal, and limited to well-trained athletes performing maximal work [47]. Extending these observations to patients may be of little value, since patients never consume O_2 at or near their maximal rate.

Published literature suggests that reduced VO_2 in postoperative and trauma patients is associated with a poor prognosis, and that increasing DO_2 by intervention (fluid boluses, administration of blood products, the use of inotropes) reduces mortality rate [48]. In contrast, other evidence indicates that the way in which DO_2 is increased is critical: volume resuscitation more effectively raises O_2 than transfusion, even though both raise DO_2.

In septic shock, VO_2 may be pathologically dependent on DO_2 [49-51]. Patients whose cardiac output (and therefore DO_2) can be increased with dobutamine [52,53] or adrenaline [54] can increase VO_2, possibly by improving specific organ perfusion [55]. However, when DO_2 is raised by increasing haemoglobin concentration by transfusion, no effect is seen on VO_2 [54-57]. In fact, when 23 critically ill patients with sepsis were transfused with stored blood, not only did the VO_2 (measured by calorimetry) fail to rise, but there was an inverse relationship between gastric mucosal pH and the age of the transfused blood [58], indicating poorer tissue oxygenation. In other studies, VO_2 failed to correlate with lactate levels in septic patients given either fluid therapy, transfusions, or dobutamine [59-61]. These studies all indicate that pathological reduction of O_2 in sepsis is due to reduced tissue perfusion, not reduced O_2 content of the perfusing blood.

Acute respiratory distress syndrome (ARDS) patients may represent another case in which O_2 uptake and utilisation do not agree: they may not increase VO_2 after increasing DO_2 [62,63]. Hanique et al. [56] studied 3 groups of patients: those with sepsis, ARDS, and hepatic failure. They increased cardiac output by volume loading to increase DO_2, measured VO_2 by calorimetry and calculated VO_2 by Fick (equation l). They found that the calculated VO_2 (Fick) increased, while the measured VO_2 (calorimetry) did not. By using an increase in VO_2 as a criterion for successful transfusion. as many as 58% of transfusions may be of questionable importance [64].

Oxygen extraction ratio (OER)

The oxygen extraction ratio is the fraction of arterial O_2 delivery extracted by tissue (equation 6). In dogs with experimental stenotic lesions in the left anterior descending coronary arteries, hearts did not raise their output in response to bleeding, showed greater lactate production, and failed at a higher haematocrit (17%) than controls (10.6%) [65]. The authors of this study concluded that in the normal heart lactate production occurs when OER $>$ 50% and Hct $<$ 10%, but in the stenotic animals OER $>$ 50% corresponded to a haematocrit $<$ 20%. Thus, an OER $>$ 50% indicated a need for transfusion, and the findings indicate that the transfusion trigger, in terms of haematocrit or haemoglobin concentration, is higher in hearts with underlying coronary ischaemia. Similar results have been reported for primates [66], and the observations are consistent with experience with patients [67].

Haemodynamic instability

In shock, reduced O_2 capacity and blood volume contraction exist at the same time. Most resuscitations are carried out first with volume expanders, then with replacement of lost red cells. However, it is not clear whether volume or O_2 capacity reduction is more important. Thus, Dietrich et al. [68] studied patients with a variety of diagnoses who had undergone volume resuscitation. They concluded that an increase of DO_2 by transfused red blood cells did increase O_2 capacity, but they could not demonstrate any benefit measured as increased O_2, decreased lactate or myocardial work. These observations lend support to the clinical dictum that in haemodynamic shock, raising the haemoglobin concentration must be accompanied or preceded by volume expansion.

Blood loss

Blood loss itself, apart from the attendant haemodynamic changes, is an important indicator of the need for transfusion. Carson et al. [42] carried out a careful study of 125 surgical patients who declined to be transfused on religious grounds and found that mortality was inversely related to haemoglobin concentration. Mortality rose from 7.1% for patients with haemoglobin concentrations over 10 g/dl to 61.5% for those with haemoglobin concentrations below 6 g/dl. Mortality was 8% for patients in whom 500 ml or less blood was lost but rose to 42.9% for those in whom loss was greater than 2000 ml.

Symptoms

Although a quantitative index of the need for a red blood cell transfusion would be optimal, in many instances, especially in cases of chronic anaemia, the decision to transfuse is based on subjective symptom evaluation. None of the subjective symptoms are uniquely indicative of anaemia per se, and so they must be evaluated in the context of the patient's total clinical presentation. However, these symptoms are of most benefit in patients in whom other, more quantitative "triggers" do not provide the clinician with a clear decision as to whether or not to transfuse. Unfortunately, many patients who require transfusions are unable to report symptoms because of their state of consciousness, or the use of sedatives or anaesthetics.

Other signs of ischaemia

It would seem that demonstration of haemoglobin-dependent oxygenation of specific tissues should be possible using modern sophisticated techniques of measurement. In general, this has not been the case. For example, when ^{19}F magnetic resonance spectroscopy was used to examine the in vivo bioenergetics in forearm muscles, no effect of increasing the haemoglobin concentration from 8.9 to 12.9 g/dl could be shown [69]. Although O_2 is needed for wound healing, deposition of new collagen requires very little of it. Jonsson et al. [70] were not able to demonstrate any correlation of haematocrit and collagen deposition in 33 postoperative surgical patients.

Summary and conclusions: Individualised transfusion triggers

The "transfusion trigger" may be not only an elusive goal, but an inappropriate one. Physiologic studies cited in this chapter have shown animals can survive with haemoglobin concentrations lower than most clinicians would permit in patients. The NIH Clinical Conference [6] recommended that a 10 g/dl haemoglobin concentration might be too high for a transfusion trigger. When the haemoglobin is between 7 and 10 g/dl many physiological and clinical data have to be considered before an intelligent decision can be made. Indeed, it might be time to abandon the concept of a "transfusion trigger" in favour of a more sophisticated individual analysis of O_2 transport.

What effect should age, sex, heart disease, sickle cell anaemia, or sepsis have on the decision to transfuse? The decision in an individual patient should be based on his/her need for augmented O_2 delivery to tissue. and the risk of not transfusing. Transfusion of blood or blood products is done for several reasons, and these should be carefully defined for each patient. The most important distinction which needs to be made is between the need for volume and the need for increased O_2 content of the arterial blood. The two do not necessarily go together: in acute haemorrhage, volume replacement may be more critical than it is in the chronically anaemic patient in which O_2 content may be of primary concern.

There is no alternative to the exercise of good clinical judgement in the decision to transfuse a patient, but this requires an understanding of the fundamental determinants of O_2 transport and the way these determinants interact and compensate for anaemia in individual patients. In approaching the decision to transfuse an individual patient, consideration must be given to each point in Table 1.

References

1. Stehling L, Simon TL. The red blood cell transfusion trigger. Physiology and clinical studies. Arch Pathol Lab Med 1994;118:429-34.
2. Goodnough LT, Verbrugge D, Vizmeg K, Riddell 4th J. Identifying elective orthopedic surgical patients transfused with amounts of blood in excess of need: the transfusion trigger revisited. Transfusion 1992; 32:648-53.
3. Levine E, Rosen A, Sehgal L, Gould S, Sehgal H, Moss G. Physiologic effects of acute anaemia: implications for a reduced transfusion trigger. Transfusion 1990;30: 11-14.
4. Greenburg, AG. A physiologic basis for red blood cell transfusion decisions. Am J Surg 1995;70(6A suppl):44S-48S.
5. Robertie PG, Gravlee GP. Safe limits of isovolemic haemodilution and recommendations for erythrocyte transfusion. Int Anesth Clin 1990;28:197-204.
6. NIH Consensus Conference. Perioperative Red Cell Transfusion. JAMA 1988;260: 2700-03.
7. Mollison PL. Blood transfusion in clinical medicine. 7th ed. Philadelphia: FA Davis, 1983.
8. Schreiber GB, MP Busch, SH Kleimnan, JJ Kovelitz, for the Retrovirus Epidemiology Donor Study. The risk of transfusion-transmitted viral infection. N Engl J Med 1996;34:1685-90.

9. Winslow, R.M. In: Rudolph AS, Rabinovici, R, Feuerstein, GZ (eds). Red Blood Cell Substitutes. New York: Marcel Dekker, 1998:37-38.
10. Baele PL, De Bruyere M, Deneys V, et al. The SANGUIS Study in Belgium: an overview. Acta Chir Belg 1994;94:69-74.
11. Friedman BA, Bums TL, Schork MA. An analysis of blood transfusion of surgical patients by sex: a question for the transfusion trigger. Transfusion 1980;20:179-88.
12. Wilkerson DK, Rosen AL, Sehgal LR, Gould SA, Sehgal HL, Moss GS. Limits of cardiac compensation in anemic baboons. Surgery 1988;103:666-70.
13. Cain SM. Oxygen delivery and uptake in dogs during anemic and hypoxic hypoxia. J Appl Physiol 1977; 42:228-34.
14. Kitchens CS. Are transfusions overrated? Surgical outcome of Jehovah's Witnesses. Am J Med 1993;94:117-19.
15. Spahn DR, Smith LR, Veronee CD, et al. Acute isovolemic haemodilution and blood transfusion. Effects on reg function and metabolism in myocardium with compromised coronary blood flow. J Thorac Cardiovasc Surg 1993;105:694-704.
16. Levy PS, Kim SJ, Eckel PK, et al. Limit to cardiac compensation during acute isovolemic haemodilution: influence of coronary stenosis. Am J Physiol 1993;265: H340-H49.
17. Christopherson R, Frank S, Norris E, Rock P, Gottlieb S, Beattie C. Low postoperative haematocrit is associated with cardiac ischemia in high-risk patients. Anesthesiology 199 l;75(3A):A99.
18. Nelson AH, Fleisher LA, Rosenbaum SH. Relationship between postoperative anaemia and cardiac morbidity in high risk vascular patients in the intensive care unit. Crit Care Med 1993;210:860-66.
19. Johnson RG, Thurer RL, Kruskall MS, et al. Comparison of two transfusion strategies after elective operations for myocardial revascularization. J Thorac Cardlovasc Surg 1992;104:307-14.
20. Dick W, Baur C, Reiff K. Which factors determine the critical haematocrit as an indication of transfusion? Anaesthesist 1992;41:1-14.
21. Wisner DH, Holcroft JW. Surgical critical care. Curr Prob Surg 1990;27:467-69.
22. Meyers RL, Paulick R-P, Rudolph CD, Rudolph AM. Cardiovascular responses to acute, severe haemorrhage in fetal sheep. J Dev Physiol 1991;15:189-97.
23. Ping Wang ZF, Ba M-CL, Ayala A, Harkema JM, Chaudry IH. Measurement of circulating blood volume in vivo after trauma-haemorrhage and haemodilution. Am J Physiol 1994;266:R368-R74.
24. Guyton AC, Jones CE, Coleman TG. Cardiac output and its regulation. 2nd ed. Philadelphia: Saunders, 1973.
25. Wasserman K, Hansen JE, Sue DY. Facilitation of oxygen consumption by lactic acidosis during exercise. News in Physiological Science 1991;6:29-34.
26. Mitzner W, Goldberg HS, Lichenstein S. Effects of thoracic blood volume changes on steady state cardiac output. Circ Res 1976;38:255-61.
27. Saxena S, Rabinowitz AP, Johnson C, Shulman IA. Iron-deficiency anaemia: a medically treatable chronic anaemia as a model for transfusion overuse. Am J Med 1993; 94:120-24.
28. Stehling L, Zauder HL. Acute normovolemic haemodilution. Transfusion 1991;31: 857-68.
29. Viele MK, Weiskopf RB. What can we learn about the need for transfusion from patients who refuse blood? The experience with Jehovah's witnesses. Transfusion 1994;34:396-401.

30. Polley JW, Berkowitz RA, McDonald TB, Cohen M, Figueroa A, Penney DW. Craniomaxillofacial surgery in the Jehovah's Witness patient. Plast Reconstr Surg 1994;93(6):1258-63.
31. Marelli TR. Use of a haemoglobin substitute in the anemic Jehovah's Witness patient. Crit Care Nurse 1994;February:31-38.
32. Newton CR, Marsh K, Peshu N, Mwangi I. Blood transfusions for severe anaemia in African children. Lancet 1992;340:916-17.
33. Faust RJ. Perioperative indications for red blood cell transfusion: has the pendulum swung too far? Mayo Clinic Proc 1993;68:512-14.
34. Winslow RM, Monge CC. Hypoxia, polycythemia, and chronic mountain sickness. Baltimore: Johns Hopkins University Press, 1987.
35. Crowell JW, Smith EE. Determination of the optimal haematocrit. J Appl Physiol 1967;22(3):501-4.
36. Roughton FJW, Forster RE. Relative importance of diffusion and chemical reaction rates in determining rate of exchange of gases in the human with special reference to true diffusing capacity of pulmonary. J Appl Physiol 1957;11:290-302.
37. Hellums JD. The resistance to oxygen transport in the capillaries relative to that in the surrounding tissue. Microvasc Res 1995;13;131-45.
38. Winslow RM. A model for red cell O_2 uptake. Int J Clin Monit Comput 1985;2:81-93.
39. Shephard AP, Granger HJ, Smith EE, Guyton AC. Local control of tissue oxygen delivery and its contribution to the regulation of cardiac output. Am J Physiol 1973;225:747-55.
40. Cordts PR, LaMonte WW, Fisher JB, et al. Poor predictive value of haematocrit and haemodynamic parameters for erythrocyte deficits after extensive elective vascular operations. Surg Gynec Obstet 1992;175:243-48.
41. Kim DA, Brecher ME, Estes TJ, Morrey BF. Relationship of haemoglobin and duration of hospitalization after total hip arthroplasty: implications for the transfusion target. Mayo Clinic Proc 1993;68:37-41.
42. Carson JL, Spence RK, Poses RM, Bonavita G. Severity of anaemia and operative mortality and morbidity. Lancet 1988;1:727-29.
43. Piiper J, Meyer M, Scheid P. Dual role of diffusion in tissue gas exchange: blood-tissue equilibration and diffusion shunt. Respir Physiol 1984;56:131-44.
44. 45. Tenney SM. A theoretical analysis of the relationships between venous blood and mean tissue oxygen pressures. Respir Physiol 1974;20:238-96.
45. Gould SA, Rosen AL, Sehgal LR, et al. O_2 extraction ratio: A physiologic indicator of transfusion need [Abstract]. Transfusion 1983;23:S416.
46. Spiess BD, Tuman KJ, McCarthy RJ, et al. Oxygen consumption and mixed venous oxygen saturation monitoring during orthotopic liver transplantation. J Clin Monit 1992;8:7-11.
47. Hoppeler YH, Noti C, Gurtner HP, et al. Limitations to VO_2max in humans after blood retransfusion. Respir Physiol 1993; 92:329-41.
48. Yu M, Levy MM, Smith P, Takiguchi SA, Miyasaki A, Myers SA. Effect of maximizing oxygen delivery on morbidity and mortality rate in critically ill patients: a prospective, randomized, controlled study. Crit Care Med 1993;21:830-38.
49. Slanetz PJ, Lee R, Page R, Jacobs Jr EE, LaRaia PJ, Vlahakes GJ. Haemoglobin blood substitutes in extended preoperative autologous blood donation: an experimental study. Surgery 1994;115:246-54.
50. Cain SM, Curtis SE. Experimental models of pathological oxygen supply dependency. Crit Care Med 1991;19:603-12.
51. Cain SM. Assessment of tissue oxygenation. Crit Care Clin 1986;2:537-50.

52. Mink RB, Pollack MM. Effect of blood transfusion on oxygen consumption in pediatric septic shock. Crit Care Med 1990;18:1087-91.
53. Lorente JA, Landin L, De Pablo R, Renes E, Rodriguez-Diaz R, Liste D. Effects of blood transfusion on oxygen transport variables in severe sepsis. Crit Care Med 1993;21:1312-18.
54. Seear M, Wensley D, MacNab A. Oxygen consumption-oxygen delivery relationship in children. J Pediatr 1993;123:208-14.
55. Silverman HJ, Tuma P. Gastric tonometry in patients with sepsis. Effects of dobutamine infusions and packed red blood cell transfusions. Chest 1992;102:184-88.
56. Hanique G, Dugemier T, Laterre PF, Dougnac A, Roeseler J, Reynaert MS. Significance of pathologic oxygen supply dependency in critically ill patients: comparison between measured and calculated methods. Intensive Care Med 1994;20:12-18.
57. Lucking SE, Williams TM, Chaten FC, Metz RI, Mickell JJ. Dependence of oxygen consumption on oxygen delivery in children with hyperdynamic septic shock and low oxygen extraction. Crit Care Med 1990;18:1316-19.
58. Marik PE, Sibbald WJ. Effect of stored-blood transfusion on oxygen delivery in patients with sepsis. JAMA 1993; 269:3024-29.
59. Steffes CP, Bender JS, Levison MA. Blood transfusion and oxygen consumption in surgical sepsis. Crit Care Med 1991;19:512-17.
60. Silverman HJ. Lack of a relationship between induced changes in oxygen consumption and changes in lactate levels. Chest 1991;100:1012-15.
61. Conrad SA, Dietrich KA, Hebert CA, Romero MD. Effect of red cell transfusion on oxygen consumption following fluid resuscitation in septic shock. Circ Shock 1990; 31:419-29.
62. Ronco JJ, Phang PT, Walley KR, Wiggs B, Fenwick JC, Russell JA. Oxygen consumption is independent of changes in oxygen delivery in adult respiratory distress syndrome. Am Rev Respir Dis 1991;143:1267-73.
63. Ronco JJ, Montaner JS, Fenwick JC, Russell JA. Pathologic dependence of oxygen consumption on oxygen delivery in respiratory failure secondary to AIDS-related Pneumocystis carinii pneumonia. Chest 1990;98:1463-66.
64. Babineau TJ, Dzik VM, Borlase BC, Baxter JK, Bistrian BR, Benotti PN. Reevaluation of current transfusion practices in patients in surgical intensive care units. Am J Surg 1992;164:22-25.
65. Levy PS, Chavez RP, Crystal GJ, et al. Oxygen extraction ratio: a valid indicator of transfusion need in 1 coronary vascular reserve? J Traum 1992;32:769-73; discussion, 773-74.
66. Wilkerson DK, Rosen AL, Gould SA, Sehgal LR, Sehgal HL, Moss GS. Whole body oxygen extraction ratio as an indicator of cardiac status in anaemia. Current Surgery 1988;45:214-17.
67. Mathru M, Kleinman B, Blakeman B, Sullivan H, Kumar P, Dries DJ. Myocardial metabolism and adaptation during extreme haemodilution in humans after coronary revascularization. Crit Care Med 1992;20:1420-25.
68. Dietrich KA, Conrad SA, Hebert CA, Levy GL, Romero MD. Cardiovascular and metabolic response to red blood cell transfusion in critically ill volume-resuscitated nonsurgical patients. Crit Care Med 1990;18:940-44.
69. Thompson CH, Kemp GJ, Taylor DJ, Ledingham JG, Radda GK, Rajagopalan B. No effect of blood transfusion on muscle metabolism. Q J Med 1992;85:897-99.
70. Jonsson K, Jensen JA, Goodson VM, et al. Tissue oxygenation, anaemia, and perfusion in relation to wound healing in surgical patients. Ann Surg 1991;214:605-13.

RECOMBINANT HUMAN ERYTHROPOIETIN – COULD IT BE USED IN A BETTER WAY?

L.T. Goodnough

Introduction

Recombinant human erythropoietin (EPO) therapy has now been approved for use in patients undergoing autologous blood donation (ABD) in Japan, the European Union, and Canada since 1993, 1994, and 1996 respectively, and for perisurgical adjuvant therapy without ABD in Canada and the US since 1966. This paper is intended to provide a framework for clinicians who will have the options of administering EPO therapy to patients undergoing surgery, and to provide a better understanding of its proper use in this setting [1].

Early clinical trials

Patients donating autologous blood under standard conditions (i.e., one blood unit weekly) [2,3] have an inadequate response of endogenous erythropoietin to blood loss anaemia, suggesting that EPO therapy might be able to facilitate autologous blood donation by enhancing compensatory erythropoiesis; this was subsequently confirmed in a clinical trial of aggressive autologous blood donation (up to six units over a three week preoperative interval), with or without EPO therapy, in patients undergoing orthopaedic surgery [4]. Subsequently clinical trials [5-8] in orthopaedic patients demonstrated that for autologous blood donors who were not anaemic (haematocrit > 39%) at first donation, no clinical benefit (defined as reduced allogeneic blood exposure) was seen with EPO therapy. Thus, for non-anaemic patients, autologous blood donation remains the standard of care if they can tolerate aggressive blood phlebotomy (i.e., up to six units over three weeks) and thereby achieve stimulation of erythropoiesis via their endogenous erythropoietin response [9].

For anaemic (haematocrit ≤ 39%) autologous blood donors, a European clinical trial demonstrated that EPO therapy reduced exposure to allogeneic blood during orthopaedic surgery when compared to placebo-treated patients [10]. However, this result was achieved with both intravenous and oral supplemental iron. A subsequent US trial with oral supplemental iron alone did not demonstrate reduced allogeneic blood transfusions when compared to placebo-treated patients [11], in large part because a substantial percentage of the patients were either severely anaemic (haematocrit < 33%) or were iron deficient.

Several studies have evaluated perisurgical EPO therapy in orthopaedic surgical patients without autologous blood procurement who were not anaemic. Both a Canadian [12] and two US studies [13,14] were able to show that EPO-treated (300 u/kg S.Q. × 14 days, beginning nine days preoperatively) patients had approximately one half the rate of exposure to allogeneic blood as the placebo-treated patients, even though the mean initial haemoglobin levels exceeded 130 g/L for patients in both studies. On the basis of these clinical trials, EPO therapy was approved for perisurgical use in Canada and the US in 1996.

Safety, dose-response, and cost

The safety of EPO therapy in patients undergoing non-cardiac surgery has been demonstrated by the equal distribution of adverse concomitant events between patients treated with EPO or placebo in over 1,000 patients participating in clinical trials. Early thrombotic events described in patients with renal failure [5] have not been seen in clinical trials of EPO in the surgical setting [6]. An analysis of the relationship between dose and response relationship of EPO therapy and red cell production has demonstrated that the EPO-stimulated erythropoiesis is independent of age and gender [15]. Red blood cell expansion in patients treated with EPO is seen with an increase in reticulocyte count by day three of treatment [4]. The equivalent of one blood unit is produced by day seven and the equivalent of five blood units produced over 28 days [5]. If three to five blood units are necessary in order to minimise allogeneic blood exposure in patients undergoing complex procedures such as orthopaedic joint replacement surgery [16,17], the preoperative interval necessary for EPO-stimulated erythropoiesis can be estimated to be three to four weeks. The costs associated with EPO therapy and the potential impact of reimbursement policies are important issues in the setting of surgical anaemias, as has been the case in medical anaemias [18,19]. Costs associated with EPO therapy may be lowered by strategies that improve the dose and response relationship. The pharmacoeconomics of subcutaneous administration is superior to intravenous administration [20]. A recent study [21] demonstrated that four weekly injections of subcutaneous EPO (600 u/kg) was less costly ($1600 in a 70 kilogram patient) but was just as effective as a daily dose of EPO (300 units per kilogram for 14 doses at a cost of $2800). However, these regimens [12-14,21] remain expensive, and when unaccompanied by autologous blood procurement, are still associated with an allogeneic exposure rate of 16-25%.

Emerging strategies

An alternative method of perioperative autologous blood procurement is acute normovolemic haemodilution (ANH). Blood is collected in standard blood bags containing anticoagulant, stored at room temperature, and reinfused after major blood loss has ceased, or sooner if indicated. The rationale for the use of haemodilution is that perisurgical red blood cell loss is reduced if whole blood is shed at a lower (25 to 30%) rather than a higher (39 to 45%) level of intraoperative haematocrit [22]. Since this blood is re-infused in the operating room, the costs of blood procurement are much lower than those of predeposited autologous blood. Two recent studies in patients undergoing radical prostatectomy concluded that moderate ANH is less costly but just as effective as autologous blood donation, resulting in an approximate allogeneic exposure rate of 20% with either technique [23,24].

One approach to enhance the efficacy of haemodilution is to couple this technique with EPO therapy. In one study, a three arm trial of moderate haemodilution with EPO therapy (1500 u/kg in three divided doses over three weeks) was compared to haemodilution alone and also to the preoperative autologous donation of three units in patients undergoing radical prostatectomy [25]. Four percent of patients treated with EPO and acute normovolemic haemodilution required allogeneic blood, compared to 16% in the other two groups. In the EPO-treated patients, mean haematocrit levels were greater than 30% throughout the surgical hospitalisation. This benefit may be clinically important, since radical prostatectomy is a procedure that is associated with a 2% risk of perioperative myocardial infarction [26]. Using this approach, the cost of three weekly doses for a 70 kg man was $1000. When the transfusion costs associated with acute haemodilution ($100) are added, the total costs may be estimated at $1100, or approximately twice the costs associated with donation of three units of autologous blood [27]. A similar regimen of EPO therapy in patients undergoing coronary artery bypass grafting (1500 u/kg S.Q. over two weeks preoperative in divided doses), coupled with "blood pooling", was also highly effective [28]. Clinical trials of reduced doses of EPO (450 u/kg × 2 and 300 u/kg × 2) compared to placebo, coupled with haemodilution, are underway in patients undergoing radical prostatectomy.

The most cost-effective us of EPO may be to simply increase the level of haematocrit (without autologous blood donation) in patients who are anaemic and who are anticipated to have substantial surgical blood losses. A target preoperative haematocrit of 45% should minimise the need for allogeneic blood transfusions, especially when accompanied by prudent transfusion practice [29,30]. Patients undergoing more complex surgeries with substantial blood needs may benefit most from a combination of EPO therapy and autologous blood procurement, such as acute normovolemic haemodilution. The minimum dose of EPO to accomplish these goals has been studied in a recent report of "very low doses" of subcutaneous EPO therapy before orthopaedic surgery [31], which found that 100 units per kilogram EPO weekly over four weeks (a total of 400 units per kilogram) was effective in stimulating preoperative erythropoiesis. For a 70 kilogram patient, this approach would require 28,000 units, for a cost of only $280.

Based on current evidence, the least costly regimen would be to administer up to four weekly subcutaneous EPO doses (starting at 100 units per kilogram with increases to 600 units per kilogram, if necessary, for evidence of a reticulocyte response). The most effective approach to minimise allogeneic blood exposure may be to combine preoperative weekly EPO therapy (two to four doses of 200 to 600 units per kilogram each) with cost-effective autologous blood procurement, such as acute normovolemic haemodilution. The challenge for surgeons, anaesthesiologists and transfusion medicine specialists will be to combine the use of EPO therapy with autologous blood procurement so that strategies are cost-equivalent to allogeneic blood transfusion.

References

1. Goodnough LT, Monk TG, Andriole GL. Erythropoietin therapy. N Engl Med 1997; 336:933-38.
2. Goodnough LT, Brittenham G. Limitations of the erythropoietic response to serial phlebotomy: implications of autologous blood donor programs. J Lab Clin Med 1990;115:28-35.
3. Kickler TS, Spivak JL. Effect of repeated whole blood donations on serum immunoreactive erythropoietin levels in autologous donors. JAMA 1988;260:65-67.
4. Goodnough LT, Rudnick S, Price TH, et al. Increased collection of autologous blood preoperatively with recombinant human erythropoietin therapy. N Engl J Med 1989; 321:1163-67.
5. Goodnough LT, Price TH, Rudnick S. Preoperative red blood cell production in patients undergoing aggressive autologous blood phlebotomy with and without erythropoietin therapy. Transfusion 1992;32:441-45.
6. Goodnough LT, Price TH and the EPO Study Group. A phase III trial of recombinant human erythropoietin therapy in non-anaemic orthopaedic patients subjected to aggressive autologous blood phlebotomy: dose, response, toxicity, and efficacy. Transfusion 1994;34:66-71.
7. Beris P, Mermillod B, Levy G, et al. Recombinant human erythropoietin as adjuvant treatment for autologous blood donation. Vox Sang 1993;65:212-18.
8. Biesma DH, Marx JJ, Kraaijenhagen RJ, Franke W, Messinger D, van der Wiel A. Lower homologous blood requirement in autologous blood donors after treatment with recombinant human erythropoietin. Lancet 1994;344:367-70.
9. Goodnough LT, Monk TG, Brecher MF. Autologous blood procurement: lessons to be learned in the last 10 years. Vox Sang 1996;71:133-41.
10. Mercuriali F, Zanella A, Barosi G, et al. Use erythropoietin to increase the volume of autologous blood donated by orthopaedic patients. Transfusion 1993;33:55-60.
11. Price TH, Goodnough LT, Vogler W, et al. The effect of recombinant erythropoietin administration on the efficacy of autologous blood donation in patients with low haematocrits. Transfusion 1996;36:29-36.
12. Canadian orthopedic perioperative erythropoietin study group. Effectiveness of perioperative recombinant human erythropoietin in elective hip replacement. Lancet 1993;341:1227-32.
13. Faris PM, Ritter MA, Abels RI. The effects of recombinant human erythropoietin on preoperative transfusion requirements in patients undergoing major orthopaedic surgery. J Bone Surg 1996;78A:62-72.
14. De Andrade JR, Jove M, Landon G, Frei D,Guilfoyle M, Young DC. Baseline hemoglobin as a predictor of risk of transfusion and response to epoietin alpha in orthopedic surgery patients. Amer J Orth 1996;25:533-42.
15. Goodnough LT, Price TH, Parvin CA, et al. Erythropoietin response to anaemia is not altered by surgery or recombinant human erythropoietin therapy. Brit J Haem 1994;87:695-99.
16. Toy PTCY, Kaplan EB, McVay PA, et al. Blood loss and replacement in total hip arthroplasty: a multicenter study. Transfusion 1992;32:63-67.

17. Goodnough LT, Vizmeg K, Marcus RE. Blood lost and transfused in patients undergoing elective orthopaedic operation. Implications for blood conservation programs. Surg Gynec Obstet 1993;176:235-38.
18. Sisk JE, Gianfrancesco FD, Costner JM. Recombinant erythropoietin and medicare payment. JAMA 199;266:247-52.
19. Doolittle RF. Biotechnology – the enormous cost of success. N Engl J Med 1991; 324:1360-62.
20. McMahon FG, Vargas R, Ryan M, et al. Pharmacokinetics and effects of recombinant human erythropoietin after intravenous and subcutaneous injections in healthy volunteers. Blood 1990;76:1718-22.
21. Goldberg MA, McCutchen JW, Jove M, et al. A safety and efficacy comparison study of two dosing regimens of erythropoietin alpha in patients undergoing major orhtopedic surgery. Amer J Ortop 1996;25:544-52.
22. Messmer K, Kreimeier M, Intagliett A. Present state of intentional hemodilution. Eur Surg Res 1986;18:254-63.
23. Monk TG, Goodnough LT, Birkmeyer JD, Brecher ME, Catalona WJ. Acute normovolemic hemodulition is a cost-effective alternative to preoperative autologous donation in patients undergoing radical retropubic prostatectomy. Transfusion 1995;35: 559-65.
24. Monk TH, Goodnough LT, Pulley DD, Brecher ME, et al. Acute normovolemic hemodilution can replace preoperative autologous blood donation as a standard of care for autologous blood procurement in patients undergoing radical prostatectomy procedures. Anesth Analg 1997;85:953-58.
25. Monk TG, Goodnough LT, Andriole GL, Colberg JW, Lemon DJ, Martin K. Preoperative recombinant human erythropoietin therapy enhances the efficacy of acute normovolemic hemodilution. Anesth Analg 1995;80:S320.
26. Andriole GL, Smith DS, Rao G, Goodnough LT, Catalona WJ. Early complications of contemporary anatomic radical retropubic prostatectomy. J Urology 1994;152: 158-60.
27. Goodnough LT, Bodner MS, Martin JW. Blood transfusion and blood conservation: cost and utilization issues. Amer J Med Qual 1994;9:172-83.
28. Sowade O, Warnke H, Scigalla P, et al. Avoidance of allogeneic blood transfusions by treatment with epoietin alpha (recombinant human erythropoietin) in patients undergoing open heart surgery. Blood 1997;89:411-18.
29. Welch GH, Meehan KR, Goodnough LT. Prudent strategies for elective red blood cell transfusion. Ann Intern Med 1992;116:393-402.
30. Goodnough LT. Blood transfusion and blood conservation practices. Flip sides of the same coin? Ann Thor Surg 1993;56:1437-41.
31. Sans T, Bofill C, Joven J, Cliville X, et al. Effectiveness of very low doses of subcutaneous recombinant human erythropoietin for autologous blood donation before orthopedic surgery. Transfusion 1996;36:822-26.

THE IMPACT OF HAEMATOPOIETIC GROWTH FACTORS ON SUPPORTIVE CARE IN CLINICAL ONCOLOGY: WITH SPECIAL ATTENTION TO POTENTIAL TUMOUR CELL CONTAMINATION IN THE STEM CELL HARVEST

C.P. Schröder[1], W.T.A. van der Graaf[1], P.H.B. Willemse[1], E. Vellenga[2], L. de Leij[3], N.H. Mulder[1], E.G.E. de Vries[1]

Haematopoietic growth factors (HGFs) are now for a number of years available for use in oncological patients. Drugs currently registered are: granulocyte colony stimulating factor (G-CSF) and granulocyte macrophage colony stimulating factor (GM-CSF) for neutrophil stimulation and erythropoietin for stimulation of erythropoiesis. With several other HGFs phase I, II and III studies have been performed or are ongoing. The new as yet unregistered compounds are often under investigation for their capacity to stimulate thrombopoiesis.

Indications for the use of neutrophil stimulating growth factor are: 1) prevention of neutropenia and its complications following chemotherapy, 2) treatment of neutropenic fever, 3) prevention or abbreviation of neutropenia during chemotherapy requiring bone marrow reconstitution and 4) peripheral stem cell harvest [1].

The prevention of neutropenia and its complications following chemotherapy.

Bacterial and fungal infection is a considerable cause of death in cancer patients [2]. Leukopenia due to multi-agent chemotherapy regimens, is associated with substantial febrile morbidity [3,4]. Infection rates increase when the peripheral blood granulocyte count falls below 0.5×10^9/L, and especially when it is less than 0.1×10^9/L or when duration of leukopenia is prolonged [5]. Haematopoietic toxicity can be decreased by chemotherapy dose reduction. However, this may have a negative effect on treatment outcome. Therefore, other means of reducing and preventing febrile leucopenia have been studied [6]. Prophylactic haematopoietic growth factors are used to reduce the incidence of febrile neutropenia, by reducing the duration of neutropenia [1,7].

In a number of phase III studies in which chemotherapy was used that induced a neutropenic fever of at least 40%, G-CSF was found to reduce the incidence of severe neutropenia, it ameliorated neutrophil nadir, reduced neutropenia duration and reduced the incidence of neutropenic fever (50%), culture positive infections and the use of antibiotics [1].

Another approach might be the use of chemoprophylaxis by the use of pro-

1. Department of Medical Oncology, University Hospital Groningen, The Netherlands.
2. Department of Haematology, University Hospital Groningen, The Netherlands.
3. Department of Immunology, University Hospital Groningen, The Netherlands.

phylactic antibiotics. Also, prophylactic antibiotics (so called chemoprophylaxis) have shown to reduce the risk of febrile morbidity [8]. Various antibiotics have been used for this purpose [9,10]. Chemoprophylaxis by quinolone-based treatment was found to be particularly effective for intestinal decontamination [11]. This way, infections with Gram negative bowel organisms, a major cause of morbidity and mortality in the leucopenic patient, can be substantially reduced [12]. Next to bacterial infections, fungi also constitute a major problem in neutropenic patients, requiring specific approaches for prevention and therapy. A number of anti-fungal agents, for instance amphotericin B, can be used for chemoprophylaxis [13,14].

In two studies comparing the use of granulocyte-stimulating growth factor (G-CSF) to G-CSF plus antibiotics [15,16], an additional beneficial effect of antibiotics was found. Furthermore, a few placebo-controlled reports on prophylactic norfloxacin or ofloxacin also clearly indicated a positive contribution in this setting [17-19]. In a retrospective study, prophylactic G-CSF was compared to prophylactic oral ciprofloxacin in ovarian cancer patients with paclitaxel induced leucopenia [20]. No difference between fever rates was observed when prophylactic G-CSF was compared to oral ciprofloxacin, but comparison with a historical control group not receiving any prophylactic agent, showed a clear benefit from prophylaxis in these patients with relatively short but deep leucopenia. In a non-randomised dose-finding study [21], early stage breast cancer patients received 5-fluorouracil (5-FU, 500 mg/m^2 intravenously), epirubicin (60 mg/m^2 IV) and cyclophosphamide (75 mg/m^2 for 14 days). Cotrimoxazol was administered prophylactically to a group of 89 consecutive patients, and fever rates decreased significantly compared to the control group not receiving prophylaxis. Currently for example in our centre a study to compare G-CSF versus quinolones is analysed. A possible disadvantage of prophylactic quinolones may be the development of resistant micro-organisms [22]. Although most data actually contradict this [23], a possible way to circumvent the risk of developing fever in immunocompromised patients would be to evaluate the efficiency of intestinal decontamination by monitoring of faecal organisms during prophylactic treatment. This way, antibiotic treatment can be altered if necessary to provide the best prophylaxis. Another option would be to limit the use of prophylaxis to those patients who have actually developed grade IV leucopenia. If chemoprophylaxis induces resistance at all, it may be limited by these precautions.

Therefore, chemoprophylaxis can be viewed as a reasonable alternative for G-CSF in preventing febrile leucopenia. However, in future studies placebo-controlled assessment of chemoprophylaxis in high risk patients would be useful.

Treatment of neutropenic fever

Randomized trials have not conclusively demonstrated a clinical benefit when G-CSF and GM-CSF are given for uncomplicated febrile neutropenia. The routine use of these factors in this setting can not be recommended. We performed a study to determine whether GM-CSF used in addition to standard inpatient antibiotic therapy shortens the period of hospitalisation due to chemotherapy-induced neutropenic fever. Patients with a haematologic (n=47) or solid tumour (n=87) who had severe neutropenia and fever were randomly assigned to receive GM-CSF 5 μg/kg/d (n=65) or placebo (n=69) in conjunction with broad-spectrum antibiotics for a minimum of 4 days and a maximum of 14 days. GM-CSF/placebo and antibiotics were stopped if the neutrophil count was greater than 1.0×10^9/L and temperature less than 37.5°C during 2 consecutive days, or for a leukocyte count ≥ 10×10^9/L, both followed by a 24-hour observation period (hospitalisation period).

Compared with placebo, GM-CSF enhanced neutrophil recovery. Median neutrophil counts at day 4 were 2.5×10^9/L (range, 0-25) in the GM-CSF arm and 1.3×10^9/L (range 0-9) in the placebo arm. No significant difference was observed with regard to median number of days with less than 1.0×10^9/L neutrophils or days of fever. The median number of days patients were hospitalised while on study was comparable in the GM-CSF and placebo groups at 6 (range 3-14) versus 7 (range 4-14). Quality-of-life scores in 90 patients demonstrated differences in favour of the placebo group. Hospital costs were higher for GM-CSF-treated patients if GM-CSF was included in the price. These results indicate that GM-CSF did not affect the number of days for resolution of fever or the hospitalisation period for this patient group, although a significant effect of GM-CSF was observed on neutrophil recovery [24].

Abbreviation of neutropenia during chemotherapy requiring bone marrow reconstitution

Patients receiving high-dose chemotherapy followed by bone marrow or peripheral stem cell reinfusion have a slightly faster neutrophil recovery if stem cell reinfusion is combined with G-CSF or GM-CSF administration [1].

Peripheral stem cell harvest

The most important role of CSFs is in the phase of peripheral blood stem cell (PBSC) mobilisation. CSFs facilitate mobilisation of haematopoietic stem cells. The advantage of PBSC transplantation following high-dose chemotherapy is that it reduces the duration of not only neutropenia but also thrombocytopenia compared to autologous bone marrow transplantation. It has been shown to shorten the duration of neutropenia and thrombocytopenia, and it reduces incidence of infections and hospital stay. Stem cell harvest before high-dose chemotherapy can also collect tumour cells from the circulation. The exact relevance for the clinic of the presence of tumour cells in the stem cell harvest is as yet unknown. Several purging methods are developed and currently in clinical trial. Ex-vivo culturing of haematopoietic stem cells in the presence of CSFs is an other way to eliminate tumour cells. Therefore, the role of tumour cell contamination is more extensively explained in this review.

Tumour cell detection

Introduction

The increased potential clinical relevance of adjuvant high-dose chemotherapy in solid tumours has raised the relevance of tumour cell contamination in bone marrow. There is increasing evidence that not only in bone marrow but also, although studies do suggest less likely, in peripheral blood stem cell harvest, tumour cell infiltration may be involved [25,26]. Early papers reported on sporadic findings of tumour contamination of solid tumours in the peripheral blood. In other studies blood was collected from cancer patients during or just after surgery and these samples often contained significant numbers of tumour cells, yet these patients do not always develop metastatic disease. Often the clinical follow up in these studies was not long [27]. It may be that the circulating tumour cells are not always viable or able to form metastases. In the animal model, however, it is shown that many viable tumour cells are shed into the circulation. So, the significance of presence of tumour cells in the circulation is as yet undetermined. The process of metastasis involves multiple host-tumour interactions and it is thought that only a few of all the circulating cells are successful in establishing metastatic colonies. Tumour cells are likely to acquire the ability to metastasise as a result of cumulative genetic changes that provide the cells with progressive metastatic capability through alterations in cell regulatory mechanisms, secretion of proteases, induction of angiogenesis, increased cellular motility and altered expression of cell adhesion molecules [28]. The ability to detect very small numbers of tumour cells may provide the clinician with an important predictive tool with respect to recurrence and might help in a better selection for adjuvant therapy.

Bone marrow micrometastases

Recently, with the availability of multiple antibodies directed against epithelial cells, it became clear that in breast carcinoma patients without signs of metastatic disease tumour cells can often be detected in the bone marrow. In breast carcinoma patients without evidence of distant metastases Redding et al. reported already in 1983 a study in 110 patients [29]. They performed immunocytochemical analysis on bone marrow smears and detected tumour cells in 28% of the samples. Bone marrow was positive in 24% of the patients who had no lymph node involvement. In a larger, identical diagnostic group of 285 patients, 27% had positive bone marrow with an antiserum raised against the epithelial membrane antigen (EMA) [30]. In following studies also the effect on prognosis was analysed. Cote et al. studied 49 patients with stage I and II operable breast cancer [31]. With a 30 months median follow up time there was an association between early recurrence and tumour infiltration of the bone marrow. Also in this study, the importance of quantifying the number of cancer cells was shown. Multivariate analysis indicated the ratio cancer cells:nucleated cells was the only significant variable for the prediction of early recurrence (>10 cells per 4×10^6 nucleated cells). Diel et al. reported in 1992 on a much larger study. In 260 patients with primary breast carcinoma bone marrow aspirates obtained from six sites of the skeleton were analysed for tumour cells [32]. After density centrifugation, cells in interphase were smeared and stained. For the immunocytologic reaction the monoclonal antibody TAG12 was used. Tumour cells could be detected in 115 (44%) of the bone marrow samples. The presence of tumour cells correlated with tumour stage, nodal stage and tumour grading. Relapses occurred especially in those with positive bone marrow. The highest prediction for distant metastases was obtained in this study by combining the nodal status, negative progesteron receptor and tumour cell presence in the bone marrow. Pantel et al. reported on the immunological detection of various markers associated with tumour progression. In cytokeratin 18 positive bone marrow from patients with cancer from the breast, gastrointestinal tract or the colon, proliferation markers Ki-67 and p120, and erb2 oncogene expression was studied. Only few cells labelled with these markers, but CK18-erb2 double labelling was associated with increased clinical stage in breast and gastrointestinal carcinoma [33]. The role of bone marrow metastases in cancer of the breast, lung, stomach and colon have been investigated in various studies [29-32,34-38]. In general, it has been shown that detection of bone marrow metastases predicts for recurrent disease, and that results have correlated with clinicopathological staging parameters.

Peripheral blood

The presence of tumour cell contamination in the peripheral blood is considered relevant because peripheral stem cell harvest and reinfusion after high-dose chemotherapy is increasingly thought to be a useful treatment for patients with high risk of tumour relapse. Also, tumour cell contamination in peripheral blood can be considered a potentially useful diagnostic tool, allowing a better selection of patients that may benefit from adjuvant chemotherapy. If a simple blood test could have prognostic value, this might be a clinically very interesting alternative to other staging methods. The detection of single tumour cells in peripheral blood or peripheral blood stem cells (PBSC) is a particular challenge. Techniques to detect these rare circulating cells should be both highly sensitive and specific.

The markers used should be indicators of tumour cell presence in the blood, not expressed by haematopoietic cells, and not shed from the tumour into the circulation. In haematological malignancies, tumour-specific qualities are available for this purpose. Gene translocation, such as t(14;18) in follicular lymphoma, were found to be accessible for molecular detection, using polymerase chain reaction (PCR) amplification [39]. The presence of t(14;18) bearing cells in bone marrow, peripheral blood stem cells and possibly peripheral blood was found to be associated with early recurrences [40-42]. Also in other haematological malignancies, specific gene translocation could be detected at a cellular level [43]. However, the cytogenetics of solid tumours are considerably more complex and less well defined than those of haematological malignancies. Mutations of either oncogenes or tumour supressor genes have been studied, but a common problem is the lack of consistency within tumour types, and the number of different mutations. For instance, p53 tumour supressor gene mutations are found throughout the open reading frame, and although 'hotspots' have been identified, even these extend over four exons. Thus, other targets have been sought. Instead of tumour specific qualities, the detection of tissue specific antigens or enzymes by reverse transcriptase-PCR (RT-PCR) has been evaluated. This approach is based on the fact that malignant cells continue to express specific marker characteristics of their tissue of origin. RT-PCR was found to be an extremely sensitive technique, allowing the detection of one tumour cell in 1×10^6-1×10^7 normal cells [44,45]. Thus, cells expressing prostatic specific antigen (PSA) were found in the peripheral blood of prostatic cancer patients without metastases [45]. Tyrosinase expression was used as a marker for melanoma cells, showing a correlation between clinical disease stage and a positive tyrosinase RT-PCR [46]. A similar result was obtained in neuroblastoma patients [47]. For breast cancer cells, specific epithelial markers were studied. Datta et al. developed a RT-PCR for keratin 19 (K19) transcripts to identify breast carcinoma cells in the peripheral blood and bone marrow of patients with breast cancer. K19 mRNA is a marker for the intermediate filament protein which is found in all normal and malignant breast cells and also in a number of simple epithelial cells and their malignant counterparts (48). In their experiment the K19 RT-PCR reliably detected 10 breast cancer cells in 1×10^8 normal peripheral blood mononuclear cells [48]. A similar experiment using also keratin filament transcripts, was earlier performed by Traweek et al. [49]. In contrast to Datta et al. they detected presence of keratin 19 activity in stromal cells (fibroblasts and endothelial cells). These stromal cells could be a possible source of keratin 19 transcripts.

Immunocytochemistry is also a widely applied technique to detect single tumour cells from solid malignancies. The detection of micrometastases in bone marrow, using antibodies against cytokeratins, has proven to be feasible and of prognostic value in breast, gastric, colorectal and lung cancer [30-33,35-39]. Immunocytochemistry is considered to be less sensitive, but more specific than molecular PCR detection [50] (although also a detection level of one tumour cell in 1×10^6 normal cells has been described [51]). Certainly, the morphological tumour cell assessment increases the specificity of this method. Sensitivity is perhaps hampered by the sample size to analyse. However, molecular detection of cellular expression of epithelial markers has recently been shown to harbour its own risks [52], particularly regarding specificity. Fifty-three control bone marrow samples were compared to 63 samples of patients with breast or prostate cancer. Commonly used markers as CK18, CEA and PSA were evaluated. Only PSA mRNA was not detected in any of the control samples, but the other markers were (CK18: 5 out of 7 control samples positive). It was stated that limiting factors in the detection of micrometastatic tumour cells by RT-PCR are: the illegitimate transcription of epithelial genes in haematological cells and the varying expression of the marker gene in micrometastatic tumour cells. The issue of low background expression of these markers in bone marrow, PBSC or peripheral blood can presumably be circumvented by quantifying the signal of the analysed sample. In our centre, a quantitative RT-PCR assay was developed for the gene encoding for the epithelial related membrane antigen EGP-2 [53]. EGP-2 is one of the most tissue specific epithelial markers known so far, and is widely expressed on almost all carcinomas derived from simple epithelia [54]. The EGP-2 molecule is not shed into the circulation. There is a monoclonal antibody available against the antigen for which this gene is encoding [55]. With the quantitative RT-PCR for EGP-2, a base-line for background signals can be established, allowing a more meaningful interpretation of RT-PCR results.

Considering the technical challenges of detecting vary rare tumour cells in peripheral blood, it is not surprising that the data on this subject are limited. In one study, the specificity issue of RT-PCR appeared to have been overcome [56]. With the detection of the maspin-transcript, tumour cell contamination was found in peripheral blood of 3 out of 9 stage IV breast cancer patients, particularly during systemic treatment. However, the role of this unusual marker remains unclear; no other research groups have validated this method so far.

Concluding, it can be said that the reports on the incidence and role of tumour cell in peripheral blood of patients with solid tumours are limited. Possibly, the low incidence and technical issues play a role in this matter. There seems to be a relation with disease stage, but for breast cancer this has not yet been clearly established. When the prognostic value of peripheral blood contamination is further evaluated, this could be a helpful tool in the allocation of therapy to poor prognostic groups. Possibly, also a disease stage amendable for immunotherapy can be distinguished. The use of cellular and molecular detection may thus be used in allocating and evaluating new clinical approaches.

Peripheral blood stem cells

Tumour cell contamination of peripheral stem cell harvest has gained considerable interest, as the number of cancer patients treated with high-dose chemotherapy and stem cell support has increased steadily over the past decade. In breast cancer patients, Ross et al. reported on a study in which paired samples of bone marrow and peripheral stem cell harvest from 48 patients were analysed with an immunocytochemical technique [25]. In cell seeding experiments with a cocktail of monoclonal antibodies, one tumour cell per 5×10^5 mononuclear cells was detected in bone marrow or peripheral stem cell harvest. Immunostained tumour cells were detected in 9.8% (13/133) peripheral stem cell specimens from 9/48 patients obtained after chemotherapy and a haematopoietic growth factor and in 62.3% (38/61) bone marrow specimens from 32/48 (66.7%) patients. It was concluded that peripheral stem cells contain fewer tumour cells than paired bone marrow specimens from patients with advanced disease and that these cells appear, based on the clonogenic assay, to be capable of clonogenic tumour growth. Brügger et al. described a study in which a small number of patients was analysed. In their immunocytochemical assay they also use a panel of monoclonal antibodies with detection of one tumour cell per 4×10^5 normal cells. They found that there was a difference in appearance of the tumour cells in the circulation after chemotherapy and haematopoietic growth factor treatment between patients without bone marrow infiltration and with bone marrow involvement. In those without tumour involvement in the bone marrow, tumour cells appeared earlier in the circulation after chemotherapy and growth factor than in those with tumour contamination of the bone marrow [26].

From this study it was clear that chemotherapy and growth factors resulted in a higher frequency of tumour cells in the circulation than without these compounds. The appearance of tumour cells in the circulation in patients with bone marrow contamination with tumour coincided with the appearance of peripheral stem cells. It was suggested that, possibly, tumour cells that metastasise to bone marrow may share some of the characteristics of haematopoietic progenitor cells, such as homing receptors/adhesion molecules. It may well be that there is a downregulation of adhesion molecules of stem cells by chemotherapy and growth factors, similar as occurs in normal maturation, but now happening at an immature stage. The fact that tumour cells can appear in the circulation without tumour cell contamination in the bone marrow suggests that either the assay to detect tumour contamination of the bone marrow was insensitive or that chemotherapy plus haematopoietic growth factors also mobilise tumour cells from other spots in the body. This raised the question whether this would also be the case in tumour types that do in general not metastasise early to the bone marrow, but in which high-dose chemotherapy is considered to be potentially useful, such as in ovarian carcinoma.

In a study addressing this issue, bone marrow and PBSC samples from 22 ovarian cancer patients were analysed. No tumour cells were found in PBSC, but 47% of bone marrow samples stained positive. The exact influence of mobilising regimes on stem cell contamination in this setting, remains to be established [57]. In breast cancer, the influence of mobilising stem cells with growth factor was compared to growth factor combined with chemotherapy [58]. Immunocytochemical detection and clonogenic assays were used. Of stage IIIb or IV breast cancer patients receiving only G-CSF, 1 of 37 peripheral blood samples, 4 of 36 bone marrow samples and 2 of 38 PBSC samples were positive. Results were similar in the group receiving GM-CSF and cyclophosphamide, implying no additional role for chemotherapy in clearing tumour cells. Recently however, a number of reports contradicting this finding were presented. In 329 breast cancer patients, mobilisation of peripheral blood stem cells with cytokine plus chemotherapy resulted in less tumour cell contamination (11.7%), than mobilisation with cytokines alone (27.8%) [59]. Also, a significant reduction of tumour cell contamination was seen when harvesting stem cells after the third course of chemotherapy for stage IV breast cancer was compared to harvesting after the first (p=0.0052) [60]. The prognostic value of immunocytochemical detection of tumour cells in bone marrow and PBSC was evaluated in a fairly large number of stage IV breast cancer patients [61]. A cocktail of anti-epithelial antibodies was used. Patients without bone marrow and PBSC contamination had a significantly longer disease free survival than others with positive bone marrow and/or PBSC (471 days vs 339 days). It was concluded that immunocytochemical staining is a useful prognostic marker for autologous stem cell transplant. Although the significance and prognostic value of the detection of tumour cells in PBSC have not yet been clarified, it seems conceivable that reinfusing tumour cells into the patient will affect the clinical outcome. Indeed, two studies [62,63] strongly support the assumption that these malignant cells reinfused after high-dose chemotherapy might contribute to relapse. In both studies grafts were marked by retroviral vectors encoding neomycin phosphotransferase or other foreign genes. These marker genes could be detected in the malignant cells in a majority of patients at relapse. These data have reinforced the need for efficient techniques for purging tumour cells from stem cell material, to reduce the risk of relapse after transplantation.

Purging

Measures to eliminate malignant cells from the graft are generally referred to as "purging " [64]. Ex vivo elimination of tumour cells is reasonable if there are no adverse effects on engraftment, haematopoietic and immune reconstitution, or other treatment outcomes. Evaluation of the efficacy of purging is difficult, as relapse may originate from residual disease in the patient as well as from malignant cells reinfused with the transplant. It is not known yet to what extent tumour cells should be depleted from the autograft, which is presumably strongly depending on the clonogenic ability of these single tumour cells.

Basically, two methods for purging have been studied: depletion of tumour cells and selection of stem cells from the graft [65]. Depletion was first studied using chemotherapy, mainly 4-hydroperoxycyclophosphamide (4-HC) [66,67]. Treatment with 4-HC clearly reduced in vitro tumour colony growth, but also colony formation and engraftment [68]. In searching for more specific purging methods, immunotherapy using monoclonal antibodies were studied. For this approach to be effective, the antibody should be specifically reactive with tumour cells. Similar as with immunocytochemical staining, this is a difficulty in solid tumours. After reacting with the antibody, additional steps are necessary to eliminate the tumour cells from the graft, either through cytotoxicity, immunotoxicity or immuno (magnetic) separation. When lymphoma cells were purged from bone marrow through an antibody-complement combination [40], a 3 to 6-log destruction was obtained. Disease free survival. was increased in patients who received purged bone marrow, compared to those who did not. In a study by Mykleburst et al., the efficiency of immunotoxins and immunomagnetic beads for purging breast cancer cells from bone marrow were compared [69]. The use of three monoclonal antibodies and immunomagnetic beads removed up to 6-log units of tumour cells. Immunotoxin efficacy was more variable, but both methods only slightly affected colony formation in bone marrow. Especially, a combination of antibodies on precoated immunobeads and two treatment cycles appears effective [64), but in these experimental settings still very high effector:target ratios are being employed. Also, these studies are performed with cell lines which are immunophenotypically well characterised. The efficacy in clinical settings with presumably a less homogeneic tumour cell population, remains to be established. Furthermore, an immunoselection method that eliminates 100% of tumour cells predictably, has not yet been described. To increase cytotoxicity, the use of cytokines has been studied. Especially the use of interleukin-2 (IL-2) in this setting seems promising. Whether IL-2 incubation of PBSC could induce tumour cell kill was studied by Verma et al. [70]. Cytotoxicity was obtained with up to 50% tumour cell kill. No adverse effect was seen on colony formation of the PBSC. If this effect can be obtained with IL-2 alone, it is tempting to speculate on an increased effect with additional monoclonal antibodies. Future possibilities also include stimulation of the graft with

GM-CSF, to induce monocyte-mediated cytotoxicity, and enhance cellular cytotoxicity [71]. Apart from increasing purging efficacy in vitro, these approaches may also contribute to a possible graft versus host effect. Residual tumour cells in the patient may thus be attacked. Post-autologous bone marrow transplantation administration of GM-CSF in vivo was shown to result in increased cytotoxicity, evaluated in vitro [72]. In a similar setting, post-transplant administration of IL-2 is currently being evaluated [73]. It will be very interesting to see whether from future studies an optimal time schedule (during mobilisation in vivo, culturing of the graft in vitro, post transplantation in vivo) and an optimal combination of cytokines and perhaps antibodies can be determined, to increase cytotoxic efficiency in this particularly interesting clinical setting. The second approach for obtaining purified stem cells is to actually select out stem cells. Systems for selecting CD34 expressing haematopoietic progenitor cells, have been evaluated and are now available for large scale purification [74,75]. Engraftment of progenitor cells is not affected by this selection procedure [75,76]. Although the CD34 antigen is not detected on tumour cells from patients with most solid tumours [74,75], a recent report indicated that tumour cells were still detectable after CD34 enrichment [77]. Therefore, it is conceivable that a combination of purging strategies including a positive selection (of CD34 positive cells) and a negative selection (of tumour cells) would be the best approach to eliminate tumour cells from the transplant. This approach however, is time- and resources consuming, and through randomized trials more insight should be gained as to the actual benefits. Another important point about selection of CD34 positive cells is that natural killer cells and T cells will be absent from the graft [65]. Whether or not this will affect clinical outcome as a result of regrowth of residual cancer cells is not known. However, it is clear that immunological methods to increase cytotoxic effects as a graft versus host (e.g. residual disease) may be greatly hampered by this depletion. The impact of residual disease in the patient after high-dose chemotherapy and stem cell support, is as yet unknown [78]. If the patient is the main source of residual tumour cells that cause relapse, this may be a rationale for adjuvant treatment with immunotherapy. The stage of minimal residual disease seems well suited for this treatment modality, as was shown by Riethmuller et al., for colorectal patients [79].

How, in the setting of stem cell transplantation this can be combined with pre-treatment of the graft to increase immunological efficiency, is of particular interest, but remains to be clarified.

Conclusion

Tumour cell detection is of particular interest in the setting of high-dose chemotherapy and peripheral blood stem cell support. It is well conceivable that reinfused tumour cells of the graft contribute to relapse, but the impact of residual disease in the patient in this setting remains to be established. A number of strategies are currently employed to purge tumour cells from stem cells. Presumably, a combination of these will be most effective in eliminating tumour cells. Short term effects of these purging procedures regarding engraftment, appear not harmful. Whether long term adverse effects will also be negligible, remains to be clarified.

References

1. Rusthoven JJ, de Vries EGE, Dale DC, Piccart M, Glaspy J, Hamilton A. Consensus of the use of neutrophil-stimulating hematopoietic growth factors in clinical practice: an international viewpoint. Int J Antimicr Agents 1997;8:263-75.
2. Scott DA, Schimpff SC. In: Klastersky J, Schimpff SC, Senn H-J (eds). Prevention of infection in cancer patients. Handbook of supportive care in Cancer New York:Marcel Dekker, Inc., 1995;45-62.
3. O'Reilly SE, Gelmon KA, Onetto N, et al. Phase I trial of recombinant human granulocyte-macrophage colony-stimulating factor derived from yeast in patients with breast cancer receiving cyclophosphamide, doxorubicin and fluorouracil. J Clin Oncol 1993;11:2411-16.
4. Lamar RE, Greco FA, Johnson DH, Murphy PB, Hainsworth JD. High-dose brief duration, multiagent chemotherapy for metastatic breast cancer. Cancer 1994;73: 1842-48.
5. Hoagland HC. Hematologic complications of cancer chemotherapy. In: Perry MC (ed). The chemotherapy source book. Baltimore: Williams and Wilkens, 1992;498-507.
6. Klastersky J. Prevention of infection in neutropenic cancer patients. Curr Opinion Oncol 1996;8:270-77.
7. Hartmann LC, Tschetter LK, Habermann TM, et al. Granulocyte colony stimulating factor in severe chemotherapy-induced afebrile neutropenla. N Engl J Med 1997; 336:1776-80.
8. Sleijfer DT, Mulder NH, de Vries-Hospers HG, et al. Infection prevention in granulocytopenic patients by selective decontamination of the digestive tract. Eur J Cancer 1980;16:859-69.
9. Warren R. Protecting neutropenic patients from bowel-derived organisms. J Hosp Infect 1991;9(suppl c):43-58.
10. De Vries-Hospers HG, Sleijfer DT, Mulder NH, et al. Bacteriological aspects of selective decontamination of the digestive tract as a method of infection prevention in granulocytopenic patients. Antimicrob Agents Chemother 1981;19:813-20.
11. Maiche AG. Use of quinolones in the immunocompromised host. Eur J Clin Microbiol Infect Dis 1991;10:361-67.
12. Bow EJ, Loewen R, Vaughan D. Reduced requirement for antibiotic therapy targeting Gram-negative organisms in febrile, neutropenic patients with cancer who are receiving antibacterial chemoprophylaxis with oral quinolones. Clin Infect Dis 1995; 20:907-12.
13. Klastersky J. Prevention and therapy of fungal infections in cancer patients:a review of recently published information. Support Care Cancer 1995;3:393-401.
14. De Vries-Hospers HG, Mulder NH, Sleijfer DT, van Saene HKF. The effect of amphotericin B lozenges on the presence and number of candida cells in the oropharynx of neutropenic leukemia patients. Infection 1982;10:71-75.
15. Gilbert C, Meisenberg B, Vredenburgh J, et al. Sequential prophylactic oral and empiric once-daily parental antibiotics for neutropenia and fever after high-dose chemotherapy and autologous bone marrow support. J Clin Oncol 1994;12:1005-11.
16. Maiche AG, Muhonen T. Granulocyte colony-stimulating factor (G-CSF) with or without a quinolone in the prevention of infection in cancer patients. Eur J Cancer 1993;10:1403-5.

17. Karp JE, Merz WG, Hendricksen C, et al. Oral norfloxacin for prevention of gram-negative bacteriaJ infections in patients with acute leukemia and granulocytopenia. Ann Intern Med 1987;106:1-7.
18. Hartlapp JH. Antimicrobial prophylaxis in immunocompromised patients. Drugs 1987;34 (suppl l):131-33.
19. DelFavero A, Menichetti F. The new fluorinated quinolones for antimicrobial prophylaxis in neutropenic patients. Eur J Cancer 1993;29A(suppl l):S2-S6.
20. Carlson JW, Fowler JM, Saltzman AK, et al. Chemoprophylaxis with oral ciprofloxacin in ovarian cancer patients receiving taxol. Gynecol Oncol 1994;55:415-20.
21. Levine MN, Bramwell K, Pritchard K, et al. The Canadian experience with intensive fluorouracil, epirubicin and cyclophosphamide in patients with early stage breast cancer. Drugs 1993;45(suppl 2):51-59.
22. Van der Auwera P, Gérain J. Use of the quinolones in the prophylaxis and treatment of granulocytopenic immunocompromised cancer patients. Drugs 1993;45(suppl 3):81-90.
23. Edlund C, Nord CE. Supression of the oropharyngeal and gastrointestinal microflora by ciprofloxacin: microbiological and clinical consequences. Scand J Infect Dis 1989;60(suppl):98-103.
24. Vellenga E, Uyl-de Groot CA, de Wit R, et al. Randomized placebo-controlled trial of granulocyte-macrophage colony-stimulating factor in patients with chemotherapy-related febrile neutropenia. J Clin Oncol 1996;14:619-27.
25. Ross AA, Cooper BW, Lazarus HM, et al. Detection and viability of tumour cells in peripheral blood cell collections from breast cancer patients using immunocytochemical and clonogenic assay techniques. Blood 1993;82:2605-10.
26. Brugger W, Bross KJ, Glatt M, Weber F, Mertelsmann R, Kanz L. Mobilization of tumour cells and hematopoietic progenitor cells into peripheral blood of patients with solid tumours. Blood 1994;83:636-40.
27. Glaves D, Huben RP, Weiss L. Haematogenous dissemination of cells from human renal adenocarcinomas. Br J Cancer 1988;57:32-35.
28. Pelkey TJ, Frierson HF, Bruns DE. Molecular and immunological detection of circulating tumour cells and micrometastases from solid tumours. Clin Chem 1996;42: 1369-81.
29. Redding WH, Monaghan P, Imrie SF, et al. Detection of micrometastases in patients with primary breast cancer. Lancet 1983;2:1271-73.
30. Berger U, Bettelheim R, Mansi JL, Easton D, Coombes RC, Neville AM. The relationship between micrometastases in the bone marrow, histopathologic features of the primary tumour in breast cancer and prognosis. Am J Clin Pathol 1988;90:1-6.
31. Cote RJ, Rosen PP, Lesser ML, Old LJ, Osborne MP. Prediction of early relapse in patients with operable breast cancer by detection of occult bone marrow micrometastases. J Clin Oncol 1991;9:1749-56.
32. Diel IJ, Kaufmann M, Goerner R, Costa SD, Kaul A, Bastert G. Detection of tumour cells in bone marrow of patients with primary breast cancer:a prognostic factor for distant metastasis. J Clin Oncol 1992;10:1534-39.
33. Pantel K, Schlimok G, Braun S, Kutter D, Lindemann F, Schaller G. Differential expression of proliferation-associated molecules in individual micrometastatic carcinoma cells. J Natl Cancer Inst 1993;85:1419-24.
34. Pantel K, Izbicki JR, Angstwurm M, et al. Immunocytological detection of bone marrow metastases in operable non-small cell lung cancer. Cancer Res 1993;53: 1027-31.
35. Pantel K, Izbicki JR, Passlick B, et al. Frequency and prognostic significance of isolated tumour cells in bone marrow of patients with non-small cell lung cancer without overt metastases. Lancet 1996;347:649-53.

36. Mansi JL, Easton D, Berger U, et al. Bone marrow metastases in primary breast cancer:prognostic significance after 6 years of follow up. Eur J Cancer 1991:27: 1552-55.
37. Schlimok G, Funke I, Pantel K, et al. Micrometastatic tumour cells in bone marrow of patients with gastric cancer: methodological aspects of detection and prognostic significance. Eur J Cancer 1991;27:1461-65.
38. Lindemann F, Schlimok G, Dirschedl P, Witte J, Riethmuller G. Prognostic significance of micrometastatic tumour cells in bone marrow of colorectal patients. Lancet 1992;340:685-89.
39. Negrin RS, Blume KG. The use of the polymerase chain reaction for the detection of minimal residual malignant disease. Blood 1991;78:255-58.
40. Gribben JG, Freedman AS, Nueberg D, et al. Immunologic purging of marrow assessed by PCR before autologous bone marrow transplantation for B-cell lymphoma. N Engl J Med 1991;325:1525-33.
41. Gribben JG, Nueberg D, Freedman AS, et al. Detection by polymerase chain reaction of residual cells with the bcl-2 translocation is associated with increased risk of relapse after autologous bone marrow transplantation for B-cell lymphoma. Blood 1993;81:3449-57.
42. Gribben JG, Nueberg D, Barber M, et al. Detection of residual lymphoma cells by polymerase chain reaction in peripheral blood is significantly less predictive than detection in bone marrow. Blood 1994;83: 3800-7.
43. Johnson PWM, Burchill SA, Selby PJ. The molecular detection of circulating tumour cells. Br J Cancer 1995;72:268-76.
44. Gerhard M, Juhl H, Kalthoff H, Shreiber HW, Wagener C, Neumaier M. Specific detection of carcinoembryonic antigen-expressing tumour cells in bone marrow aspirates by polymerase chain reaction. J Clin Oncol 1994;12:725-29.
45. Ghossein RA, Sher HI, Gerald WL, Kelley WK, Curley T, Amsterdam A. Detection of circulating tumour cells in patients with localized and metastatic prostatic carcinoma: clinical implications. J Clin Oncol 1995;13:1195-200.
46. Vormwald-Dogan V, Nickel P, Willemse M, Thome M, Tilgen W. Prevalence of melanoma cells in peripheral blood of patiens with malignant-melanoma stage I-IV-detection by polymerase chain reaction. J Invest Dermatol 1994:103:400-5.
47. Mattano LA, Moss TJ, Emerson SG. Sensitive detection of rare circulating neuroblastoma cells by the reverse transcriptase-polymerase chain reaction. Cancer Res 1992;52:4701-5.
48. Datta YH, Adams PT, Drobyski WR, Ethier SP, Terry VH. Sensitive detection of occult breast cancer by the reverse-transcriptase polymerase chain reaction. J Clin Oncol 1994;12:475-82.
49. Traweek ST, Liu J, Battifora H. Keratin gene expression in non-epithelial tissues. Detection with polymerase chain reaction. Am J Pathol 1993;142:1111-18.
50. Dwenger A, Lindemann A, Mertelsmann R. Minimal residual disease:detection, clinical relevance and treatment strategies. J Hematother 1996;5:537-48.
51. Osborne MP, Wong GY, Asina S, Old LJ, Cote RJ, Rosen PP. Sensitivity of immunoeytochemical detection of breast cancer cells in human bone marrow. Cancer Res 1991;51:2706-9.
52. Zippelius A, Kufer P, Honold G, et al. Limitations of reverse-transcriptase polymerase chain reaction analyses for detection of micrometastatic epithelial cells in bone marrow. J Clin Oncol 1997;15:2701-8.
53. Helfrich W, Ten Poele R, Meersma GJ, et al. A quantitative reverse transcriptase polymerase chain reaction-based assay to detect carcinoma cells in peripheral blood. Br J Cancer 1997;76:29-35.

54. De Leij L, Helfrich W, Stein R, Mattes ML SCLC cluster 2 antibodies detect the pancarcinom/epithelial glycoprotein EGP-2. Int J Cancer 1994;8:60-63.
55. Helfrich W, Wittop Koning P, The TH, de Leij L. Epitope mapping of SCLC cluster 2 MABs and generation of antibodies directed against new EGP-2 epitopes. Int J Cancer 1994;8:64-69.
56. Luppi M, Morselli M, Bandieri E, et al. Sensitive detection of circulating breast cancer dells by reverse-transcriptase polymerase chain reaction of maspin gene. Ann Oncol 1997;7:619-24.
57. Ross AA, Miller GW, Moss TJ, et al. Immunocytochemical detection of tumour cells in bone marrow and peripheral blood stem cell collections from patients with ovarian cancer. Bone Marrow Transpl 1995;15:929-33.
58. Passos-Coehlo, Ross AA, Kahn DJ. Similar breast cancer cell contamination of single-day peripheral-blood progenitor-cell collections obtained after priming with hematopoietic growth factor alone or after cyclophosphamide followed by growth factor. J Clin Oncol 1996;14:2569-75.
59. Meagher RC, Moss TJ, Cooper B, et al. Association of mobilization regimen on tumour contamination of stem cell products (PBSC) taken from patients with stage IV breast cancer. Proc Am Soc Clin Oncol 1997;16:415.
60. Glück S, Ross AA, Layton TJ, et al. Detection of breast cancer cells in the apheresis products (AP) and their potential clinical significance. Proc Am Soc Clin Oncol 1997; 16:392.
61. Moss TJ, Cooper B, Kennedy MJ, et al. The prognostic value of immunocytochemical (ICC) analysis on bone marrow (BM) and stem cell products (PBSC) taken from patients with stage IV breast cancer undergoing autologous transplant (ABMT) therapy. Proc Am Soc Clin Oncol 1997;16:317.
62. Brenner MK, Rill DR, Moen RC, et al. Gene-marking to trace origin of relapse after autologous bone-marrow transplantation. Lancet 1993;341:85-86.
63. Deisseroth AB, Zu Z, Claxton D. Genetic marking shows that Ph + cells present in autologous transplants of chronic myelogenous leukemia (CML) contribute to relapse after autologous bone marrow in CML. Blood 1994;83:3068-76.
64. Champlin R. Purging: elimination of malignant cells from autologous blood or marrow transplants. Curr Opin Oncol 1996;8:79-83.
65. Kvalheim G, Wang MY, Pharo A, et al. Purging of tumour cells from leucapheresis products: experimental and clinical aspects. J Hematother 1996;5:427-36.
66. Passos-Coelho J, Ross AA, Davis JM, et al. Bone marrow micrometastases in chemotherapy-responsive advanced breast cancer:effect of ex vivo purging with 4-hydroperoxy-cyclophosphamide. Cancer Res 1994;54:2366-71.
67. Anderson IC, Shpall EJ, Leslie DS, et al. Elimination of malignant clonogenic breast cancer cells from human bone marrow. Cancer Res 1989;49:4659-64.
68. Vredenburgh J, Shpall EJ, Ross M, et al. Immunopharmacologic bone marrow purging and high-dose chemotherapy with autologous bone marrow for patients with metastatic breast cancer. Proc Am Soc Clin Oncol 1992;11:58.
69. Mykleburst AT, Godal A, Juell S, Pharo A, Fodstad T. Comparison of two antibody based methods for elimination of breast cancer cells from human bone marrow. Cancer Res 1994;54:209-14.
70. Verma UN, Areman E, Dickerson SA, Kotula PL, Sacher R, Mazumder A. Interleukin-2 activation of chemotherapy and growth factor-mobilized peripheral blood stem cells for generation of cytotoxic effectors. Bone Marrow Transpl 1995;15:199-206.
71. Wing EJ, Mitchell Magee D, Whiteside TL, Kaplan S, Shadduck RK. Recombinant human granulocyte-macrophage colony-stimulating factor enhances monocyte cytotoxicity and secretion of tumour necrosis factor alpha and interferon in cancer patients. Blood 1989;73:643-46.

72. Nagler A, Shurt I, Barak V, Fabian I. Granulocyte-macrophage colony-stimulating factor dependent monocyte-mediated cytotoxicity post-autologous bone marrow transplantation. Leuk Res 1996;20:637-43.
73. Beyunes MC, Higuchi C, York A, et al. Immunotherapy with interleukin-2 with or without lymphokine-activated killer cells after autologous bone marrow transplantation for malignant lymphoma: a feasibility trial. Bone Marrow Transpl 1995;16:283-88.
74. Sphall EJ, Stemmer SM, Bearman SI, Myers S, Purdy M, Jones RB. New strategies in marrow purging for breast cancer patients receiving high-dose chemotherapy with autologous bone marrow transplantation. Breast Cancer Res Treatm 1993;26:S19-S23.
75. Berendson PJ, Bensinger WI, Hill RS, et al. Engraftment after infusion of CD34+ marrow cells in patients with breast cancer or neuroblastoma. Blood 1991;77:1717-22.
76. Dunbar CE, Cottler-Fox M, O'Shaughnessy JA, et al. Retrovirally marked CD34-enriched peripheral blood and bone marrow cells contribute to long-term engraftment after autologous transplantation. Blood 1995;85:3048-57.
77. Mapara MY, Körner IJ, Hildebrandt M, et al. Monitoring of tumour cell purging after highly efficient immunomagnetic selection of CD34 cells from leukapheresis products in breast cancer patients: comparison of immunocytochemical tumour cell staining and reverse transcriptase-polymerase chain reaction. Blood 1997;89:337-44.
78. Pantel K, Felber E, Schlimok G. Detection and characterization of residual disease in breast cancer. J Hematother 1994;3:315-22.
79. Riethmüller G, Schneider-Gädicke, Schlimnok G, et al. Randomised trial of monoclonal antibody for adjuvant therapy of resected Dukes' C colorectal carcinoma. Lancet 1994;343:1177-83.

THE DEVELOPMENT OF SYNTHOCYTES™, A NOVEL PLATELET SUBSTITUTE

S.M. Middleton

Introduction

A novel platelet substitute Synthocytes™ is being developed for the treatment and prevention of bleeding in acute thrombocytopenia. Synthocytes™ are composed of microcapsules of human serum albumin (HSA) to which human fibrinogen is immobilised. The product is manufactured using virally inactivated human blood derived proteins and is formulated as a sterile pyrogen free lyophilised preparation. The potential advantages of Synthocytes™ over platelet transfusion include a reduced risk of blood borne virus transmission, no risk of alloimmunogenic reactions, an increased shelf life and therefore a more cost effective, more easily managed therapy.

Synthocytes™ – Production and product characteristics

Clinical grade HSA is atomised under pressure in a spray drier to produce microcapsules. Spray drying parameters are controlled to produce microcapsules with a mean volume diameter 3-4 micron (Figure 1). Soluble fibrinogen is subsequently immobilised to the microcapsules and the final product lyophilised. An outline of the characteristics of Synthocytes™ is shown in Table 1. The mean volume size of the microcapsules and the restriction of numbers of microcapsules in excess of 6 micron ensures the passage of the product across the pulmonary bed following intravenous injection. It can also be seen that the amount of fibrinogen bound to the microcapsules represents less than 1% of the total protein.

The efficacy of Synthocytes™

Synthocytes™ have been administered to rabbits rendered thrombocytopenic using anti-platelet antibodies. A goat anti-rabbit platelet antibody [1] was injected into anaesthetised rabbits. Groups of rabbits (n=6) were subsequently dosed with Synthocytes™, control HSA microcapsules (i.e. with no fibrinogen) or saline. Template bleeding times were performed in the rabbit ear [2]. The results of this experiment are shown in Figure 2. As can be seen, following the antibody injection, the normal bleeding time of the rabbit of approximately

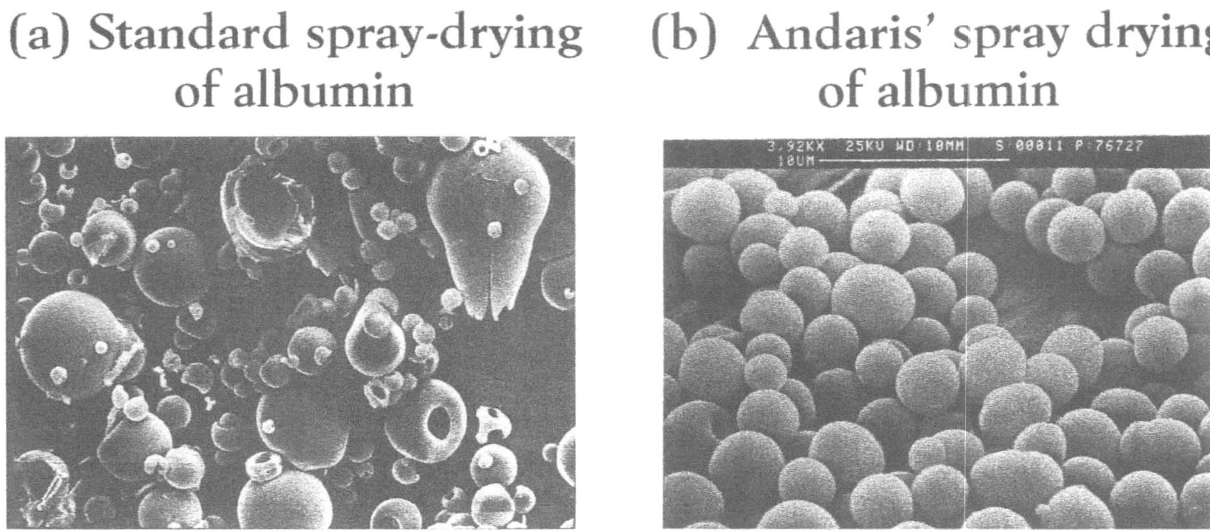

Figure 1. Standard spray-drying of albumin compared with Andaris' spray-drying.

Table 1. Synthocytes™ summary of product characteristics

Product characterisation	
Microcapsule number	1500×10^6/ml
Microcapsule size	3.5-4,5 µm
> 6.0 µm	< 2%
Total protein	20 mg/ml
Fibrinogen concentration	< 1% total protein

2 minutes became significantly prolonged to in excess of 20 minutes, which corresponded to a reduction in platelet level to $10\text{-}20\times10^9$/L. Following the injection of Synthocytes™ at doses of 1 ml/kg and 0.5 ml/kg, the bleeding time was significantly reduced to approximately 5 and 7 minutes respectively, for up to 75 minutes, which was the duration of the experiment. By contrast, the control HSA microcapsules or saline at doses of 1 ml/kg had no effect on the prolonged bleeding time. There was no change in the platelet count in any of the animals following injection of Synthocytes™ or controls.

The interaction of Synthocytes™ with platelets on a collagen surface

The interaction of Synthocytes™ with platelets is being studied using a perfusion chamber [3]. In a preliminary study, Synthocytes™ and control HSA microcapsules (i.e. no fibrinogen) were mixed with normal citrated blood and perfused over a collagen III surface [4]. Platelet deposition was observed using image analysis; and following perfusion with Synthocytes™ enhanced surface coverage was observed which was not seen in the control groups. A scanning electron micrograph of the perfused surface shows Synthocytes™ incorporated into the thrombus formed on the collagen surface (Figure 3). This was not seen with the control microcapsules.

Effect of Synthocytes™ on thrombus growth in a rabbit jugular vein thrombosis model

Synthocytes™ have been studied with respect to the potential for thrombus growth in an experimental model for rabbit jugular vein thrombosis. Non-radioactive thrombi were formed in the jugular veins of the rabbit and ^{125}I-labelled fibrinogen was injected systemically. The accretion of radiolabelled fibrinogen onto the preformed non-radioactive thrombi represented thrombus growth. Rabbit blood was mixed with human thrombin and 0.25 M was injected in an isolated jugular vein segment. After 30 minutes of ageing of the thrombus the blood flow was restored by removing the clamps and ^{125}I-labelled fibrinogen was injected systemically. Synthocytes™ 1 ml/kg, control HSA microcapsules 1 ml/kg or saline 1 ml/kg were administered by a bolus intravenous dose 30 minutes after thrombus formation. Two hours after the start of the study the thrombi were removed and the experiment was terminated.

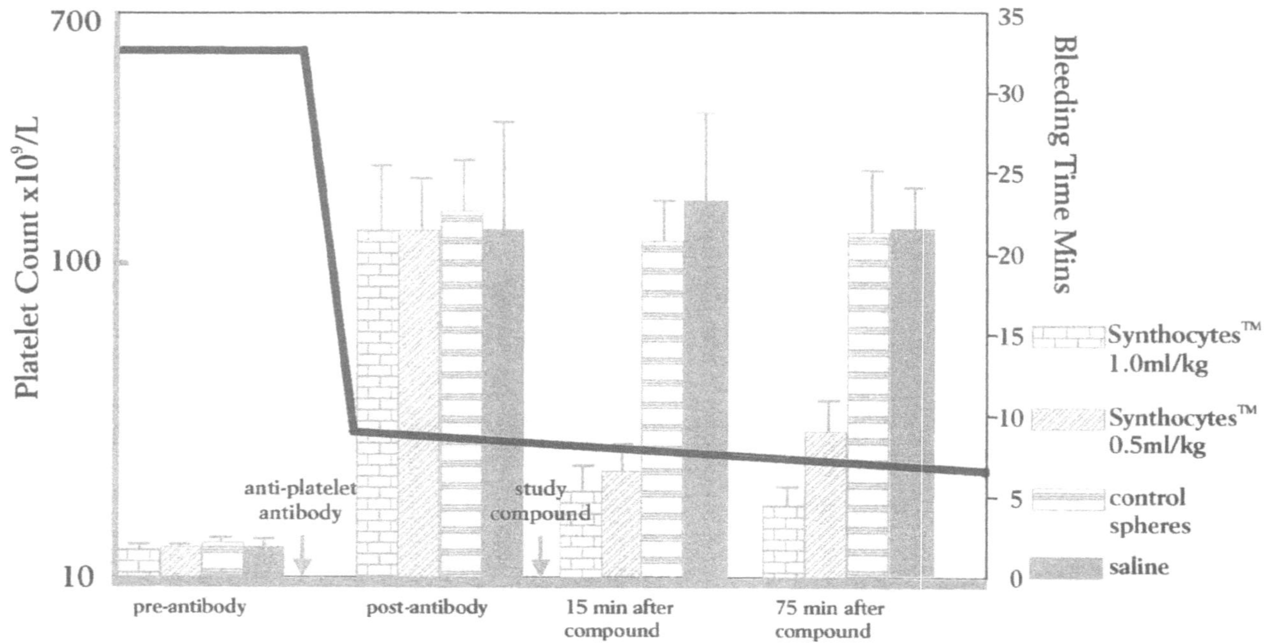

Figure 2. The effect of Synthocytes™ on bleeding time in thrombocytopenic rabbits.

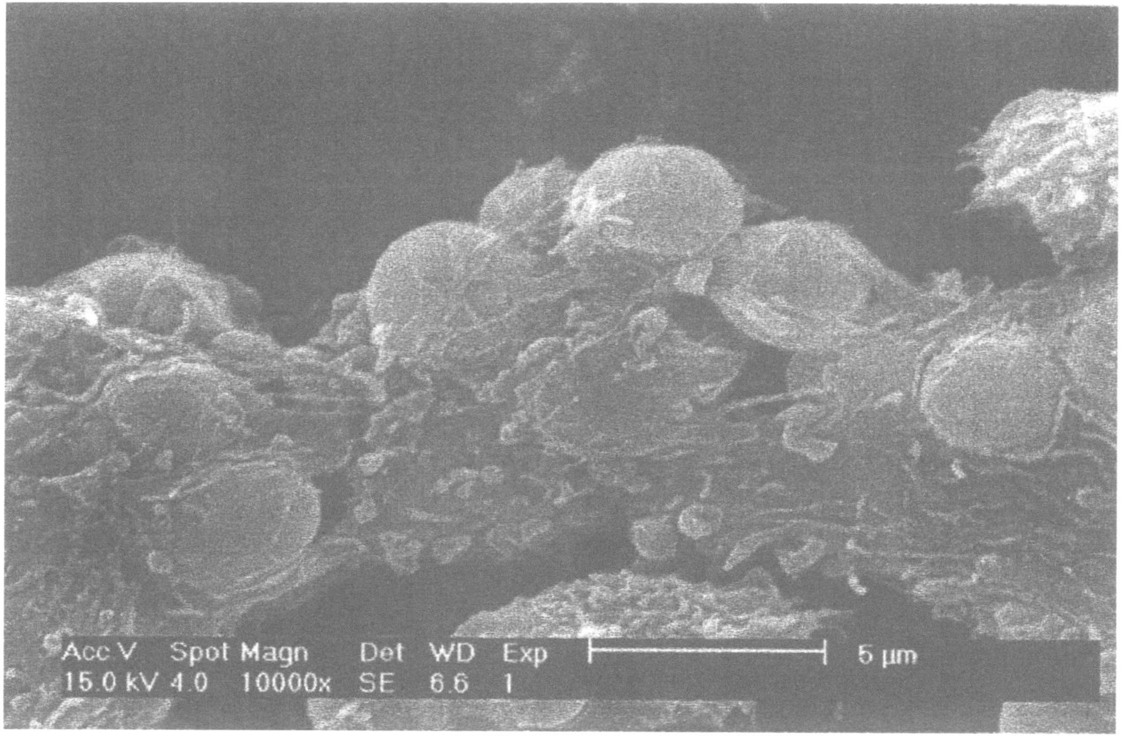

Figure 3. A scanning electron micrograph showing the interaction of Synthocytes™ and platelets.

Thrombus growth was determined by measuring the accretion of ^{125}I-labelled fibrinogen onto the preformed non-radioactive thrombi, as related to plasma radioactivity.

The results are shown in Table 2. As can be seen, the infusion of Synthocytes™ did not result in a statistically significant effect on thrombus growth as compared with HSA control microcapsules or saline. It was concluded that there was no evidence of the potential for thrombogenicity associated with the injection of Synthocytes™ in this preliminary experiment.

Table 2. The effect of Synthocytes™ on thrombus growth in a rabbit model

Percentage initial thrombus growth		
Synthocytes™ 1 ml/kg	**Control HSA microcapsules 1 ml/kg**	**Saline 1 ml/kg**
50.3 ± 5	49.6 ± 7	46.6 ± 6
p = NS with ANOVA	p = NS with ANOVA	

Summary

A platelet substitute, Synthocytes™, which are prepared by immobilising human fibrinogen to HSA microcapsules is currently being developed. Results from initial in vitro and in vivo studies are sufficiently encouraging that the product is now undergoing further preclinical studies prior to commencing studies in man.

References

1. Sullam PM ,Frank U, Yeaman MR, Tauber MG, Bayer AS, Chambers HF. Effect of thrombocytopenia on the early course of streptococcal endocarditis. J Inf Dis 1993; 168:910-14.
2. Levi M. Written communication. 1997.
3. Sakariassen KS, Aarts PAMM, de Groot PhG, Houdijk WP, Sixma JJ. A perfusion chamber developed to investigate platelet interaction in flowing blood with human vessel wall cells, their extracellular matrix and purified components. J Lab Clin Med 1983;102:522-35.
4. De Groot PhG. Written communication. 1997.

RECENT DEVELOPMENTS IN THE CONSTRUCTION OF BISPECIFIC ANTIBODIES

W. Helfrich, B.J. Kroesen, G. Molema, L. de Leij

Introduction

Current systemic anti-cancer therapies largely depend upon the cytotoxic effect of the drug(s) on tumour cells versus a more restricted cytotoxic effect on non-tumour cells. This inherently limited targeting specificity may lead to unacceptable toxicity at therapeutic doses, thus restricting the available "therapeutic window". Already at the beginning of this century Ehrlich envisioned that immunoglobulins (Ig) or antibodies (Ab) can specifically deliver cytotoxic reagents to tumour cells to eradicate these cells. This idea was called the "magic bullet" concept [1].

In the normal immune response Abs can be regarded as flexible, soluble "adapters", i.e. in addition to a fine-tuned recognition of almost any antigenic structure on a foreign body, they can recruit powerful effector functions as mediated by e.g. the complement system or the various myeloid effector cells like monocytes, macrophages, and granulocytes. In addition, they can activate dendritic cells and NK cells. The effector functions mediated in this way include complement lysis, phagocytosis, Ab dependent cellular cytotoxicity (ADCC), superoxide release, and cytokine production.

In the field of cancer therapy, murine monoclonal antibodies (MAbs) with their predefined specificity were initially seen as offering new hopes for cure. Indeed, during the past decade a large number of different MAbs have been used successfully as a vehicle for delivery of a variety of agents to tumour cells including radionuclides for imaging purposes, therapeutic radioisotopes, drugs, toxins, cytokines, and enzymes. However, due to the "Fc-FcR" incompatibility, most murine MAbs are unable to activate genuine immune effector pathways such as complement fixation and ADCC. In addition, when applied in vivo such MAbs must compete with high concentrations of the normally present human antibodies for binding to e.g. the high-affinity-type I Fc receptors (FcγRI, CD64) on myeloid effector cells resulting in an usually low level of therapeutic benefit in the treatment of human malignancies,

Experience with the use of murine MAbs to treat human diseases has also shown that these molecules are usually highly immunogenic to the extent that the evoked human anti-mouse antibody (HAMA) responses can block the therapeutic effect [2]. Enzymatically derived antibody fragments such as $F(ab')_2$ or

Fab may have lower immunogenicity and have the advantage of a more rapid biodistribution However their lack of an Fc portion render Fab and $F(ab')_2$ without natural effector function.

Tumour associated target antigens

To date, for obvious reasons, the specific immunologic recognition of tumour cells by murine MAb largely depends on targeting to tumour associated antigens (TAA) rather than to tumour specific antigens (TSA). The identification and charterization of tumour associated antigens has provided several candidate target antigens as previously reviewed [3]. The present article will reflect only briefly on two TAA that have been extensively studied as target antigens in human carcinoma therapy, EGP2 and Her/neu antigen.

The epithelial glyco-protein-2 (EGP2, also known as the CO17-1A antigen, EpCam, or KSA) is a 38 kDa transmembrane tumour associated antigen that is abundantly expressed on a variety of human carcinomas [4]. EGP2 is not expressed on any of the blood cells, cells of the lymphoreticular system, and the cells of the connective, muscular, skeletal and nervous tissue [5-9]. Since EGP2 is not shed into the circulation, this glycoprotein is widely regarded as a suitable target antigen for imaging and immunotherapy of human carcinomas. Several anti-EGP2 antibodies like 17-1A, KS 1/4, and MOC31 (developed by our own lab) have been studied in clinical trials [10-12]. Anti-EGP2 MAbs have been conjugated to a wide variety of chemical drugs, including doxorubicin, methotrexate, and vinca alkaloids, in order to increase tumour selectivity of these agents [11,13-15].The results of these studies confirmed the potential of using antibodies to EGP2 in antibody mediated therapy of human carcinomas.

Another widely used target antigen is the product of the *erb*B-2 or HER2/neu oncogen. The HER2/neu antigen is a 185 kDa ($p185^{neu}$) transmembrane protein that has tyrosine-kinase activity and whose amplified expression on the cell surface can be a cofactor in the process of malignant transformation. Overexpression of HER2/neu is strongly correlated with progression of human ovarian and breast carcinomas [16].

Tumour vascular antigens as immunotherapeutical target

Another promising approach in solid tumour therapy is to target therapeutical antibodies to tumour vasculature rather than to the tumour cells themselves which are outside the bloodstream. The approach aims to construct immunoconjugates that selectively occlude the vasculature of solid tumours by the induction of local blood coagulation (clotting). This will disrupt the blood supply to tumour cells leading to nutrient- and oxygen deprivation (infarction) and thus to rapid and massive tumour cell death. Selective occlusion of tumour vasculature was recently tested as a therapy for solid tumours in a mouse model [17]. The formation of blood clots within the tumour vessels was initiated by targeting a truncated, soluble tissue factor (tTF) to an experimentally induced marker on tumour vascular endothelial cells. This tTF had limited ability to initiate thrombosis when free in the circulation, but became an effective and selective thrombogen when targeted to the surface of endothelial cells. Targeting of the tTF to tumour located endothelial cells was accomplished by employing a bispecific antibody (see below) harbouring within one molecule a specificity against tTF and a specificity against the induced endothelial marker. Intravenous administration of the bispecific antibody-tTF complex to mice with s.c. neuroblastomas resulted in complete tumour regressions in 38 percent of the mice. For clinical application, this strategy will require the identification of target molecules that are selectively present on tumour vascular endothelium. The search for such target molecules is ongoing.

Bispecific antibodies

A promising approach to increase the immunological effectiveness of therapy with MAbs is the use of bispecific antibodies (BsAb). BsAb that bind to both triggering molecules on cytotoxic effector cells and surface tumour antigens on target cells can induce the entire cytotoxic effector cell population to kill target cells expressing the relevant tumour antigen. In other words, the use of bispecific antibodies enables the retargeting of large populations of predefined effector cells to cells expressing a predefined target antigen.

If BsAbs are to be used in vivo, they must be pure, homogeneous proteins. Dependent on the way of preparing and isolation of a bispecific antibody preparation (see below) this could be a difficult task. In addition such a preparation should contain bispecific antibodies that lack Fc domains, since, by interacting with FcγR on various cell types, this could induce premature triggering, lysis, or sequestration of effector cells. Whole BsAb can be converted into $F(ab')_2$ fragments by limited pepsin digestion of the Fc domain (see fig. 1). This procedure however suffers from the fact that it can produce non-specific hydrolysis which can inactivate a substantial percentage of the antibody preparation. Another potential drawback which should be kept in mind is that the interaction of a BsAb with its targets is monovalent, which means that this binding is substantially weaker due to the reduced avidity effect when compared to parental Ab where each of the two arms are identical and the antigen binding site on each arm recognises the same antigen.

Retargeting myeloid immune effector cells

BsAb with combined specificity for human Fc-receptors (FcR) (CD16, CD32, CD64, CD89) and TAAs like the HER2/neu oncogene product have been described [18]. FcR are expressed on many different myeloid effector cells like monocytes, macrophages, dendritic cells, NK cells, and neutrophils and generally function as a trigger molecule for ADCC, phagocytosis, and cytokine release. The anti-FcR specificity of the above BsAb are however directed to an epitope outside the Ig ligand binding site on the FcR molecule and are thus able to activate myeloid effector cells even in the presence of high concentrations of other immunoglobulins. In vitro and in vivo data demonstrated that these BsAb

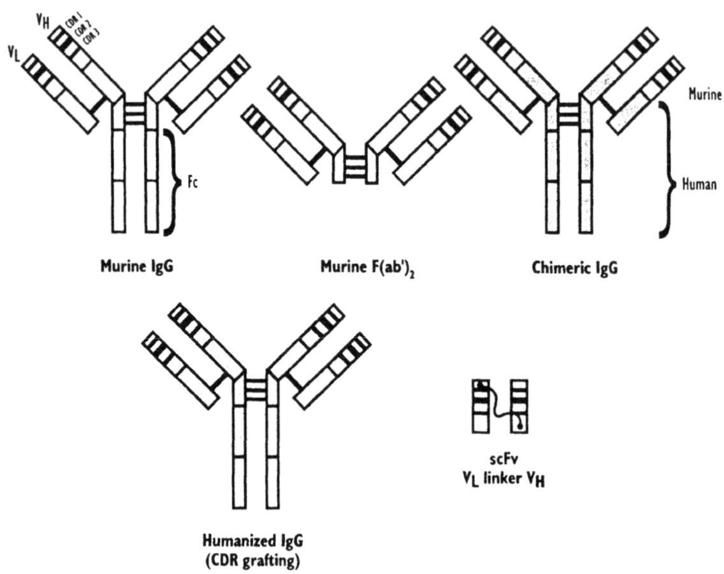

Figure 1. Antibody engineering.

Enzymatically derived murine $F(ab')_2$ fragments show rapid biodistribution and are expected to be of lower immunogenicity but lack natural effector functions. Chimeric versions of murine MAb can be constructed where the variable chains of the original murine MAb are combined with the constant domains of human Ig to enhance effector functions and reduce the HAMA response. Alternatively, the six hypervariable loops (CDRS) forming the antigen binding site of a murine antibody can be transplanted into a human framework resulting in a CDR grafted or humanised antibody. Recombinant DNA technology has been used to construct single chain Fv fragments (scFv). ScFvs consist of only the variable light chain (VL) and variable heavy chain (VH) domains covalently connected by a flexible typically 15 residue linker. Due to their relative small size (approximately 26 kDa), scFvs have rapid pharmacokinetics and can show a strongly improved solid tumour penetration in vivo.

are able to retarget myeloid effector cells and facilitate ADCC and phagocytosis of HER2/neu-positive targets and stimulate release of monocyte/macrophage-derived cytokines [19]. Based on these encouraging preclinical observations, phase I/II studies have been undertaken in women with breast or ovarian cancer, and men with prostate cancer.

Retargeting cytotoxic T-cells

By using bispecific antibodies with a specificity for both the signal transducing CD3ε chain of the TCR/CD3 complex on T-cells and EGP2 on tumours, $CD8^+$ cytotoxic T lymphocytes (CTL) (and to a lesser extent $CD4^+$ T-cells) can be activated and specifically redirected against various EGP2 positive carcinoma

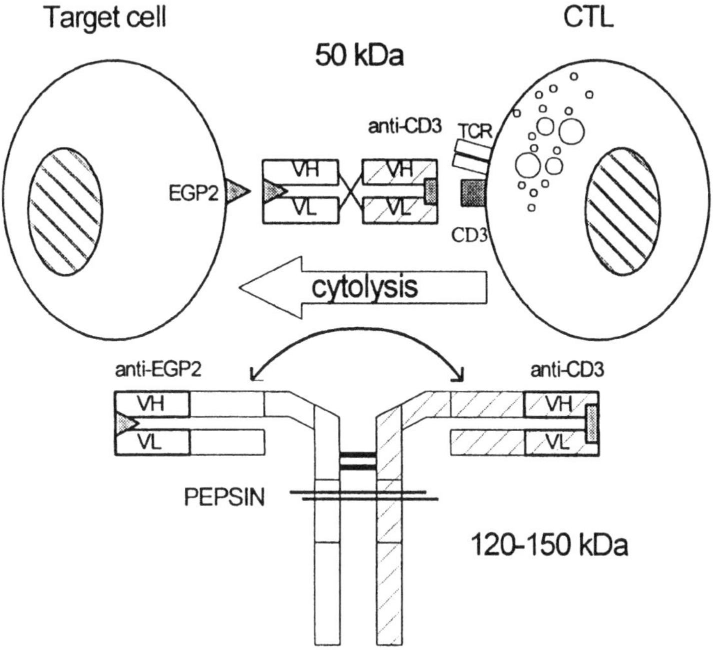

Figure 2. Retargeting of human lymphoid effector cells using BsAb.
By using bispecific antibodies with a specificity for both the signal transducing CD3ε chain of the TCR/CD3 complex on T-cells and the tumour associated antigen EGP2 on tumours, $CD8^+$ cytotoxic T lymphocytes (CTL) (and to a lesser extent $CD4^+$ T-cells) can be activated and specifically redirected against various EGP2 positive carcinoma cells in a non-MHC restricted manner.

cells in a non-NHC restricted manner (Fig. 2). Indeed clinical trials suggest that T-cell retargeting BsAb may offer considerable promise for therapeutic applications [20-22]. Previously, we studied a hybrid-hybridoma derived bispecific antibody combining the high affinity anti-EGP2 MAb MOC31 with an anti-CD3 MAb (BIS1 = anti-EGP2×anti-CD3), in a local application study [22] and subsequently in a phase 1 clinical study in which BISl $F(ab')_2$ was intravenously applied in renal cell cancer patients receiving subcutaneous IL-2 [21]. Furthermore, the effectiveness of this BsAb mediating cellular anti-tumour activity was evaluated in vitro and in vivo in an immunocompetent rat tumour model [23]. These studies indicated the efficacy of BIS1 in BsAb mediated immunotherapy, but also showed that systemic treatment of bulky disease is ineffective.

Production of bispecific antibodies

Bispecific antibodies (BsAb) have traditionally been prepared by fusing two hybridoma cell lines to produce a hybrid-hybridoma or "quadroma". If a quadroma is constructed, several pairings of heavy- and light-chains can be found in the intracellularly assembled and subsequently secreted IgG molecules.

Hence, quadroma cell lines can potentially produce all these possible antibody assemblies simultaneously. By random assortment of light and heavy chains, theoretically only 10% of the antibody combinations produced by a quadroma cell form the desired BsAb. Other manufacturing techniques basically rely upon chemical procedures to first disassemble, and then reassemble two antibodies to make an antibody composed of both parent MAb. This procedure does produce BsAb, but often in low yield and mostly without consistency in how the two parts of the antibodies are joined. Elaborated methods have been established to purify the desired BsAb away from the other mixed molecular Ab species formed using these procedures. Nevertheless, both of these approaches present challenges with respect to yield and purity of formed BsAb products, which generally hamper their clinical evaluation. Problems related to the production and purification of BsAb are currently being solved through molecular genetic approaches as will be discussed later.

Recombinant DNA technology

In addition to the immunogenicity of rodent based MAb, the relatively large size of Ig molecules in general (typically 150 kDa) is anticipated to reduce its efficacy especially in solid tumour therapy. Recombinant DNA technology can be exploited to deal with these problems and has been used to not only manipulate the size, but also shape, affinity, and immunogenicity of the Ab molecule. Chimeric versions of murine MAb can be constructed where the variable chains of the original murine MAb are combined with the constant domains of human Ig to enhance effector functions and reduce the chance of a HAMA response to occur. Alternatively, the six hypervariable loops (CDRS) forming the antigen binding site of a murine antibody can be transplanted into a human framework resulting in a CDR grafted or humanised antibody (Fig. 1)

Single Fv antibody fragments

In addition to modified complete Ig molecules, recombinant DNA technology has been used to construct small antibody-like molecules called single chain Fv fragments (scFv) [24]. ScFvs are recombinant antibody fragments consisting of only the variable light chain (VL,) and variable heavy chain (VH) domains covalently connected by a flexible polypeptide linker typically composed of 15 amino acid residues: (Glycine$_4$Serine)$_3$ (Fig. l). Due to their relative small size (approximately 26 kDa), scFvs have rapid pharmacokinetics and can show a strongly improved solid tumour penetration in vivo. Murine scFv fragments can be produced by PCR based gene assembly using mRNA templates isolated from the corresponding hybridoma cell line [25]. Functional expression (display) of scFv proteins on the surface of bacteriophage has widely been exploited to select for scFv that have retained the binding properties similar to those of the MAb from which they were derived. The inherent advantage of phage display technology is its direct link of DNA sequence to protein function [26]. Large numbers of clones can be rapidly screened for antigen binding, making it the method of choice for hybridoma Ig cloning. It is clear that molecular cloning and sequencing of scFv's forms the basis for further antibody engineering and modelling.

Phage display library

As an alternative to immunisation and hybridoma construction procedures, it has proven to be possible to construct large (synthetic) human antibody gene repertoires entirely in vitro. This procedure generates a huge library of recombinant filamentous bacteriophages that express hundreds of millions of different human scFvs on their tips fused to the phage minor coat protein III [27,28]. The scFvs displayed by these phages can show antigen binding activity and phages of the desired binding characteristics and specificity can be selected by panning on antigen. The selected phage (including the genetic information of the displayed scFv inside) can be rescued and grown after each round of panning after which the "enriched" phage library is subjected to selection again so that even very rare phages ($<1/10^8$) can be isolate. Using this strategy human antibody fragments have been isolated with specificities against foreign and self antigens [26,29,30]. Recently, we screened two large human synthetic phage-antibodies for scFv fragments specific for EGP2 using either a synthetic EGP2 peptide or a recombinant EGP2 molecule. After iterating rounds of selection, phages were identified that showed specific reactivity with their selective antigen in an ELISA assay. Unfortunately, none of the selected scFv's showed reactivity with native EGP2 as is present in carcinoma tissue specimens (unpublished results).

For clinical application scFv must have affinities in the nano, or possibly in picomolar range. Selection of such presumably very rare scFv will require the construction of phage display libraries of extremely large functional complexity combined with very sophisticated screening procedures. Alternatively, affinity maturation can be done from a selected specificity by employing directed mutagenesis or chain-shuffling procedures.

Recombinant bispecific antibody formats

Recombinant DNA technology has also been used to manipulate the size and shape of BsAb. To this end several approaches can be followed, some of which will be discussed briefly below.

Firstly, scFv molecules have been modified to express a C-terminal cysteine by which they can be crosslinked to a similarly modified scFv with another specificity using conventional sulphide reactive crosslinkers.

Secondly, by genetically interconnecting two different scFv constructs with a flexible linker, so-called bispecific single chain Fv fragment ($Bs(scFv)_2$) have been generated [31-33]. $Bs(scFv)_2$ molecules have the advantage that post-production modification such as chemical coupling is no longer needed. However, when expressed in *E. coli* $Bs(scFv)_2$ tend to form aggregates which generally have to be isolated and refolded from inclusion bodies. The construction of a functional murine $Bs(scFv)_2$ with specificity for human CD3 and EGP2 has

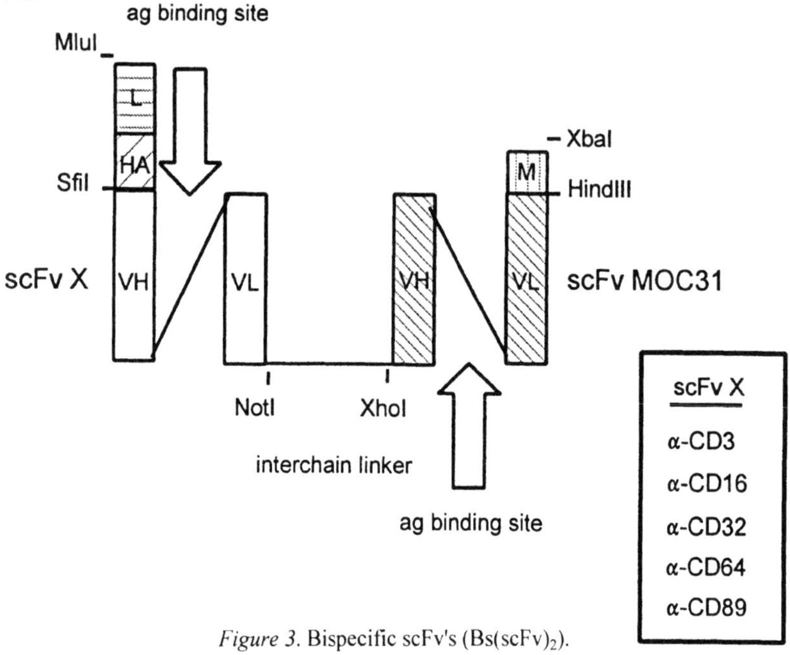

Figure 3. Bispecific scFv's (Bs(scFv)$_2$).

Shown is the cloning cassette of a mammalian expression plasmid that allows for rapid construction and expression of Bs(scFv)$_2$. The first scFv specificity, designated as scFv X, can be conveniently inserted as a SfiI-NotI restriction enzyme fragment. The second specificity, here shown is the anti-EGP2 scFv MOC31, can also be exchanged for other specificities. This plasmid contains the CW promoter and the neomycin resistance gene for high and stable expression of the encoded Bs(scFv)$_2$ in mammalian cell lines. L = leader, HA = haemagglutinin A tag, M = Myc tag, both tags are for detection purposes. Arrows indicate the dual antigen binding site.

been described by Mack et al. 1995 [34,35]. This construct could be expressed to high levels in mammalian (CHO) cells as a fully functional protein, while its expression in *E. coli* resulted in a non-functional protein. Recently, we have constructed a mammalian expression plasmid that allows for rapid construction and expression of Bs(scFv)$_2$ by cassette cloning of the desired scFvs specificities (Fig. 3). This plasmid contains the CMV promoter and the neomycin resistance gene for high and stable expression of the encoded Bs(scFv)$_2$ in mammalian cell lines. Using this plasmid we have recently constructed a number of Bs(scFv)$_2$ including one with dual specificity for the murine CD3ε-chain and EGP2 for evaluation of Bs(scFv)$_2$ therapy in an EGP2 transgenic-mouse tumour model. Furthermore, we constructed a Bs(scFv)$_2$ with dual specificity for the human CD16 (FcγRIII) and EGP2. For both Bs(scFv)$_2$ bispecificity has been established. Assessment of their cytotoxic potential is currently under investigation.

A third approach has been the use of the self-association properties of various protein subunits genetically engineered to antibody fragments. Kostelny et al.

[36] used peptides derived from the Fos and Jun leucine zipper proteins to generate bispecific heterodimers. This technique takes advantage of the property of these transcription factors to spontaneously form stable Fos-Jun heterodimers. Two different scFv fusion proteins are constructed either containing a Fos or a Jun dimerisation domain. Upon expression, Fos-Fos and Jun-Jun homodimers are formed which can be monomerised by mild reduction. Subsequent mixing and oxidation of equimolar quantities of scFv-Fos and scFv-Jun monomeric fragments will preferentially yield bispecific Fos-Jun zippered antibody fragments with high recovery yields up to 60%. To further minimise the size of these antibody constructs, pepsin digestion can be applied to remove part of the Fos-Jun zipper.

Non-covalent bispecific scFv dimers or diabodies

The most recent approach to produce dimeric scFv has been to exploit the tendency of scFv to spontaneously form non-covalent dimers. These recently described molecules are known as diabodies [37,38]. Diabodies are a new class of dimeric antibody fragments formed by non-covalent cross-pairing of two single-chain variable fragment (scFv) molecules. Each chain consists of a VH domain connected to a VL variable domain using a linker that is too short to allow intra-chain pairing between complementary domains. Instead, two chains dimerise to form two binding sites, thus forming a bivalent monospecific dimer (see Fig. 4A). Diabodies can also be engineered to harbour two different antigen-binding sites. Subsequently, for a bispecific diabody (made from antibodies A and B), the first chain is assembled from the VH domain of antibody A and the VL domain of antibody B (and the second chain from the VH domain of antibody B and the VL domain of antibody A). Co-expression of the two chains (VH_A-VL_B, VH_B-VL_A) from a dicistronic expression construct (Fig. 4B) in *E. coli* leads to assembly of bispecific diabodies in the periplasmic space. Unlike in other bispecific antibodies, the two antigen-binding sites in diabodies are at opposite ends of the molecule and separated by an average of only ~6.5 nm (less than half the distance in IgG) [39]. Holliger et al, 1996 [40] observed an increased potency of their bispecific diabody in in vitro CD3 retargeted cytolysis using an idiotypic marker on a mouse B-cell lymphoma when compared to an analogous hybrid-hybridoma bispecific antibody. These workers suggest that in bispecific diabody mediated cytolysis the distance (~6.5 nm) between target and cytolytic cells resembles the distance of the natural interaction of the antigen-presenting MHC molecules on target cells with the specific T-cell receptors of the effector cells. A tighter effector-target cell interface may thus lead to a higher local concentration of the cytotoxic cocktail release from the crosslinked CTLs. The typical molecular weight of a diabody is only approximately 52 kDa, which is similar to the size of a Fab' fragment. Due to this relatively small size, diabodies are expected to show rapid pharmacokinetics and improved tumour penetration in vivo [41]. Additionally, diabodies can be expressed by secretion from bacterial cultures which is in contrast to the single-chain bispecific scFv fragments which generally have to be refolded from inclusion bodies.

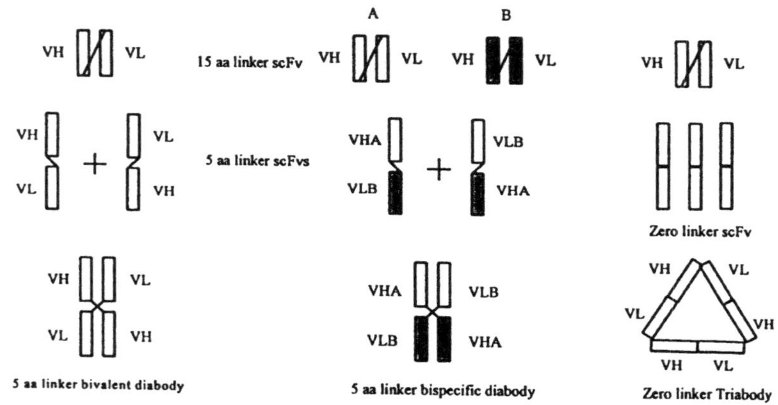

4A 4B 4C

Figure 4A. Diabody.

Diabodies are a new class of dimeric antibody fragments formed by non-covalent cross-pairing of two single-chain variable fragment (scFv) molecules. Each chain consists of VH domain connected to a VL variable domain using a linker that is too short to allow intra-chain pairing between complementary domains. Instead, two chains dimerise to form two binding sites, thus forming a bivalent monospecific dimer.

Figure 4B. Bispecific diabody.

For a bispecific diabody (made from antibodies A and B), the first chain is assembled from the VH domain of antibody A and the VL domain of antibody B (and the second chain from the VH domain of antibody B and the VL domain of antibody A). Co-expression of the two chains (VH_A-VL_B, VH_B-VL_A) from a dicistronic expression construct in *E. coli* leads to assembly of bispecific diabodies in the periplasmic space.

Figure 4C. Triabody.

Triabodies can be formed from a limited number of zero-linker scFv's. Triabodies have three Fv heads with the polypeptides arranged in a cyclic, head-to-tail fashion. Monospecific triabodies show an increased antigen binding affinity due to an increased avidity. The construction of combinatorial triabodies derived from two or three zero-linker scFvs of different specificities may offer the possibility of constructing therapeutic molecules with novel multifunctional affinity and effector characteristics (not shown here).

Recently, we reported on the construction and characterisation of a recombinant bispecific antibody in the diabody format potentially suitable for human therapy (Helfrich et al. Int J Cancer). In this work we have aimed to construct a small and partially humanised recombinant diabody molecule with dual specificity for both EGP2 and the signal transducing CD3ε-chain of TCR/CD3 complex. The murine anti-EGP2 (MOC31) scFv and the humanised anti-CD3 (Ucht1v9) scFv were cast into a diabody format (designated Dia5v9) using a short 5 amino acid Gly_4Ser linker between VH's and VL's (see Fig. 2). Purification of the poly-histidine tagged Dia5v9 was achieved from extracts of protease deficient *E. coli* by IMAC (immobilised metal ion affinity chromatography). The Dia5v9 diabody showed strong binding to both EGP2 and CD3 expressed on transfected cells. The in vitro efficacy of Dia5v9 in mediating tumour cell lysis by IL-2 activated human T-cells appeared to be similar to the hybrid hybridoma derived $BsF(ab')_2$ BISI (anti-EGP2/anti-CD3) in a standard 4hr ^{51}Cr release assay. The binding kinetics of diabody Dia5v9 for the target cell antigen EGP2 showed an off-rate of 7.27 +/– 0.04×10^{-4} s^{-1} which was about 2-fold faster than that of the parental scFv MOC31 (3.4×10^{-4} s^{-1}).

To further reduce the size of the diabody, and thereby increase its rigidity, the 5 amino acid linker between VH and VL was omitted by connecting the VH and VL domains of each chain directly, yielding the zero-linker diabody Dia0v9. However, the zero-linker diabody Dia0v9 showed no immunoreactivity, possibly due to too much intermolecular strain.

Diabody Dia5v9 stability in PBS appeared to be very high with no significant reduction in immunoreactivity after >12 months storage at 4°C. Moreover, the diabody immunoreactivity was resistant to multiple freeze/thaw cycles. Stability in human serum however appeared to be reduced. The stability of Dia5v9 may be improved further by the provision of one or two disulphide bridges between the VH-VL pairs [42].

In collaboration with other laboratories, we currently are constructing a series bispecific diabodies that are suitable for retargeting myeloid effector cells via CD16, CD32, CD64, and CD89 towards EGP2 positive carcinoma cells. For the diabody harbouring CD16 and EGP2 specificities the bispecific binding has been demonstrated. We envision that simultaneous or successive targeting of myeloid en lymphoid effector cells might synergise the immunotherapeutic effect (Fig. 5).

Bispecific diabodies are an attractive new class bispecific antibody fragments that in theory are relatively simple to construct. However, until now there are only few examples of biologically functional bispecific diabodies potentially suitable for T-cell retargeted tumour therapy in human carcinoma [43]. The Dia5v9 diabody is the first example of a biologically active and partially humanised T-cell redirecting bispecific diabody directed against EGP2. Interestingly, our attempts to incorporated the anti-CD3 scFv derived from the OKT3 hybridoma failed, possibly indicating that only a limited subset of scFvs can be recasted into the diabody format yielding a functional molecule.

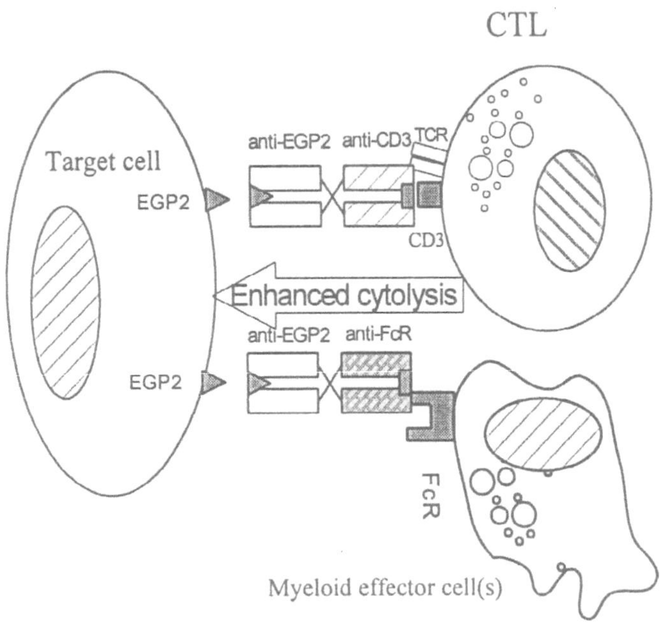

Figure 5. Simultaneous or successive targeting of myeloid and lymphoid effector cells might synergise the immunotherapeutic effect (see text for details). Shown are diagrams for a diabody harbouring FcR and EGP2 specificities and for a diabody harbouring CD3 and EGP2 specificities.

Conclusions and future perspectives

BsAb can accommodate portions of two separate Abs into a single cancer-fighting molecule. Understanding of current limitations in the construction and application of traditional BsAb has initiated the design of strategies to overcome these problems, i.e. through recombinant DNA technology various predefined bispecific antibody formats can be designed, e.g. via the use of leucine zippers, the construction of single chain bispecifics or more recently bispecific diabodies.

Following the lead of diabody construction also the formation of similarly designed trimers has been described recently [44]. These so called triabodies have three Fv heads with the polypeptides arranged in a cyclic, head-to-tail fashion (see Fig. 4C). Monospecic triabodies show an increased antigen binding affinity due to an increased avidity. However, the forming of triabodies appears to be dependent on the particular scFv chosen and the precise choice of contact residues for the VH and VL. Nevertheless, the construction of combinatorial triabodies derived from two or three zero-linker scFvs of different specificities may offer the possibility of constructing therapeutic molecules with novel multifunctional affinity and effector characteristics.

BsAbs recognise and bind cancer cells with one "arm" of the antibody. A major challenge appears to be how to effectively use the other "arm" to simultaneously activate and draw cytotoxic cells to the site of the tumour in vivo. To be effective, the antigen on the effector cells must be able to trigger signal transduction for cytotoxicity upon binding the antibody. Such antigens include subunits of the T-cell receptor or a subunit of the CD3 complex on cytotoxic T-cells, as well as Fc-receptors on natural killer cells and monocytes. However, it is known that for an adequate activation and function of these immune cells a more complicated array of immune response accessory signals have to be delivered. E.g. one of the problems with immunotherapy appears to be to artificially deliver adequate costimulation to redirected T-cells in order to prevent anergy or apoptosis.

To solve this problem one possibility might be to first induce a local inflammation reaction at the site of the tumour possibly through the use of a bispecific antibody that redirects and activates tumour resident myeloid effector cells that subsequently will locally produce proinflammatory cytokines and chemokines. As a result the endothelium near the tumour might become activated, leading to an influx of a.o. lymphoid effector cells, like CTL harnessed with anti-CD3 based BsAb.

The concept of using a bispecific antibody to direct a patient's immune cells against cancer is still a challenging prospect. Over the last few years this concept has been studied extensively both in preclinical models and in a number of phase I clinical trials. Promising pre-clinical results have been reported using tumour models in which diverse immune effector cell populations have been used. Nevertheless, lessons can be learnt from new insights in tumour cell biology and basic immunology. More and more details are becoming revealed on how tumour cells can actively evade and/or modulate the immune system. It is tempting to speculate that cancer might not be solely the result of malignant transformation of deceased cells but might well be interconnected to subtle, yet not revealed defects of the immune surveillance system. It is anticipated that these findings can be translated into clinical experience eventually leading to better results. The use of protein engineering has permitted entirely new designs for BsAbs based on antigen-binding fragments such as scFv fragments as building blocks rather than whole antibodies. The next years will be marked by increasing knowledge on possibilities for the production of novel high grade bispecific antibody reagents in quantities enough to allow experimental and clinical testing.

Acknowledgements

The author would like to acknowledge the excellent assistance of Lidia Westers, Baukje Elzinga, Gwenny Fuhler, Renske van der Hoeven, and Jelleke Dokter-Fokkens.

References

1. Kaminski MS, Zasadny KR, Francis IR, et al. Radioimmunotherapy of B-cell lymphoma with [131] anti-B1 (anti-CD20) antibody. N Engl J Med 1993;329:459-65.
2. Schroff RW, Foon KA, Beatty SM, Oldham RK, Morgan AC Jr. Human anti-murine immunoglobulin responses in patients receiving monoclonal antibody therapy. Cancer Res 1985;45:879-85.
3. De Leij L. Tumor and differentiation antigens. In: Bertino JR (ed). Encyclopedia of Cancer. San Diego: Academic Press Inc. 1997:p1818-39.
4. De Leij L, Helfrich W, Stein F, Mattes MJ. SCLC-cluster-2 antibodies detect the pancarcinoma/epithelial glycoprotein EGP-2. Int J Cancer 1994;57(suppl 8):60-63.
5. Momburg F, Moldenhauer G, Hammerling GJ, Moller P. Immunohistochemical study of the expression of a Mr 34,000 human epithelium-specific surface glycoprotein in normal and malignant tissues. Cancer Res 1987;47:2883-91.
6. Edwards DP, Grzyb KT, Dressler LG. Monoclonal antibody identification and characterization of a Mr 43,000 membrane glycoprotein associated with human breast cancer. Cancer Res 1986;46:1306-17.
7. Varki NM, Reisfeld PA, Walker LE. Antigens associated with a human lung adenocarcinoma defined by monoclonal antibodies. Cancer Res 1984;44:681-87 .
8. Bumol TF, Marder P, DeHerdt SV, Borowitz MJ, Apelgren LD. Characterization of the human tumor and normal tissue reactivity of the KSI/4 monoclonal antibody. Hybridoma 1988;7:407-15.
9. Spurr NK, Durbin H, Sheer D, Parkar M, Bobrow L, Bodmer WF. Characterization and chromosomal assignment of a human cell surface antigen defined by the monoclonal antibody AUAI. Int J Cancer 1986;38:631-36.
10. Riethmuller G, Schneider-Gadicke E, Schlimok G, et al. Randomised trial of monoclonal antibody for adjuvant therapy of resected Dukes' C colorectal carcinoma. German Cancer Aid 17-IA Study Group [see comments]. Lancet 1994;343:1177-83.
11. Elias DJ, Ibrschowitz L, Kline LE, et al. Phase 1 clinical comparative study of monoclonal antibody KS 1/4 and KS 1/4-methotrexate immunconjugate in patients with non-small cell lung carcinoma. Cancer Res 1990;50:4154-59.
12. Kosterink J, De Jonge M, Smith E, et al. Pharmacokinetics and scintigraphy of indium-111-DTPA-MOC-31 in small-cell lung carcinoma. J Nucl Med 1995;36:2356-62.
13. Spearman ME, Goodwin RM, Kau D. Disposition of the monoclonal antibody-vinca alkaloid conjugate, KS1/4-DAVLB (LY256787), in Fischer 344 rats and rhesus monkeys. Drug Metab Dispos Biol Fate Chem 1987;15:640-47.
14. Apelgren LD, Zimmerman DL, Briggs SL, Bumol TF. Antitumor activity of the monoclonal antibody-Vinca alkaloid immunoconjugate LY203725 (KS1/4-4-desacetylvinblastine-3-carboxhydrazide) in a nude mouse model of human ovarian cancer. Cancer Res 1990;50:3540-44.
15. Schneck D, Butler F, Dugan W, et al. Disposition of a murine monoclonal antibody vinca conjugate (KS1/4-DAVLB) in patients with adenocarcinomas. Clin Pharmacol Ther 1990;47:36-41.
16. Carter P, Rodrigues ML, Lewis GD, Figari I, Shalaby N1R. Towards an immunotherapy for p185HER2 overexpressing tumors. Adv Exp Med Biol 1994;353:83-94.
17. Huang X, Molema G, King S, Watkins L, Edgington TS, Thorpe PE. Tumor infarction in mice by antibody-directed targeting of tissue factor to tumor vasculature. Science 1997;275:547-50.
18. Digiesi G, Giacomini P, Fraioli R, et al. Production and characterization of murine mabs to the extracellular domain of human neu oncogene product GP185HER2. Hybridoma 1992;11:519-27.

19. Heijnen IA, Van de Winkel JG. A human Fc gamma RI/CD64 transgenic model for in vivo analysis of (bispecific) antibody therapeutics. J Hematother 1995;4(5):351-56.
20. Fanger MW, Morganelli PM, Guyre PM. Bispecific antibodies. Crit Rev Immunol 1992;12(3-4):101-24.
21. Kroesen BJ, Buter J, Sleijfer DT, et al. Phase I study of intravenously applied bispecific antibody in renal cell cancer patients receiving subcutaneous interleukin 2. Br J Cancer 1994;70:652-61.
22. Kroesen BJ, ter Haar A, Spakman H, et al. Local antitumour treatment in carcinoma patients with bispecific-monoclonal-antibody-redirected T cells. Cancer Immunol Immunother 1993;37:400-7.
23. Kroesen BJ, Helfrich W, Bakker A, et al. Reduction of EGP-2-positive pulmonary metastases by bispecific-antibody-redirected T cells in an immunocompetent rat model. Int J Cancer 1995;61:812-18.
24. McCafferty J, Griffiths AD, Winter G, Chiswell DJ. Phage antibodies: filamentous phage displaying antibody variable domains. Nature 1990;348:552-54.
25. Orlandi R, Gussow DH, Jones PT, Winter G. Cloning immunoglobulin variable domains for expression by the polymerase chain reaction. Proc Natl Acad Sci USA 1989;86:3833-37.
26. Hoogenboom M Griffiths AD, Johnson KS, Chisweil DJ, Hudson P, Winter G. Multi-subunit proteins on the surface of filamentous phage: methodologies for displaying antibody (Fab) heavy and light chains. Nucleic Acids Res 1991;19:4133-37.
27. Clackson T, Hoogenboom M Griffiths AD, Winter G. Making antibody fragments using phage display libraries. Nature 1991;352:624-28.
28. Winter G, Griffiths AD, Hawkins RE, Hoogenboom HR. Making antibodies by phage display technology. Annu Rev Immunol 1994;12:433-55.
29. Marks JD, Hoogenboom M Bonnert TP, McCafferty J, Griffiths AD, Winter G. By-passing immunization. Human antibodies from V-gene libraries displayed on phage. J Mol Biol 1991;222:581-97.
30. Hoogenboom HR, Winter G. By-passing immunisation. Human antibodies from synthetic repertoires of germline VH gene segments rearranged in vitro. J Mol Biol 1992;227:381-88.
31. Gruber M, Schodin BA, Wilson ER, Kranz DM. Efficient tumor cell lysis mediated by a bispecific single chain antibody expressed in Escherichia coli. J Immunol 1994;152:5368-74.
32. Traunecker A, Lanzavecchia A, Karjalainen K. Bispecific single chain molecules (Janusins) target cytotoxic lymphocytes on HIV infected cells. EMBO J 1991;10: 3655-59.
33. Jost CR, Titus JA, Kurucz I, Segal DM. A single-chain bispecific Fv-2 molecule produced in mammalian cells redirects lysis by activated CTL. Molecular Immunology 1996;33:211-19.
34. Mack M, Riethmuller G, Kufer P. A small bispecific antibody construct expressed as a functional single-chain molecule with high tumor cell cytotoxicity. Proc Natl Acad Sci USA 1995;92:7021-25.
35. Mack M, Gruber P, Schmidt S, Riethmuller G, Kufer P. Biologic properties of a bispecific single-chain antibody directed against 17-1A (EpCAM) and CD3: tumor cell-dependent T cell stimulation and cytotoxic activity. J Immunol 1997;1997 Apr15;158:3965-70.
36. Roder JC, Cole SP, Kozbor D. The EBV-hybridoma technique. Methods Enzymol 1986;121:140-67.

37. Whitlow M, Filpula D, Rollence ML, Feng SL, Wood JF. Multivalent Fvs: characterization of single-chain Fv oligomers and preparation of a bispecific Fv. Protein Eng 1994;7:1017-26.
38. Holliger P, Prospero T, Winter G. "Diabodies": small bivalent and bispecific antibody fragments. Proc Natl Acad Sci USA 1993;90:6444-48.
39. Perisic 0, Webb PA, Holliger P, Winter G, Williams RL. Crystal structure of a diabody, a bivalent antibody fragment. Structure 1994;2:1217-26.
40. Holliger P, Brissinck J, Williams RL, Thielemans K, Winter G. Specific killing of lymphoma cells by cytotoxic T-cells mediated by a bispecific diabody. Protein Eng 1996;9:299-305.
41. Wu AM, Chen W, Raubitschek A, Tumor localization of anti-CEA single-chain Fvs: improved targetting by non-covalent dimers. Immunotechnology. Immunotechnology 1996;221-36.
42. Fitzgerald K, Holliger P, Winter G. Improved tumour targeting by disulphide stabilized diabodies expressed in Pichia pastoris. Protein Eng 1997;10:1221-25.
43. Zhu Z, Zapata G, Shalaby R, Snedecor B, Chen H, Carter P. High level secretion of a humanized bispecific diabody from Escherichia coli. Bio-Technology 1996;(New York):192-96.
44. Iliades P, Kortt AA, Hudson PJ. Triabodies: Single chain Fv fragments without a linker form trivalent trimers. Febs Letters 1997;409:437-41.

RE-APPRAISING THE WASTE STATUS OF BUFFY COATS: NATURAL HUMAN INTERFERON

D.M. Nicolson

"We shall not cease from exploration and the end of all our exploring will be to arrive where we started and know the place for the first time."

T.S. Elliot

Some thirty years have passed since Isaacs and Linderman discovered natural human interferon in 1957. Many other cytokines have been discovered since that time yet a complete understanding of the full importance of interferons has to be reached. Even a brief review of current scientific publications demonstrates the extensive interest in the clinical applications of natural alpha interferon therapy.

Alpha interferon is produced by a number of different white blood cells in varying degrees [1], however, myelomonocytic cells [2] are the best producers. There are in excess of 13 different alpha interferon subtypes [3] with molecular weights in the range of 17.5-27.6 kD under reducing conditions on SDS-PAGE [4]. A number of subtypes have variants many of which are expressed at very low levels in the general population [5]. Some of the subtypes are glycosylated [6]. The 13 alpha interferon genes along with a beta interferon gene, an omega interferon gene and some pseudogenes are located on chromosome 9 in the human.

Katschinski et al. [7] conducted studies to determine the genetic control of alpha interferon production in humans. They concluded that some individuals were high producers and some were low and that there was no correlation with HLA genotype. They also stated that in general interferon production decreases with age and varies significantly between individuals. This agreed with work done in the 1980's [8] which related increasing age and lower interferon production to increased susceptibility to viral infections and malignant diseases. Other researchers are evaluating the clinical value of measuring a patient's ability to produce interferon to determine immune status in a number of disease states [9].

Interferon elicits its effects through binding to a multisubunit type I interferon receptor which is present on a large number of cells [10]. Binding to the receptor results in signal transduction and kinase activation [11]. This results in three main biological effects:

- Antiviral [12].
- Anti-proliferative [13].
- Immunomodulatory [14].

There are extensive supporting publications for all of the aforementioned general effects of alpha interferon.

These three main biological effects have been utilised in a number of therapeutic applications:

- 1986 licensed Hairy cell leukaemia.
- 1988 licensed Genital warts.
- 1988 licensed Kaposi sarcoma.
- 1991 licensed Hepatitis C.
- 1992 licensed Hepatitis B.

A large number of other potential indications are currently being examined including HIV and multiple sclerosis [15]. Interferon is also widely used in the therapy of chronic myelogenous leukaemia.

In Annual Reviews of Immunology 1993 [17] is stated: "The reasons for the complexity of the IFN alpha gene system remain unclear but recent studies suggest that the different IFN alpha species effect distinct arrays of biological responses in different cells". Although the biological activity profile of each subtype has not been fully defined it has been shown that their receptor binding characteristics vary and that the strength of receptor interaction helps determine the predominant biological effect: anti-viral or anti-proliferative. On the basis that alpha interferon subtypes can exhibit subtle differences in biological activity there is reason to believe that a mixture of subtypes may exert a slightly different effect than a single subtype such as those contained in recombinant preparations.

Another difference between natural human interferon alpha and recombinant interferon alpha is the lack of immunogenicity by the natural products. Neutralising antibodies to recombinant interferons have been widely reported [18] and a significant proportion of patients treated with recombinant interferon alpha develop neutralising antibodies that makes the recombinant treatment ineffective. In many cases re-treatment of patients with neutralising antibodies to recombinant interferon with natural alpha interferon is successful [19].

So, natural human interferon has some significant differences from recombinant interferon one of which has already been shown to be of clinical importance. Natural interferon is produced by peripheral blood mononuclear cells (PBMC's). There are a large number of indications where interferon may have clinical benefits.

The same cells that represent a useful raw material for interferon production are currently considered as a waste material by most transfusion services. Indeed there is a general trend to remove PBMC's wherever possible [20], this was one of the topics discussed at last year's conference[1]. The reduction of PBMC's can reduce complications like: nonhaemolytic febrile transfusion reactions, alloimmunisation and refractoriness to platelet transfusion and immunomodulation [21]. One method used to assess the health of PBMC's in buffy coats or other blood fractions is vital staining and FACS analysis. Using propidium iodine we have found PBMC's can remain viable for considerable periods of time in a buffy coat environment.

It is these unwanted cells that Viragen can use to produce natural interferon alpha utilising our proprietary culture and purification technologies. Our first European production facility was opened in July of 1997 in Edinburgh Scotland. It will initially process buffy coats provided by the Scottish National Blood Transfusion Service who are our joint venture partners in that country. Despite being discovered three decades ago natural alpha interferon remains one of the most therapeutically interesting and significant cytokines.

Acknowledgements

Scottish National Blood Transfusion Service, National Scientific Laboratory. Dr. Nicola Williams, Dr. Ray Ziai.

References

1. Greenway AL, Hertzog PJ, Devenish RJ, Linnane AW. Constitutive and virus induced interferon production by peripheral blood leukocytes. Exp Hematol 1995;23: 229-35.
2. Akerlund K, Bjork L, Fehinger T, Pohl G, Andersson J, Andersson U. Sendai virus-induces ifn-alpha production analysed by immunocytochemistry and computerized image analysis. Scand J Immunol 1996;44:345-53.
3. Dent CL, Gewert DR. A regulatory domain within the virus response element of the interferon alpha 1 gene acts as a transcriptional repressor sequence and determinant of cell specific gene expression. Eur J Biochem 1996:236:895-903.
4. Zoon KC, Miller D, Bekisz J, et al. Purification and characterisation of multiple components of human lymphoblastoid interferon alpha. J Biol Chem 1992;267: 15210-16.
5. Hussain M, Gill DS, Liao MJ, Testa D. Interferon alpha 8B is the only variant of interferon alpha 8 identified in a large human population. J Interferon Cytokines Res 1996;16:523-29.
6. Shirono H, Koga J, Uemura H, Matsuo A. Identification of glycosylated subtypes of interferon alpha produced by human leukocytes. Biosci Biotechnol Biochem 1994; 58:1714-15.
7. Katschinski DM, Neustock P, Kluter H, Kirchner H. Influence of various factors on interferon alpha production in cultures of human leukocytes. 1994;14:105-10.
8. Abb J, Abb H, Deinhardt F. Age related decline of human interferon alpha and interferon gamma production. Blut 1984;48:285-90.

---

1. Cytokines and Growth Factors in Blood Transfusion. Smit Sibinga Cth, Das PC, Löwenberg, eds. Kluwer Academic Publ. Dordrecht/Boston/Lancaster, 1997.

9. Uno K, Nakano K, Maruo N, et al. Determination of interferon alpha producing capacity in whole blood cultures from patients with various diseases and healthy persons. J Interferon Cytokines Res 1996;16:911-18.
10. Domanski P, Colamonici OR. The type 1 interferon receptor. The long and the sort of it. Cytokine Growth Factor Rev 1996;7:1143-51.
11. Chislain J, Sussman G, Goelz S, Ling LE, Fish EN. Configuration of the interferon alpha/beta receptor complex determines the context of the biological response. J Biol Chem 1995;270:21785-92.
12. Crance JM, Leveque F, Chousterman S, Jouan A, Trepo C, Deloince R. Antiviral activity of recombinant interferon alpha on hepatitis A virus replication in human livers. Antiviral Res 1995;28:69-80.
13. Iacopino F, Robustelli Della Cuna G, Sica G. Natural interferon alpha activity in hormone sensitive, hormone resistant and autonomous human breast cancer cell lines. Int J Cancer 1997;71:1103-8.
14. Corssmit EP, Heijligenberg R, Hack CE, Endert E, Sauerwein HP, Romijn JA. Effects of interferon alpha (IFN alpha) administration on leucocytes in healthy humans. Clin Exp Immunol 1997;107:359-63.
15. Squillacote D, Martinez M, Sheramata W. Natural alpha interferon in multiple sclerosis: results of three preliminary series. J Int Medial Res 1996;24:246-57.
16. Lauta VM. Interferon and chronic melogenous leukemia. Med Oncol 1995;12:41-46.
17. Farrar MA, Schreiber RD. The molecular cell biology of interferon gamma and its receptor. Ann Rev Immunol 1993;11:571-611.
18. Nolte KU, Gunther G. Von Wussow P. Epitopes recognized by neutralizing therapy-induced human anti interferon alpha antibodies are localised within the N terminal functional domain of recombinant interferon alpha 2. Eur J Immunol 1996;26:155-59.
19. Milella M, Antonelli G, Santantonio T, et al. Treatment with natural IFN of hepatitis C patients with or without antibodies to recombinant IFN. Hepatogastroenterology 1995;42:201-4.
20. Muylle L. The role of cytokines in blood transfusion reactions. Blood Rev 1995; 9:77-85.
21. Higgins VL. Leukocyte reduced blood components: patients benefits and practical applications. Oncol Nurs Forum 1996;23:659-67.

DISCUSSION

C.R. Valeri, H.J.C. de Wit

C.Th. Smit Sibinga, Groningen, NL: Dr. de Vries, you have not been requesting granulocyte concentrates for years now. Might it be possible to further shorten the thrombocytopenic phase through the direct injection of a cocktail of cytokines and TPO or do you foresee a possibility in expanding autologous stem cells, lineaging them and giving them back together with the pluripotent stem cells.

E.G.E. de Vries, Groningen, NL: This is probably the big problem; there have been studies in which people had the courage to inject growth factors together with chemotherapy. If you do that you increase toxicity of chemotherapy, probably because you bring stem cells into cycling which are then affected by chemotherapy, so people do not dare to do that anymore. Despite all the growth factors that do affect thrombopoiesis it really takes days before you see any effect on thrombopoiesis which is not so bizarre because the platelets have to go through all the stages, while G-CSF is a much later acting cytokine. Probably combination of the various thrombopoietic growth factors will help and I am really somewhat worried about the side-effects in the clinic. People are at the moment rather excited about IL11 which has proven efficacy on platelet transfusions. But if you look at the side effects then you would only give it to a patient if you really need it. It is not a gentle way of supportive treatment to my opinion. So, what we would like is giving a bone marrow or stem cell transplantation need no platelet transfusions anymore after seven days. But I think it is still too early now.

C.Th. Smit Sibinga: So, the first option is not really the option to go for: the immediate injection of cytokines even not after chemotherapy because of interference with the cytostatic regime.

E.G.E. de Vries: Yes, you cannot give that at the same time. So, you have to wait until the drug has phased out.

C.Th. Smit Sibinga: So, the other option transplanting back both pluripotent as well as specifically committed stem cells would be the solution.

E.G.E. de Vries: Well, that is one way. However, all this is going to be very expensive. Another problem is that using combinations of cytokines is at the moment not very easy in the clinic because experimental drugs are not allowed to be used. In general they come from different companies which is another logistic problem. What is quite interesting although it is a little bit too early to predict how it is going to be applied in the clinic, but in the laboratory several companies are really reshaping these haematopoietic growth factors and try to create new molecules that do not have this toxicity profile, do have more efficacy and if that is successful in a few years it may be much easier.

C.R. Valeri, Boston, MA, USA: Dr. de Vries, are you convinced that the peripheral blood mononuclear cell is as good as the bone marrow mononuclear cell? The second question is: what is the minimum number of mononuclear cells that you would recommend to be reinfused for engraftment?

E.G.E. de Vries: At the moment the idea is that peripheral stem cells will be as good as bone marrow transplants. In the Netherlands the haematologists conduct a randomised study. I am not worried about the short term effect of bone marrow or peripheral stem cell transplantation, because peripheral stem cell transplantation is really great because for the patients do better. What is probably something that we should be worried about is the long term effect on the quality of the bone marrow. We know for example in a breast cancer study that if you have to retreat those patients with chemotherapy that is almost impossible; from a haematopoietic point of view they cannot handle that well enough. The other thing is that we do have quite a number of patients that never get normal blood counts back and quite some patients that have relatively few platelets which is kind of a logistic problem. For example in our breast cancer study we have young ladies often from one family; they want to have their ovaries removed, want to have a breast removed (the good one) and that really poses us for problems. So, when we only did bone marrow transplant we had the same problems. It is just that people are so excited about the peripheral stem cell transplant, but scientifically it would be good still to compare.

C.R. Valeri: What about the number of cells? Do you have a minimum number?

E.G.E. de Vries: The cut-off point more or less advised to use is 5×10^{6}/kg but we are not sure that 2½ and 3×10^{6}/kg will do as well. There is still the chance that the bag will break or some unpleasant thing will happen. We tend to do another harvest if we do not feel sure enough.

J.P. AuBuchon, Lebanon, NH, USA: A theoretical question. Dr. Winslow,. I do not disagree with your reading of the literature that 35% seems to be the best haematocrit delivery of oxygen for a patient. Could you offer any theoretical conjecture to why most of us have a haematocrit above 40% and evolutionarily why are we there? Is it to have a safeguard against being attacked by a tiger and bleeding out, so we can still stay above that 35%? Is 35% enough? Should not we even try to get higher possibly in some patients?

R.M. Winslow, San Diego, CA, USA: I do not think there is any way to provide a very satisfying answer to the question, but from a biological point of view many things are different about us now than they were even a century ago. Humans probably evolved in a very different sort of situation than we find ourselves in now with regard to nutrition, life-span and many other things. People are bigger now than they used to be. To me, the sensible answer is that the system is designed for an optimum at around 35. Now we are better nourished, healthier and things are different. When you look at it simply from any one of a number of theoretical points of view, that number of 35 keeps coming back. If you go from 35 to 45 because of the exponential nature of the viscosity curve, you probably lose something in blood flow and viscosity. I am sorry I cannot give you a better answer. The system is probably designed for 35 and we find ourselves in a very different situation now.

H. Boralessa, Brentwood, UK: Following on about this optimum haemoglobin now most anaesthetists and surgeons accept a haemoglobin of 10 and a haematocrit of 30 and anaesthetists accept a lower level of haemoglobin and haematocrit. Now having heard your lecture about the optimum haemoglobin how should we go, should we advise them to amend to an optimal haemoglobin or a safe low haemoglobin to reduce the transfusion requirements?

R.M. Winslow: I try to be careful not to say that the goal should be 35, merely to say if you observe nature, what you see is that nature seems to like that number of 35. That is not to say that that is where we need to be, because the system is variable over some range. It varies from patient to patient and from situation to situation. So, I think there are two separate, distinct questions. One is what is the optimum and the other is how low can you go before getting into trouble.

J.C. Fratantoni, Rockville, MD, USA: Dr. Middleton, you alluded to the attempt some years ago to develop a platelet substitute based on red cells. Can you tell us what is different about your product and why it should work.

S. Middleton, Nottingham, UK: The first reports were actually on fibrinogen and then went on to RGG. No, we have a lot of work yet to prove how this product is actually working. We have not yet confirmed the mechanism of action and that still remains to be done. So, I think time will tell.

C.Th. Smit Sibinga: Another question. What do you know at this point in time about the disappearance and the metabolism of these microspheres.

S. Middleton: We know from the mother microcapsules that they seem to be broken down ultimately in the liver as albumin. When you raise antibodies to these spheres in animals the antibodies do not show any difference from human serum albumin. So, it looks very similar to that protein and apparently is broken down in the liver as albumin.

C.Th. Smit Sibinga: Thank you very much. A question to Prof. de Leij about his fascinating presentation. Do you think that the diabody approach would be suitable for the production eventually of specific immunoglobulins not so much for targeting tumour cells. For instance in the area of anti-D, anti-CMV or anti-tetanus or do you see a future with the hybridoma technology to get these kind of proteins synthesised.

L. de Leij, Groningen, NL: Yes, I guess this diabody approach will be useful for all purposes where you have to attach one antigen to the other. So for instance if you want to clear a substance (say antigen A) from the circulation it may be quite useful to make a diabody against antigen A and against an antigen on the mononuclear system. For instance if you target this to Fc receptors then you can really get a good clearance. So, everywhere you want to attach one antigen to the other, it will be a very fine approach.

H.J.C. de Wit, Leeuwarden, NL: Dr. Goodnough, I understood the most economic and effective approach to autologous transfusion is low-dose erythropoietin and pre-haemodilution. As you use a very low-dose of erythropoietin cannot we think of triggering a natural stimulus for erythropoietin. I could think of prescribing cigarettes for 14 days, but that might not be a good idea; could there be another idea to stimulate that bit of the natural production of erythropoietin 14 days or 4 weeks before an operation.

L.T. Goodnough, St. Louis, MO, USA: There are certainly a lot of ways to do it. You could put someone in a hypoxic chamber for instance periodically and you could probably do it with little risk. It reminds me I was in Bolivia talking to a group that we were treating post MI patients by moving them actually to high altitude and watching their haemoglobins come back. This sounded crazy but there were some pretty good clinical data that they had reduced reinfarctions when they did that. So, maybe it is not a crazy idea. I do not know how you would design the trial although.

C.R. Valeri: I would like to ask dr. Goodnough to comment on the use of iron when EPO is given. Does the platelet count increase following the administration of EPO?

L.T. Goodnough: The iron question is kind of a complex question for me; it has taken me about 10 years to get a handle on this. I concluded that one of the ironies is that the drug is approved for use in anaemic patients, but when you use EPO that way you are starting behind in a good 30% of these anaemic or frankly iron deficient patients, the rest of them having anaemia because of a chronic disease. That is why we need to use such high doses of EPO to show a clinical effect and it is just too costly. The alternative strategy would be to take patients who seemingly are not at risk, such as patients with normal haematocrits undergoing radical prostatectomy. But because of the nature of the surgical procedure they have still a substantial risk of allogeneic exposure. So there you have the luxury of starting in iron replete individuals with normal bone marrow, with a relatively low dose and a cost effective approach. In that setting all patients were supplemented with oral iron over the two week period of time. The role of oral iron or the role of storage iron seems to be just to maintain iron saturation. We know from the 1950's when Bill Crosby[1] and others did aggressive phlebotomy studies in patients with haemochromatosis that you can accelerate erythropoiesis by a factor of 9 when you maintain iron saturation. In prostatectomy patients with normal iron stores and oral iron supplementation you can increase erythropoiesis by a factor 3 or 4 not 9. So, it seems we have a lot of room to improve with innovative strategies such as intravenous iron therapy especially in the patients who are starting out at risk already because they are anaemic or because they are iron depleted. I think there is emerging a role for intravenous iron supplementation in that setting. Your second question is what happens to platelets. We know that from our autologous blood donor studies when you stimulate the bone marrow either with endogenous erythropoietin or exogenous erythropoietin and perhaps in the setting of blood loss it is well known that you have a reactive form of thrombocytosis. So, the platelet count goes up statistically in both placebo treated patients. These platelet counts are well within the range of normal and I do not believe that the thrombocytosis associated in that setting has anything to do with the risk of thrombosis in the surgical setting.

J.C. Fratantoni: Dr. Nicolson, when interleukin was first approved of in the 80's it was being manufactured from buffy coats from leukocytes that were collected from regular donors. The natural material was being made from buffy coats and there is an enormous amount of that material generated every year. What are you considering: buffy coats from whole blood donors or different sources?

D.M. Nicolson, Penicuik, UK: Well, I believe that every transfusion service in the world at the moment discards its buffy coats. They are a part of the donation for which there is no direct therapeutic use for at this time. Viragen, however, can use this waste material to produce natural alpha interferon. There is a growing understanding of the complexity of natural alpha interferon; which exists not as a single molecule but many molecules with varying interactions and potential clinical benefits. Although recombinant single subtype alpha interferon can be effective, a percentage of patients can develop neutralising antibodies to the recombinant protein. We have spent many years developing proprietary technology in terms of interferon superinduction and purification. Our process was designed to produce natural alpha interferon in a cost effective manner using buffy coats as a raw material. We intend to create partner-ships with blood transfusion agencies where we bring the technology and they provide the raw material: the buffy coats. It is our hope that through effective partner-

1. Crosby WM. Treatment of haemochromatosis by energetic phlebotomy. One patient's response to the letting of 55 litres of blood in 11 months. Br J Haematol 1958;4:82-88.

ships the availability of alpha interferon therapy to a variety of patient groups will be increased.

J.C. Fratantoni: Dr. Winslow, you indicated that the clinical evaluation for transfusion involved many complex variables. Someone who has a computer might be tempted to feel that you can write an algorithm and have a simple way of determining when or where not to give a transfusion. Are we smart enough to do that, are we smart enough to write a programme together or is there something we have to wait for?

R.M. Winslow: We are always smart enough to write a programme; the question is "is it useful". In fact, some of the calculations I showed you were from such a programme, but the transfusion problem is that you transfuse. What you are really doing is you are preparing for some event like the haemorrhage, and you cannot really predict what that is going to be. You really want to know what the size of that oxygen reserve is in the individual patient and in order to do that you have to know a lot about all the different oxygen transport systems. Invasive studies are really overwhelming to do that.

C.Th. Smit Sibinga: Dr. Nicolson, what is known about the consistency of subtype mosaics from individual to individual and in one individual over time?

The question relates actually to the donors, and how much the variability is or how consistent the sub-type mosaics are.

D.M. Nicolson: I stated that there were in excess of 13 different alpha interferon subtypes. If you include subtype variants this can increase to about 30. I mentioned the variants of alpha 7: 7a, 7b and 7c. Hussain et al. conducted PCR studies on 28,000 donors[2]. They found that interferon alpha 7a was the predominant variant of alpha 7. The same situation was found when alpha 14 and alpha 21 were analysed. The very low occurrence of subtype variants in the general population means that subtype variation between buffy coats is not a major issue for us.

C.Th. Smit Sibinga: Does the ageing of the interferon producing cells in the buffycoat affect the sub-type pattern?

D.M. Nicolson: We have not seen that and I have not looked into that myself. We see stable expression patterns at the moment in our particular culture system. If we moved out with our production limits we may see some change; although we have not explored whether this is something which may happen.

---

2. Hussain M, Gibbs DS, Liao MJ, Testa D. Interferon alpha 8B is the only variant of interferon alpha 8 identified in a large human population. J Interferon Cytokine Res 1996;16:523-29.

C.Th. Smit Sibinga: The 48-54 hr limit you showed, how are you going to deal with the logistics; I assume that that is a time that you need to have a vital buffycoat in the plant to be further processed.

D.M. Nicolson: Essentially, we feel that as long as the mononuclear cells are healthy they can be used for interferon production. These experiments were conducted on one type of buffy coat preparation. We can use buffy coats that are plasma rich or plasma depleted in our process. In fact we tend to get buffy coats in Europe that are so plasma depleted that I am not sure they can be classified as "fluid", yet even these buffy coats can be used to produce interferon. So from the results presented time only becomes a potential issue 54 hours post donation.

C.Th. Smit Sibinga: Dr. Goodnough, you changed for obvious reasons the last bit of the title when you started. I asked you to talk about how could EPO be used better, you said I am going to present the best way. Is this the end of the story of EPO or do you see further improvement? In other words would there be other fields in medicine where you think there is a justifiable applicability of EPO to come up. I am not talking about the sports indications.

L.T. Goodnough: Well I think a large part of the story from my point of view starts and stops with use in the surgical arena, because we feel that probably about 25% of blood transfused in the US and perhaps elsewhere is in the elective surgical setting. So it is a huge, huge area especially if we are all convinced that as we approach zero risk blood transfusion perhaps what will drive blood conservation is the concept of inventory. If there really is going to be a chronic global shortage of blood then the elective surgical situation is exactly the place where you would want to emphasise blood conservation. Of course I do not mean to ignore the vast array of medical anaemias for which erythropoietin world-wide has many applications, but I have always been especially fond of the elective surgical setting for reasons of inventory importance, if nothing else.

A. Lust, Aalst, B: Dr. Winslow, you seem very fond of upcoming oxygen carriers, haemoglobin solutions. When do you expect them and what will be their influence on biochemistry parameters. On what haemoglobin level will we work at that moment? We will have haemoglobinaemia and haemoglobinuria and to what extent will these obscure our biochemistry parameters.

R.M. Winslow: I think your question was how are we going to follow the haemoglobin concentration and how are we going to decide something about the adequacy of haemoglobin concentration.

A. Lust: It might interfere with a lot of other parameters.

R.M. Winslow: I will make two comments: first, all of the companies that have been involved in clinical trials with haemoglobin solutions have to go through an extensive revalidation of many serum chemistries and various biochemical tests. It is not a small thing because in many tests, enzyme assays are optical measurements in which haemoglobin interferes. The other comment is how do we, if we have cell free haemoglobin which transports oxygen in a different way fundamentally, assess the adequacy of oxygenation. I think that is a very difficult question because total haemoglobin may not have the same meaning when we have cell free haemoglobin as it does when we have red cell haemoglobin, and I do not think there is an answer to that yet. I think that is something that will have to be addressed when these products become available in the next year or two.

A. Lust: In what time do you expect that it will become clinically available for us.

R.M. Winslow: I have been asked that question for 15 years. I always say five years, and I stay with that answer. If you listen to what the companies are saying, Baxter claims that they will have the product on the market within a year. I just report what I hear, but I think it is likely that there may be some solutions in limited availability for limited applications within the next year or two.

C.R. Valeri: Dr. Middleton, when the fibrinogen albumin microcapsule is radiolabelled, what happens to the radioisotope associated with fibrinogen and albumin molecules?

S. Middleton: We have done that experiment and they appeared to be distributed in the same manner.

C.R. Valeri: Did the radioisotope labels provide similar results?

S. Middleton: I do not want to go into the linkage at this point, we have another technology for linking the fibrinogen to spheres, it appears to be quite stable .

C.R. Valeri: What happens if you use fibrinogen without the microsphere in your model?

S. Middleton: We have not done that.

L.T. Goodnough: What is the source of the fibrinogen that you are using; where do you get that?

S. Middleton: I cannot tell you exactly where I get it; we are obtaining from a fractionator. It is virus inactivated and it comes with very good credentials.

L.T. Goodnough: So ultimately if it were to be used clinically it would come from a pooled source.

S. Middleton: It would, but it would have been through two viral inactivating procedures, SD and heating and the albumin is clinically heated.

L.T. Goodnough: Another comment is that it appears to have a relatively short biologic period of activities so that presumably if you give it to a patient with chronic thrombocytopenia you would have to give it probably every six hours; it would be a pharmacologic intervention every six hours or so.

S. Middleton: The first results are shown in rabbits indicating that it was circulating for 48 hours. In the second experiment the animals were anaesthetised and therefore that experiment was terminated after six hours; we have no information yet about the length of time. We know that in normal rabbits we are still recovering activity at 24 hours.

L.T. Goodnough: The point I want to make is that I find it especially attractive in the area of open heart surgery if there is an acquired platelet disorder that gives you bleeding over a relatively circumscript period. Perhaps the ultimate value of this kind of an approach would be in that surgical setting rather than in a chronic thrombocytopenic patient.

S. Middleton: One of the reasons we want to get into human subjects as soon as possible is to determine how it circulates in humans, because in rabbits that have been treated with an antibody or with a radiation it is difficult really to extrapolate.

H.J.C. de Wit: I would only comment that I would be very anxious to know what is the critical dose. Did you see any of thrombotic side-effects in rabbits or did you determine a critical dose where those side-effects begin.

S. Middleton: We have not yet gone to the top maximum tolerated dose we still are doing this experiments.

III. ALTERNATIVE APPROACHES IN CLINICAL PRACTICE

VOLUME: A MATTER OF REPLACEMENT

P.L. Baele, MD, B. Fraselle, MD, J.M. Gouverneur, MD, M. de Kock, MD PhD

Introduction

Massive fluid losses or shifts are mostly associated with trauma, burns and surgery. They are prominent features of anaphylactic or septic shocks and in some forms of acute pancreatitis. They can be encountered in obstetrics and gastrointestinal bleeds. Less frequent causes of hypovolemia include acute removal of ascitis, haemodialysis, low pressure pulmonary oedema. All these patients need quick restoration of their circulating volume and oncotic pressure. Many solutions are available nowadays to deal with acute hypovolemia [1].

Globally speaking the vast majority of those situations occur or may occur in surgical patients. This paper will therefore focus on surgical cases.

Available products and their recent evolution

Whole blood

Whole blood has disappeared from our therapeutic armamentarium, and fractionation of blood into its components is now the rule. Concentrated red cells resuspended in a variety of conservation solutions are the usual oxygen-carrying fluid available. Over the last years a trend has emerged towards removing leukocytes either soon after collecting blood or at the time of transfusion. As a result of fractionation and further processing, current red cell suspensions now barely contain any plasma and perfusion of adequate volumes of fluid must accompany their transfusion. Furthermore coagulation factors, especially fibrinogen, must be supplied at an earlier stage [2].

Plasma

The natural complement of red cells is plasma. Obtained from centrifugation of whole blood or through plasmapheresis, it always comes from blood donors. Therefore it has the potential like whole blood to transmit blood borne viruses (with the exception of intracellular viruses such as CMV). It is thus illogical to collect whole blood, then separate it into red cell concentrates and plasma. Only to re-assemble red cells and plasma from different donors at the time of transfusion. Such practice, sometimes called "reconstitution" of whole blood, must be strongly discouraged because it exposes the recipient to the risk of two donors instead of one. To preserve clotting factors plasma must be frozen soon after collection and slowly thawed at 37°C prior to transfusion. This makes the use of plasma impractical in emergencies, and restricts its use to facilities with capabilities for cold storage and appropriate thawing.

Due to the infection risk and to the cost of preparation and storage, the indications of fresh frozen plasma are limited to the treatment of coagulation defects for which no other therapy is available. Such consensus had already been reached by the NIH in 1985 [3].

Since the emergence of AIDS, many countries have adopted virus-inactivated fresh frozen plasma. The inactivation process usually involves successive contact with a solvent and a detergent. This ensures the destruction of all viruses with a lipid capsule. Viruses with a proteic capsule such as hepatitis A and parvovirus B19 are unaffected and can still be transmitted.

Due to its complexity, virus inactivation is only performed on large quantities of plasma coming from thousands of donors at a time, called "pools", yielding "batches" of final products. Obviously, this changes fundamentally the contents of "a unit of fresh frozen plasma". Although each donor is selected according to strict eligibility criteria for blood donors, and each donation must be tested for transmissible diseases, it remains true that the theoretical chances are real to include a contaminated unit in the batch. Like stable blood products, virus-inactivated fresh frozen plasma should now be considered at high risk for contamination by (new) viruses resistant to current virus-inactivation techniques. Therefore ascending and descending traceability of all plasma transfusions and donations must be ensured. This means that for each transfusion the unit's (batch) identification number must be documented in the patients' surgical file and that for every unit the name of the recipient must be known to the blood bank. It also means that all donors of a pool and corresponding batch must be identified by the transfusion centre (or manufacturer) which processed it. Finally, some countries have added to these precautions the obligation to follow up all recipients of blood products in extensive haemovigilance programmes.

Stable solutions of albumin and plasma proteins

When the active properties of coagulation factors are not to be preserved, it is relatively easy to prepare virus-free plasma by pasteurisation. Stable solutions of plasma proteins (SSPP) have been available for many years in many countries and were prepared from batches of several thousands of donations. These sometimes included plasma obtained from centrifugation of outdated whole blood and therefore could contain high concentrations of cytokines and other vasoactive molecules liberated by ageing or activated leukocytes and platelets. Severe vasoplegic reactions have been described. Over the years these preparations have increased in purity as the source of plasma progressively shifted towards fresh donations.

Albumin solutions are usually available in 5% and 20% concentrations and are obtained by resuspending in normosaline albumin extracted from plasma by physicochemical methods. Some commercial solutions used human placentas as source of albumin, instead of plasma from well-informed voluntary donors. This practice has recently been out-lawed by several countries, mainly on the grounds that full traceability could not be guaranteed.

Albumine solutions are purer than SSPP solutions: they usually contain at least 99% albumin, while SSPP contains 15 to 25% of other proteins such as immunoglobulins. Some patients carry atypical IgA or are deficient in IgA and may present an anaphylactic reaction when exposed to normal IgA in SSPP.

The cost of albumin and plasma protein solutions is high. Furthermore many countries lack expensive processing plants to produce them. Availability and cost are therefore major determinants in their use.

It must be added that no prospective randomized study has ever demonstrated their efficacy is terms of patient outcome. In particular a recent study involving more than 400 intensive care patients failed to show any advantage of albumin solutions as compared to gelatin solution in terms of renal failure, pulmonary function, length of stay or mortality, despite higher levels of circulating proteins [4-5].

Several countries have held consensus conferences concerning the good use of albumin. They mostly agree in that albumin solutions should never be used as first line therapy, except in neonates, for whom normal levels of albumin are critical to carry and neutralise bilirubin [6-10].

Crystalloids

Crystalloids freely and immediately diffuse into the extravascular and intracellular space. Due to their very short intravascular stay (a few minutes) they are of little help to correct acute hypovolemic states. They are totally devoid of anaphylactic and viral risks.

Hyperosmolar crystalloid solutions have been used in the management of trauma patients since more than sixty years but have enjoyed renewed interest over the last five years. Up to 4 ml per kg of hypertonic (up to 7.5% NaCl) or hyperoncotic solutions are highly effective in normalising cardiovascular function, due to the rapid mobilisation of fluid from the extravascular compartment. This beneficial effect lasts for about two hours and can be measured in terms of improved cardiac output and volemia, after which further infusions of colloids or crystalloid are needed to maintain this result. The direct effect on cardiac myocytes is still controversial, but coronary blood flow improves probably because of a direct dilation of its large conduction vessels [11]. Hypertonic solution has been found to exert a favourable influence on neurologic outcome provided the blood-brain barrier is intact at the time of infusion. This may result from a decreased tendency towards cerebral oedema [12]. Potentially deleterious effects include rapid hypernatremia which can cause central pontine myelinolysis in patients starting with low serum sodium concentrations. Dilutional hypokalemia can provoke cardiac rhythm disturbances especially in patients treated with digoxin. Finally fluid overload remains a potential risk in patients with a poor cardiac function. Phlebitis is frequent when infusing hyperosmolar solution via a peripheral vein. Solutions combining high sodium concentrations with dextran 70 or hydroxyethylstarches have reached the stage of clinical trials. In conclusion in selected circumstances hypertonic solutions are a valuable fluid replacement therapy for the treatment of acute hypovolemia [1,13,14].

Artificial colloids

Artificial colloids are now considered as first choice therapy when volemia and oncotic pressure must be acutely restored. They can be grouped in four major classes: dextrans, gelatins, hydroxyethylstarches, and perfluorocarbons.

Dextrans are synthetic polysaccharides. Most popular solutions have mean molecular weights of 40.000 or 70.000 daltons. They interfere with platelet aggregation and increase fibrinolysis and are therefore used in the prevention of perioperative thrombosis and embolism. The importance of their antiplatelet action severely limits the amounts that can be administered [15]. They interfere with blood group testing, which may create a serious problem in emergency situations. As they share common sequences with widespread bacterial products, they can trigger severe anaphylactoid reactions which can be prevented by prior administration of short-chain (low molecular weight) dextrans. They are no longer used as first line volume replacement solutions.

Gelatins are polypeptides from animal – usually bovine – origin. The production process usually involves heat-inactivation of viruses. Their molecular weight varies around 35.000, which means that a substantial part of these molecules can escape through the glomerules or leak into the extravascular space. Their vascular half-life is rather short (3 to 6 hours). As any foreign molecule, they can trigger severe anaphylactic or anaphylactoid reactions, though less often than dextrans. They are otherwise well tolerated and there seems to be no maximal daily dose. Their very low cost, good tolerance, good stability, and short half-life have made them popular for transient volume replacement in operating rooms and emergency rooms alike.

Hydroxyethylstarches (HES) are more recent manufactured molecules from amylopectin i.e. from vegetal origin. They can provoke anaphylactoid reactions. HES are macromolecular polymers of hydroxyethylated glucose molecules linked by alpha-1.4 bonds. HES solutions may be characterised by their hydroxyl substitution ratio, their molecular weight and their concentration. A degree of substitution of 0.5 means that 5 out of 10 molecules of glucose are substituted with hydroxyethyl groups. The lower the degree of substitution, the faster these huge polymers are degraded by serum alpha amylases, down to smaller molecules which interfere less with haemostasis. The higher the molecular weight, the longer the intravenous persistence, but the lower the potential for expanding circulatory volume: more numerous small molecules will attract more water from the extravascular space. Finally, at equal molecular weight, the higher the concentration the higher the oncotic power of the solution. The initial preparations had a high mean molecular weight (450.000) and high substitution ratio (0.7); they also exhibited a strong and prolonged activity against the Von Willebrand part of factor VIII, which resulted in latent hypocoagulability, haematoma formation in surgical wounds and increased transfusion needs. More recent hydroxyethylstarches with a lower molecular weight (200.000) and substitution ratio (0.5) seem devoid of such side-effects. Manufacturers still advocate not to exceed the dosis of 30 to 40 $ml/kg^{-1}/day^{-1}$. New HES solutions feature a long intravascular half life (12 hours or more) and at a concentration of 6% they can even serve as plasma expanders by attracting water from the extravascular space. They are more expensive than gelatins but much less than plasma proteins or albumin solutions.

Perfluorocarbons are molecules with a high affinity for oxygen. Besides they come as hyperosmolar solutions which gives them potentially a supplemental value in shock. Unfortunately current solutions do not come in a ready to use form, carry only limited amounts of oxygen and are trapped for months in the reticuloendothelial system instead of being excreted. Waiting for better molecules and preparations, the clinician's interest for perfluorocarbons remains only theoretical at the time being.

Conclusions

All colloid solutions exhibit to various degrees some common properties (oncotic expansion of the vascular space, prolonged intravascular half-life), so that they can be used as "plasma substitutes". Unfortunately they all can provoke anaphylactoid reactions, sometimes even severe ones. Because plasma protein solutions are much more expensive and may also provoke severe reactions, artificial colloids are now considered first line therapy in acute hypovolemic states, except in neonates and infants. Anaphylactic reactions occurring during pregnancy, up to the moment of birth, can have catastrophic results for the baby. Therefore the administration of any foreign molecule that is not vitally needed should be avoided until the baby is safely born. This includes all colloids and blood products, except in extreme situations. If a colloid must be given before birth, purified albumin should be preferred.

Recent trends in the use of colloids

The SANGUIS study reported transfusion practices in more than 7.000 elective surgical cases operated in 1990 and 1991 [16-18]. The study also collected data concerning plasma and artificial colloids. The principal findings were the following: there was no consensus concerning the use of any of those products, 16% of patients received whole blood, 12% received plasma, 22% received albumin or plasma protein solutions, 35% received artificial colloids.

Plasma

Plasma transfusion rates ranged from 0 to 100% of patients for procedures such as abdominal aneurysmectomy or coronary bypass. Wide variations were found within the same countries, and sometimes also within hospitals for comparable procedures such as hemicolectomy and abdominal aneurysmectomy. For very few plasma transfusions (26%) evidence of laboratory coagulation testing could be found; in only 12% of plasma recipients the prothrombin time was less than 60% of control. Many plasma units were administered without adequate (traceable) documentation in the surgical files. In many centres plasma was transfused to each patient who had been given three units of red cells, which means "reconstitution" was still a common practice. In some places liquid

Table 1. Main features of commonly used colloid solutions

	Viral risk	i.v. persistence (hours)	i.v. distribution	Interference with haemostasis	Anaphylactic risk	Relative cost per volume unit	Recommended max. daily dosis
FFP	+++	6-12	100	+	+	17	None
FFP v.i.	+?	6-12	100	+	+	43	None
Albumine 20%	0?	6-12	100	0	0	110	None
SSPP	0?	6-12	80	0	+	19	None
Dextran 70	0	6-12	100	––	++	3	1.5 g/kg^{-1}
HES 200,000/0.5	0	>12	1000	–	+	3.5	30 ml/kg^{-1}
Gelatins	0?	4	50	0	+	1.5	None
Crystalloids	0	<<1	25	0	0	1	None

or recovered (not fresh frozen) plasma was liberally used as volume therapy: it represented 39% of the total volume of plasma transfused in the study. Finally some surgeons also gave plasma postoperatively at the rate of one unit a day for its alleged "healing properties". Globally, the median dosis of plasma was two units, which is insufficient to correct a serious coagulation defect, the only accepted indication for plasma transfusion. The conclusion of the study was therefore that plasma was rarely given for the right reasons and even more rarely in adequate dosage. It is hoped that recent consensus conferences and a large distribution of the results of studies like this will succeed in reducing unnecessary plasma transfusions and resulting costs.

Stable solutions of albumin and plasma proteins

Administration of albumin and plasma protein solutions was even more variable. However their use also depended heavily on local availability: countries like Greece or Portugal depending on import of such products almost never reported their use. About half the total amount of albumin was given to the 15% of patients enrolled in Belgium. The financial implications of such practices are obvious and matter of serious consideration.

Artificial colloids

Artificial colloids were available and used in all countries. However, huge variations (usually from 0 to 100% of patients) between hospitals could be documented for most procedures. Surprisingly those hospitals using more plasma also used more albumin and more artificial colloids. It seemed that patients could be managed in a "dry" fashion (i.e. without colloid solutions) in some places and needed much more volume in others, despite similar red cell transfusions, and similar hematocrits at admission and at discharge. Furthermore no pattern could be found in the selection of colloids for any procedure. It all happened as if the specific properties of each solution had no importance: there only were "dextran teams", "gelatin teams", etc. with a large dominance of the market by gelatins, at the time of the study. Median infused volumes were usually low: e.g. 500 ml for HES, 1000 ml for gelatin and 2000 ml for dextrans (Belgian data). However, for dextrans and HES the upper range of doses given in one single day extended well over the maximum doses recommended by the manufacturers. Artificial colloids were thus globally under-utilised but the limits to their use were also largely unknown.

Over the last five years most european countries have tightened their guidelines concerning transfusion practice. Under the combined pressure of AIDS lawsuits, consensus conferences, new guidelines and large studies about transfusion practice a significant decrease in the consumption of blood products has taken place, especially whole blood and plasma. Albumin and SSPP consumptions are decreasing sharply in the places which used them most. It is unclear whether artificial colloids will fill in the gap. New HES solutions are increasing their share of the market, to the expense of gelatins. Most centres report no difference in global morbidity or mortality in association with current changes, but few controlled studies have yet been published.

a)

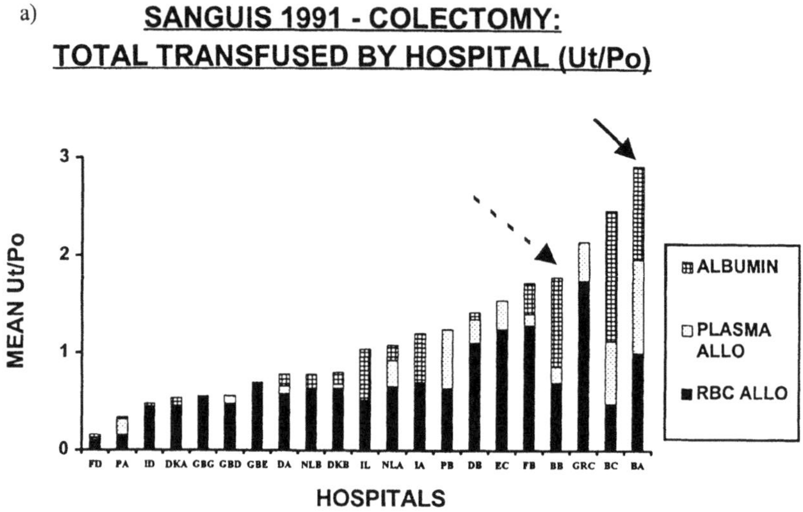

b)

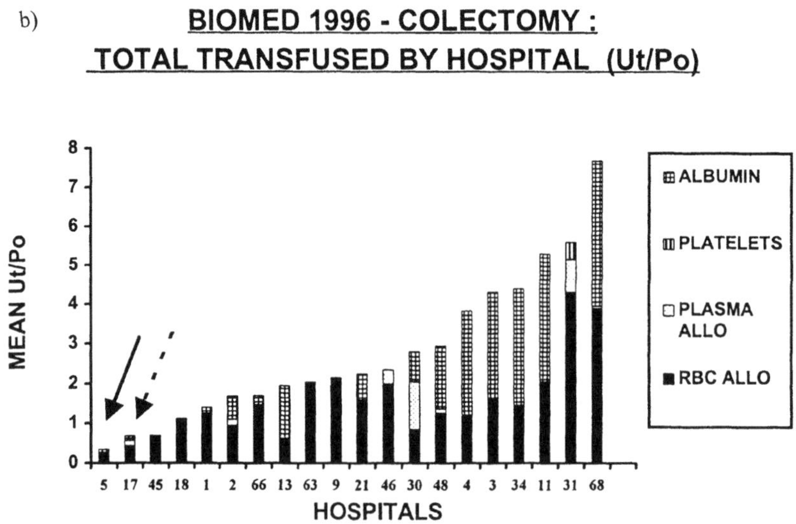

Figure 1. Utilisation of transfusion resources for elective hemicolectomy by participating centres: a) during het SANGUIS study (1991, European teaching hospitals); and b) during the Belgium Biomed Transfusion Study (1996, all types of acute care hospitals). Note the relative places of centre BA (black arrow) and BB (dashed arrow), involved in both studies.

Controlling vascular space rather than its contents

In 1996 a large scale observational study was undertaken in Belgium, using a simplified version of the SANGUIS methodology (Biomed Belgium Transfusion Study: personal communication). Sixty seven general as well as teaching hospitals enrolled more than 3000 surgical patients. In some hospitals the similar methodologies allowed for comparisons between the results obtained by the same teams five years apart. One example will be cited to illustrate how a radical change in resuscitation strategy affected consumption of blood products (Figure l). In 1991 centre BA was at the high end of blood consumption in the SANGUIS study. Its anaesthetic technique was based on neuroleptanalgesia with supplemental inhalational anaesthesia when needed.

In 1996 the same team (same surgeons, same anaesthesiologists) using the same surgical technique was at the lowest extreme of the more recent study. In the meantime the following changes had been made in the standard intraoperative patient management: a peridural catheter was inserted before induction of anaesthesia, a non steroidal anti-inflammatory drug was given before incision (Diclofenac 1 mg/kg), and clonidine was given as a continuous infusion (1 to 2 mcg/kg/hr) after an initial loading dose (4 mcg/kg) infused prior to incision.

Peridural injection of local anaesthetics provokes a sympathic bloc and vasodilatation in the affected metameres. As such this technique provokes systemic hypotension which is classically treated with active vascular filling. Abdominal surgery is often associated with brutal bouts of vasoplegia heralded by facial flushing during surgical manipulations of the mesenteries and abdominal viscerae. The released inflammation mediators are thought to be responsible for the constitution of a so-called "third sector" by massive fluid leakage from the microvasculature to the interstitial tissue. The usual way of dealing with this phenomenon has been further infusion of fluids. The resulting haemodilution will lead to increased red cell transfusions during the haemorrhagic phase of surgery.

Several strategies may be used to prevent and/or counteract this unwelcome chain of events. First, anti-inflammatory drugs have been proven effective to prevent the vasoplegic phenomena induced by surgical manipulation of the viscera [19]. Second, clonidine, an α_2 agonist, has been proven safe and effective in reducing pressure surges during major surgery ("alpine surgery") [20]. It is also an effective splanchnic and cutaneous vasoconstrictor acting mainly on small venous capacitance vessels, thereby reducing volemic needs [21].

The central effect of α_2 agonists results in potentiation of opioids and general anaesthetics such as halogenated vapours [22]. By this action they reduce the intra and postoperative need for these products in a dramatic way and thus their vasodilatory effects.

Finally, if hypotension still occurs without bleeding, e.g. during the installation phase of peridural anaesthesia, it can be counteracted with slow infusion of catecholamines such as norepinephrine or a mixture of epinephrine and norepinephrine (in patients receiving α_2 agonists their doses should be reduced). A slow infusion of vasopressin can also be used for the same purpose.

Postoperative pain control with a peridural infusion of opioids and low concentrations of local anaesthetics (e.g. bupivacaine 0.125%) contributes to the haemodynamic stability, along with the use of an α_2 agonist. Stable vascular conditions prevent secondary bleeding and tissue oedema formation, therefore further reducing the need for vascular filling with either colloids or crystalloid, and transfusion of blood products. Figure 1 also features another hospital (BB) which participated to both studies. Although the specific changes in strategies are not known to the authors of this paper, a similar and dramatic decrease in blood product consumption occurred between 1991 and 1996 in that centre too. These examples illustrate both the impact of benchmarking-type studies and the possibility to address the issue of volume replacement in different ways.

Conclusions

Various products are now available as plasma substitutes. All are reasonably inexpensive and safe in comparison with blood derived products. The latter should therefore be given only when specific indications warrant their use. As stable blood products are still mostly obtained from thousands of pooled donations, they should be handled according to strict haemovigilance rules which include thorough documentation of every step, down to the transfusion itself, to allow for ascending and descending traceability.

The SANGUIS study showed that much progress remains to be made in everyday clinical practice to achieve a cost-effective and safe management of acute blood losses and volume shifts during elective surgery. Later studies performed during abdominal surgery showed that this goal could be achieved by preventing intraoperative vasodilatation, and its associated fluid shifts, using a combination of epidural anaesthesia, IV administration of a non-steroidal inflammatory drug along with the α_2 agonist clonidine. Further research is needed before applying this strategy to other types of surgical procedures. Very small doses of IV vasoconstrictors should be tried before resorting to fluid infusion to control systemic hypotension unaccompanied by blood loss. One should keep in mind that acting on the vessel wall may be as effective as increasing vascular contents to control blood pressure and cardiac output.

References

1. Vincent J.L. Fluids for Resuscitation. Brit J of Anaesthesia 1991;67:185-93.
2. Hiippala ST, Myllylä GJ, Vahtera EM. Hemostatic factors and replacement of major blood loss with plasma-poor cell concentrates. Anesth Analg, 1995;81:360-65.
3. Consensus Conference. Office of medical applications of research. National Institute of Health, Bethesda. Fresh Frozen Plasma: Indications and risks. JAMA 1987; 257,13:1777-80.
4. Stockwell M, Soni N, Riley B. Colloid solutions in the critically ill. A randomised comparison of albumin and polygenine. 1: Outcome and duration of stay in the intensive care unit. Anesthesia 1992;47:3-6.
5. Stockwell M, Scott A, Day A, Riley B, Soni N. Colloid solutions in the critically ill. A randomised comparison of albumin and polygenine. 2: Serum albumin concentration and incidences of pulmonary oedema and acute renal failure. Anaesthesia 1992; 47:7-9.

6. Conference de Consensus 22 et 23 avril 1994. Les perfusions d'albumine humaine et les produits de substitution. Ministère de la Santé Publique et de l'Environnement, Conseil Supérieur d'Hygiène, Commission des Médicaments of Arch. Public Health 1994;52:289-468.
7. Durand-Zaleski I, Bonnet F, Rochant H, Bierling P, Lemaire F. Usefulness of consensus conferences: the case of albumin. Lancet. 1992;2340:1388-90.
8. Nicholls MD, Whyte G. Red cell, plasma and albumin transfusion decision triggers. Anaesth Intens Care 1993;21:156-62.
9. Vermeulen LC Jr, Ratko TA, Erstad BL, Brecher ME, Matuszewcki KA. A paradigm for consensus. The University Hospital Consortium guidelines for the use of albumin, nonprotein colloid, and crystalloid solutions. Arch Intern Med 1995;155:373 –79.
10. Subcommittee of the Victorian Drug Usage Advisory Committee. Human albumin solutions: consensus statements for use in selected clinical situations. Med J Aust 1992;1570:340-43
11. Crystal GJ, Gurevicius J, Kim SJ, Eckel PK, Ismail EF, Salem MR. Effect of hypertonic saline solutions in the coronary circulation. Circ Shock 1994;42:27-38.
12. Favre JB, Ravussin P, Chiolero R, Bissonnette B. Hypertonic solutions and intracranial pressure. Schweiz Med Wochenschr 1996; 126:1635-43.
13. Younes RN, Aun F, Accioly CQ, Casale LP, Szajnbok I, Birolini D. Hypertonic solutions in the treatment of hypovolemic shock: a prospective, randomized study in patients admitted to the emergency room. Surgery 1992;111:380-85.
14. Younes RN, Aun F, Ching CT, et al. Prognostic factors to predict outcome following the administration of hypertonic/hyperoncotic solution in hypovolemic patients. Shock 1997;7:79-83.
15. Boldt J, Knothe C, Zickmann B, Andres P, Dapper F, Hempelmann G. Influence of different intravascular volume therapies on platelet function in patients undergoing cardlopulmonary bypass. Anesth Analg 1993;76:1185-90.
16. Sirchia G, Giovanette, Baele Ph, et al. In: Sirchia G, Giovanetti AM, McClelland DBL, Fracchia GN (eds). Safe and good use of blood in surgery (SANGUIS). European Commission, DG XII Medical Research, Medicine and Health ISBN 92-826-4118-X;1994.
17. The SANGUIS study group. Use of blood products for elective surgery in 43 European hospitals. Transf Med 1994;4:251-68.
18. The Belgium SANGUIS study group: Baele, De Buryère, Deneys et al. Results of the SANGUIS study in Belgium. Special issue of the Acta Chirurgica Belgica 1994; 94(Suppl):5-61.
19. Hudson JC, Wunn H, O'Donnell TF, et al. Ibuprofen pretreatment inhibits prostacyclin release during abdominal exploration in aortic surgery. Anesthesiology 1990;72: 443-49.
20. De Kock M, Versailles H, Colinet B, Karthaeuser R, Scholtes J.L. Epidemiology of the adverse hemodynamic events occuring during "clonidine anesthesia": a prospective open trial of intraoperative intravenous clonidine. J Clin Anesth 1995;7:403-10.
21. Dubols P, De Kock M, Laterre PF. Effects of IV clonidine as an adjunct to anesthesia during orthotopic liver transplantations. Anesthesiology 1997;87(3A):A84.
22. De Kock M. The association of clonidine with an opioid is a major step toward the "ideal opioid" analgesia. Thesis. Université Catholique de Louvain, 1995:p155.

THE MANAGEMENT OF ANAEMIA IN THE SURGICAL PATIENT: WHAT'S NEW?

R.K. Spence

The traditional belief of surgeons that allogeneic blood is an effective and safe therapy with minimal risks has been challenged by a heightened awareness of the problems of transfusion reactions, disease transmission and immunomodulation related to red blood cell transfusion. Surgeons have responded to these challenges by reassessing the reasons for transfusion, increasing the use of autologous blood, modifying surgical techniques to reduce blood loss, and employing various drugs to reduce transfusion need. Current practice policies recommend that elective transfusion of allogeneic blood should be viewed as an outcome to be avoided in surgical patients [1]. Each time we reach this goal, our patients' safety and outcomes will be improved. Of primary importance is the need for the surgeon to change from a casual approach to allogeneic blood transfusion to one characterised by thoughtful planning.

Surgical anaemia

Anaemia may present a problem to the surgeon at any time in the perioperative period. Malnourished, iron-deficient patients may present in need of surgery; anaemia of blood loss may be an unwanted complication of any surgical procedure. If anaemia is discovered during preoperative investigations, the surgeon must decide if the level of anaemia and the risk of blood loss from the planned procedure are of enough merit to warrant action. If they are and if surgery can be postponed, the surgeon can use oral iron to correct the anaemia. Oral iron therapy should also be used in patients undergoing autologous predonation of blood and those receiving erythropoietin [2]. If surgery cannot be delayed or in those with severe, life-threatening levels of anaemia, the use of intravenous iron dextran may be considered an option [3]. Iron dextran may produce anaphylaxis and should be used according to dosage instructions issued by manufacturers [4]. Polysaccharide forms may be better tolerated than dextran preparations.

Recombinant human erythropoietin (Procrit) (Ortho Biotech, Raritan, NJ) has been proven to increase red cell mass in patients with anaemia caused by both renal failure and chronic disease [5,6]. The drug has also shown usefulness in stimulating autologous blood donation and is approved for this use in patients undergoing orthopaedic procedures [7,8]. rHuEPO is useful in the treatment of acute anaemia in Jehovah's Witness patients [9].

Allogeneic blood

If the need to intervene is urgent, the surgeon may need to resort to allogeneic blood transfusion. The incidence of transfusion transmitted diseases from allogeneic blood has been reduced by the use of patient screening and specific antigen tests. Allogeneic blood can be made even safer through the use of leukocyte reduction filters. Leukoreduction filters can limit the number of white blood cells transfused with packed red cells, thereby limiting the potential for febrile reactions, exposure to leukocyte-borne viruses such as CMV, and the consequences of immunosuppression [10, 11].

Allogeneic blood risks

A variety of animal and human studies have demonstrated systemic immunomodulation caused by allogeneic blood transfusion [12-15]. Both cellular and humoral factors seem to play a role. Macrophage function is altered following allogeneic blood transfusion, resulting in decreases in migratory capabilities and both eicosanoid and interleukin-2 production. Lymphocyte responses to both antigen and mitogen are suppressed, suppressor cell activity is increased with concomitant declines in helper:suppressor cell ratios. Both an increased susceptibility to bacterial infection and increased mortality following allogeneic blood transfusion have been reported. Post-surgical infections may be increased by as much as 30% following allogeneic blood transfusion. Patients transfused during surgery for cancer may have a decreased disease free interval and shortened survival. Although these clinical findings are controversial, the surgeon should be aware of the potential risks of transfusion-induced immunosuppression. This potential risk can be eliminated either by avoiding allogeneic blood transfusion or by reduction of leukocytes with leukodepletion filters when allogeneic blood is necessary.

The transfusion decision

The surgeon must pay close attention to the reasons for and results of transfusion. Surgical transfusion practices have evolved rapidly in recent years in response to the recognition of new risks of transfusions, technologic innovation, and changing demands for blood. Practice guidelines for surgical blood management were developed in 1995 by an expert panel of physicians to aid surgeons in their decision making regarding red cell transfusion [1]. These policies are based on the understanding that red cell transfusion should be given only when there is a documented need to increase oxygen delivery in those patients who are unable to meet demands through normal cardiopulmonary mechanisms. The primary function of red blood cells is the transport of oxygen to tissues. Therefore, any red cell transfusion should be physiologic, i.e., to provide the additional oxygen delivery needed to correct or protect against the development of tissue hypoxia [16-18].

New information about the impact of clinical factors on the transfusion decision will allow us to develop transfusion triggers based on patient factors, not just haemoglobin values. The effect of transfusion is influenced by a number of variables including haemoglobin concentration, respiratory status, peripheral organ perfusion, coronary artery disease, beta blocker therapy, base excess, lactate, etc. Well-meaning attempts to improve oxygen delivery by transfusing red blood cells to attain a haemoglobin of 10 gm/dL or greater may be futile if these parameters are overlooked. Our continued efforts to understand the dynamics of oxygen transport in the variety of patients we treat will pave the way for improved transfusion outcomes.

Understanding the physiologic response to anaemia is essential to making rational transfusion decisions. The heart provides the primary response to surgical anaemia by increasing cardiac output through either an increase in heart rate or an increase in stroke volume [18]. Since the heart extracts approximately 80% of the oxygen delivered under normal conditions, its ability to increase output is limited by its ability to increase its oxygen consumption.

Cardiac oxygen extraction is improved by increasing coronary flow. To this the coronary arteries must dilate. In the presence of coronary artery disease, the heart may be unable to provide the work needed to increase total body oxygen delivery without risk to the myocardium. Continued demands on the stressed heart to provide oxygen may come at the expense of conversion to an anaerobic metabolic state and eventual subendocardial infarction.

Surgeons are learning of the dangers of relying on haemoglobin levels alone as a basis for transfusion. Multiple clinical factors that may affect the transfusion decision should be assessed in each patient on a case-by-case basis [17]. This assessment should include a history and physical examination, a review of pertinent laboratory data, consideration of the operation planned and expectant blood loss, and analysis of risk factors that may contribute to increased morbidity and mortality [19].

Patients with known cardiopulmonary disease are at increased risk of perioperative complications if their haemoglobin levels are maintained in the 7-8 gm/dL range. A haemoglobin level that is acceptable for one patient at one specific time may not be appropriate for another. Although a postoperative haemoglobin level of 7-8 gm/dL may be adequate for most healthy, young patients with no risk factors, haemoglobin levels may need to be higher than 7-8 gm/dL in patients with cardiopulmonary disease and other risk factors. Recent information from Carson, et al. demonstrated that the non-transfused Jehovah's Witness patient with cardiopulmonary disease is at increased risk of dying as haemoglobin drops below 10 gm/dL [19]. Emerging information such as this will help make surgeons more aware of the risks of both overtransfusion and undertransfusion if haemoglobin alone is used as a transfusion trigger.

Autologous blood

The use of autologous blood is not a new concept to surgeons. This alternative to allogeneic blood transfusion has been used for several years in orthopaedic and cardiac surgery in the form of predonated autologous blood (PAD) and in urologic procedures in the form of acute normovolemic haemodilution (ANH). Preoperative autologous donation of blood is considered a standard of care for elective orthopaedic procedures and radical prostatectomy [1,20,21].

Recent approval of erythropoietin as an adjunct to predonation should stimulate increased use of these alternatives. An analysis of predonation capabilities in patients scheduled for elective orthopaedic procedures demonstrated that patients at risk for subsequent allogeneic blood transfusion were those who were anaemic at the time of their first autologous blood donation and those who were required to donation four or more units of blood [22]. Low endogenous erythropoietin levels at the time of the initial encounter have also been shown to prevent completion of a planned predonation. [23] To address this problem, Goodnough, et al. treated a group of non-anaemic patients with 600 u/kg of rHuEPO intravenously twice weekly [24]. When compared to placebo-treated control patients, the rHuEPO patients donated 41% more red cell volume. Subsequent clinical trials of non-anaemic patients have shown little benefit with the use of rHuEPO given in doses ranging from 150 u/kg to 600 u/kg to stimulate predonation with aggressive predonation protocols [25].

Biesma, et al. used rHuEPO therapy to reduce overall exposure to allogeneic blood transfusion when predonation was limited to only two units of blood [26].

Subsequent studies of the impact of rHuEPO focused on the anaemic surgical patient, i.e., the patient with a haematocrit in the 39-40% at the time of initial predonation. Mercuriali and European colleagues demonstrated a reduction in allogeneic blood use in orthopaedic patients with the use of preoperative rHuEPO and intravenous iron in a randomized, clinical trial [27]. In a similar United States study, allogeneic blood transfusion was required in 31% of placebo-treated patients compared to 20% of rHuEPO-treated patients [28]. Although this difference did not reach statistical significance, the rHuEPO-treated patients did demonstrate the ability to donate more autologous units (4.5 vs. 3.0; $p<0.001$) and to increase their production of red cells (688 vs. 353 ml over baseline; $p<0.05$). These studies have shown that rHuEPO therapy coupled with iron administration can make autologous predonation a successful option for many anaemic surgical patients who would otherwise need allogeneic blood transfusion.

Successful autologous predonation depends on adequate time for donation, a haemoglobin level greater than 11.0 gm/dl, absence of significant patient disease, i.e., severe aortic stenosis or active angina, selection of appropriate patients and both patient and physician co-operation [29-32]. The ideal patient for PAD is one who has a need for blood transfusion in the perioperative period with a window of two or more weeks before surgery to donate. Freezing of PAD blood may be an option for those patients who need more time.

The majority of patients can successfully complete a predonation programme without incident. An increased incidence of reactions is associated with donor age under 17 years, weight over 110 lbs., female gender and a history of previous reactions. Newer approaches to PAD can help minimise symptoms and make the process applicable to more patients. Phlebotomy is now being performed in select blood centres using apheresis machines. This process reduces the volume loss associated with standard blood donations. As a consequence, patients can donate more packed red cells with less risk of adverse events. These approaches require additional logistics and medical expertise that add to the cost of autologous predonation.

Goodnough and colleagues have championed the use of acute normovolemic haemodilution as an alternative to allogeneic blood transfusion in the patient undergoing radical prostatectomy [33]. Their recent analysis of rHuEPO therapy as an adjunct to acute normovolemic haemodilution has shown that erythropoietin is effective both in preventing exposure to allogeneic blood and in increasing production of red blood cells. [34]. Acute normovolemic haemodilution (ANH) is an alternative to PAD that eliminates many of the objections to the process. Acute normovolemic haemodilution is the process of removing and temporarily storing blood just before or immediately after the induction of anaesthesia and replacing volume losses with either crystalloid or colloid solutions [32]. The removal of one to four units is possible in the patient with a normal haematocrit and results in a post-dilutional haematocrit of 20 to 30% [35]. The advantages of acute normovolemic haemodilution include an improvement in tissue perfusion secondary to decreased viscosity and loss of fewer red cells from bleeding. A major disadvantage of haemodilution is the need for an experienced anaesthesiologist or perfusionist. Haemodilution can be performed safely in most patients, with the only contraindications being anaemia, which limits the amount of blood that can be removed, and cardiac disease. Because of its advantages over PAD, ANH is being used more and more often in patients at risk of surgical blood loss.

Autologous blood may also be obtained through the collection and reinfusion of blood shed in the perioperative period, that is, autotransfusion [36]. Intraoperative autotransfusion can be performed with systems that either collect blood directly, anticoagulate it and reinfuse it through filters or systems that collect the blood, wash it and reinfuse a packed red cell product [37]. Systems without washing capability collect shed blood via a suction wand or wound drainage catheter. Heparin or citrate-phosphate-dextrose anticoagulant must be added to the collection chamber. The collected blood is returned to the patient through a filter, relying on this as the only means of preparing the blood. Filters are capable of removing large debris, e.g., bone chips in orthopaedic cases and smaller particulate matter up 260 microns, e.g., cellular fragments. Following filtration, the salvaged blood represents "red cells suspended in plasma", containing platelets, fibrinogen and clotting factors. Unwashed blood may contain vasoactive contaminants, activated clotting factors, fibrin degradation products and free haemoglobin, all of which can be dangerous. Unwashed blood appears to be safe if transfusion is limited to small quantities and to appropriate circumstances.

Systems that wash blood and concentrate the red cells have the advantage of providing a cleaner product, free of the contaminants found in unwashed blood. With these devices, blood is collected from the operative field, filtered, anticoagulated, temporarily stored in a reservoir, and then washed for return. The advantage of portability previously found only with systems that did not wash blood has been added to washer devices. The machines used are mounted on wheels, allowing easy movement from the operating room to the recovery room or ICU. Smaller washing bowls permit collection of volumes as small as 100 ml. Collection chambers have been modified to portable, smaller sizes using a "collect first" philosophy.

Surgical technique

Surgeons are relearning Halstedian principles of gentle tissue handling, anatomic dissection and minimisation of blood loss in all operations. The surgeon should enter the operating room with the goal of preventing as much blood loss as possible by maintaining careful surgical homeostasis [1]. Transfusion need in surgery is clearly tied to blood loss; it follows that reduction of operative blood loss should minimise the need for transfusion. Any blood not shed is blood that does not have to be replaced.

Technical factors and operative approach have a critical effect on blood loss in most procedures. Surgical approaches, e.g., vascular isolation and temporary occlusion, may be modified to reduce operative blood loss in liver resection [38]. New methods of localising and dissecting hepatic tissues using a water jet dissector and microwave tissue coagulation have shown success in decreasing blood loss [39-41]. Joint repair and replacement procedures frequently lead to transfusion. Arthroscopic repair, when feasible, results in significantly less blood loss [42]. Modifications of total knee arthroplasty to close the surgically-created defect reduces perioperative blood loss [43]. Simple measures may have a dramatic impact on blood loss. Levy and Marmar found the use of cold compression following total knee arthroplasty significantly reduced blood loss when compared to a control group of patients. Total blood loss with compression was 1298 ml compared to 1908 ml in the control group, a difference of 610 mls [44].

Major vascular operations are associated with both large-scale and rapid haemorrhage. Bleeding from oesophageal varices can be particularly lethal. The use of transjugular intrahepatic portosystemic shunt (TIPS) in the treatment of variceal haemorrhage has been reviewed recently by McCormick, et al. [45]. The authors note that the shunt can be inserted successfully in 90% of patients and that TIPS can reduce blood transfusion requirements in bleeding patients. The mortality, from variceal bleeding remains high in spite of aggressive medical and interventional therapy. Orloff's extensive experience in treating patients with variceal bleeding points out that success may be obtained not just by modifying operative technique but by moving quickly to the operating room to prevent further haemorrhage [46].

The nineties saw the introduction of intraluminal stents and grafts in the treatment of large vessel disease, especially the abdominal aortic aneurysm. Two groups have reported their early clinical experience with the use of endoluminal techniques to place grafts and stent-graft devices, showing that major abdominal aortic surgical repair can be accomplished while reducing blood loss [47,48]. These techniques, although in their infancy and in need of further clinical trials, hold great promise for decreasing the need for blood transfusion in vascular surgery.

The success of laparoscopic cholecystectomy has encouraged surgeons to develop similar, alternative approaches to many operations that previously required incision into the chest or abdomen. In many cases, laparoscopic techniques are easier on patients by producing smaller incisions, more rapid recovery and shorter hospital stays. Laparoscopic techniques in surgery do much to minimise the need for transfusion. The improved visualisation of the operative field, coupled with the knowledge that extra care must be taken in dissection through a minimal-access port, has lead to a reduction in blood loss from laparoscopic procedures when compared to open techniques.

Senagore, et al. compared 140 elective cooling resections for both benign and malignant disease, with 102 patients undergoing open procedures and 38 laparoscopic [49]. Blood loss was significantly less with the laparoscopic approach, 157±19 ml compared to 687±54 ml for the open cases. Adrenalectomy has been performed through the laparoscope with varying results. Go, et al. report a reduction in mean blood loss with laparoscopic adrenalectomy performed in 7 patients [50]. Blood loss was between 40 to 500 ml (mean 217.2 ml) –less than one unit of blood. Suzuki, et al. have described results with 12 patients who underwent laparoscopic adrenalectomy [51]. Three of these patients had massive bleeding because of technical problems. Vietz, et al. describe a minimally-invasive technique of hysterectomy – pelviscopic intrafascial hysterectomy – that leaves the vascularised extrafascial tissue around the cervix intact and minimises blood loss [52]. Average haemoglobin drop in their group of 60 patients was 1.8 gm/dL. Arbogast, et al. have reported on the use of laparoscopic-assisted hysterectomy as an alternative to open techniques [53].

Electrocautery has been used successfully for many years to control intraoperative small vessel bleeding. It is particularly effective in well-vascularised regions such as the head and neck. Tan, et al. studied over 500 cases of primary tonsillectomy and adenoidectomy and found that the use of scalpel dissection was associated with more intraoperative bleeding and a greater risk of postoperative haemorrhage than the use of cautery [54]. The use of the laser may either reduce or increase bleeding depending on the disease being treated and the operation being performed. Wyman and Rogers performed a prospective, randomized trial in forty women undergoing modified radical mastectomy using a neodymium yttrium-aluminium-garnet laser scalpel compared to a conventional scalpel [55]. Operative blood loss was significantly less with the laser (149 vs. 421 ml) but the mean operating time was approximately 25 minutes longer, leading the authors to question the use of the laser scalpel. Tchabo, et al. compared 422 patients equally divided into two groups who underwent cervical conisation, 217 with laser and 205 with the cold knife [56]. Use of the cold knife was associated with less intraoperative blood loss. Bhatta, et al. conducted a study of various cutting techniques used to perform ovarian wedge resections in rabbits [57]. Scalpel, electrocautery, continuous and pulsed CO_2 and YAG lasers were employed. Electrocautery, CO_2 laser, continuous Nd:YAG laser, and pulsed Ho:YAG laser produced minimal or no bleeding whereas both scalpel and pulsed Er:YAG laser lead to bleeding that required homeostatic measures.

Pharmacologic agents

The choice of anaesthetic agent and technique may have an effect on surgical blood loss. Blackwell, et al. studied the effect on blood loss of general anaesthesia with isoflurane inhalation in 13 patients versus monitored sedation with a continuous intravenous infusion of propofol in 12 similar patients undergoing endoscopic sinus surgery [58]. Blood loss in the isoflurane group was 251 ml compared to a 101 ml loss in the propofol group ($p<.01$).

Locally-acting agents that encourage clotting, e.g., fibrin glue, collagen, topical thrombin, may be helpful in maintaining homeostasis [59]. Antifibrinolytic drugs, such as aprotinin, EACA, DDAVP, and tranexamic acid may be helpful in reducing blood loss, especially during cardiac surgery [60].

Perioperative rHuEPO has been used in both anaemic and nonaenemic patients either in anticipation of or following surgical blood loss. Early experience with erythropoietin in Jehovah's Witness patients demonstrated its superiority to haematinics alone in restoring red cell mass following haemorrhage. Atabek, et al. reported results of erythropoietin therapy using either 150 U/kg or 300 U/kg three times a week in conjunction with intravenous iron replacement in Jehovah's Witnesses with post-surgical, severe anaemia (Hct <25%) [9]. Results in twenty patients treated with this combination were compared to a similar group of twenty patients who received only intravenous iron. Haematocrit after one week was significantly higher in the rHuEPO-treated group – 19.3% vs. 12.5%. Haematocrit continued to rise during the second week of therapy. Other authors have reported success with erythropoietin in the severely anaemic Jehovah's Witness [61,62].

Severe anaemia need not be the only reason for using erythropoietin in the perioperative setting. Ravikumar, et al. recently reported the effectiveness of preoperative erythropoietin as a primary alternative to allogeneic blood transfusion in patients scheduled for cancer surgery with normal hematocrits and low to moderate expected blood loss [63]. Twelve patients received 600 IU/kg of subcutaneous erythropoietin per week starting three weeks before surgery along with oral iron. All showed increases in haematocrit from a baseline of 30-43%, typically 8-10%. Following surgery, hematocrits returned to baseline. All patients avoided allogeneic blood transfusion. Although this study contains only a small number of patients and is anecdotal, it demonstrates a future, significant role for perisurgical erythropoietin use as a means of providing for expected surgical blood loss. The increase in red cell mass provided by erythropoietin was essentially equivalent to that lost in the operating room. By making more red blood cells before surgery, the patients were able to tolerate anticipated losses without being exposed to the risks of allogeneic blood.

Three separate studies of preoperative erythropoietin therapy, two in orthopaedic surgery and one in cardiac, have demonstrated the usefulness of rHuEPO in the avoidance of allogeneic blood. Fourteen daily, subcutaneous doses of 300 IU/kg rHuEPO started ten days before surgery were compared to a similar regimen using placebo (N = 77 rHuEPO and N = 78 placebo) in patients scheduled for elective primary or revision hip arthroplasty in a multicentre Canadian trial

[64]. Only 24% of rHuEPO-treated patients received allogeneic blood compared to 42% in the placebo-treated group. Faris, et al. reported similar results for a multicentre, United States trial of 200 patients undergoing elective joint replacement [65]. The study protocol was the same as the Canadian study except that rHuEPO was given for 15 days rather than 14. 54% of 67 placebo-treated patients were transfused with allogeneic blood compared to only 17% of 54 rHuEPO-treated patients. A third study of patients undergoing coronary artery bypass reported similar results with a variable dose of either 150 IU/kg or 300 IU/kg rHuEPO given over 8 days before surgery [66]. These three studies clearly demonstrate the utility of erythropoietin as a stand-alone alternative to allogeneic blood transfusion in patients at risk of significant surgical blood loss.

Perioperative use of erythropoietin requires attention to detail in terms of iron replacement and dosage. Erythropoietin rapidly depletes iron stores and will have little effect if used without adequate iron therapy. This is especially true in the patient who has suffered recent blood loss and has depleted iron stores [67]. The timing of erythropoietin dosing has an effect on erythropoiesis as well. Breymann and colleagues recently reported that intravenous erythropoietin was more effective in increasing haematocrit in healthy volunteers when administered at 72-hour intervals rather than within 24 hours [68].

This brief review was focussed on recent changes and emerging trends in surgery directed at preventing or controlling operative blood loss, thereby reducing the need for transfusion. Surgeons are responding to the need to reassess the transfusion trigger, increase the use of autologous blood, modify surgical techniques to reduce blood loss, and employ various drugs to reduce transfusion need.

Some patients, such as the Jehovah's Witness, may refuse allogeneic blood. The challenges of operating on these patients when they are anaemic are significant, but success can be attained. Bloodless medicine and surgery have come out of obscurity over the last five years to become a driving force in the practice of medicine today. Continued growth of bloodless surgery centres provides appropriate care for those patients who refuse blood transfusion. The majority of surgeons have incorporated into their practices some of the alternatives developed to avoid the risks of the use of allogeneic blood. Surgeons continue to revise operative procedures and revisit old drugs to reduce operative blood loss. Laparoscopic surgery avoids blood loss in many operations. Attention to detail and careful planning of the surgical procedure helps prevent blood loss, thereby reducing the need for transfusion.

Industry also has responded to our needs by developing new alternatives. The arrival of erythropoietin signals a paradigm shift in our thinking about blood banking. We can now use the patient as his/her blood bank, rather than relying on an external supplier of red blood cells. Erythropoietin coupled with iron replacement promotes replenishment of the red cell mass both before surgery as an adjunct to autologous blood use or after surgery to replace lost blood. Familiar drugs such as vasopressin and the antifibrinolytics have found new life in preventing blood loss. Fibrin sealants derived from human-only products are in clinical trials, as are both perfluorocarbons and haemoglobin-based oxygen carriers, i.e., blood substitutes. Recombinant technology coupled with gene manipulation will produce more human-like products in the near future.

References

1. Spence RK for the Blood Management Practice Guidelines Conference, Surgical Red Blood Cell Transfusion Practice Policies, Am J Surg 1995;170:6A(Suppl):3S-12S.
2. Van Wyck DB. Iron management during recombinant human erythropoietin therapy. Am J Kidney Dis 1989;14(2 Suppl l):9-13.
3. Tasaki T, Ohto H, Noguchi M, et al. Iron and erythropoietin measurement in autologous blood donors with anemia: implications for management. Transfusion 1994;34: 337-43.
4. Ashby EC. Total dose iron-dextran infusions in general surgery. Lancet 1967;2:807-9.
5. Nissenson AR. Erythropoietin treatment in peritoneal dialysis patients. Perit Dial Int 1994;14(Suppl 3):S63-9.
6. Spivak JL. Recombinant human erythropoietin and the anemia of cancer [editorial]. Blood 1994;84:997-1004.
7. Goodnough LT, Price TH, Friedman KD, et al. A phase III trial of recombinant human erythropoietin therapy in nonanemic orthopedic patients subjected to aggressive removal of blood for autologous use: dose, response, toxicity, and efficacy. Transfusion 1994;34:66-71.
8. Beris P, Mermillod B, Levy G, et al. Recombinant human erythropoietin as adjuvant treatment for autologous blood donation. A prospective study. Vox Sang 1993;65: 212-18.
9. Atabek U, Alvarez R, Pello MJ, et al. Erythropoietin Accelerates Heamtocrit Recovery in Post-Surgical Anemia. Amer Surg 1994;61:74-77.
10. Popovsky MA. Quality of blood components filtered before storage and at the beside: implications for transfusion practice. Transfusion 1996;36:470-74.
11. Higgins VL. Leukocyte-reduced blood components: patient benefits and practical applications. Oncol Nurs Forum 1996;23:659-67.
12. Bradley J. The blood transfusion effect: experimental aspects. Immunology Letters. 1991;29:127-32.
13. Klein HG. Immunologic aspects of blood transfusion. Semin Oncol 1994;21 (Suppl 3):16-20.
14. Triulzi D, Blumberg N, Heal J. Association of transfusion with postoperative bacterial infection. Crit Rev Clin Lab Sci 1990;28:95-107.
15. Blumberg N, Heal J. Transfusion-induced immunomodulation and its possible role in cancer recurrence and perioperative bacterial infection. Yale J Biol Med 1990;63: 429-33.
16. Practice strategies for elective red blood cell transfusion. Ann Int Med 1992;116: 403-6.
17. Perioperative red cell transfusion. NIH Consensus Development Conference Statement. Bethesda, MD: NIH, 1988:1-17.
18. Gerson Greenberg A. A physiologic basis for red blood cell transfusion decisions. Am J Surg 1995;170(6A Suppl):44S-48S.
19. Carson, JL. Morbidity risk assessment in the surgically anemic patient. Am J Surg 1995;170:6A (Suppl):32S-36S.
20. Goodnough LT, Grishaber JE, Birkmeyer JD, et al. Efficacy and cost-effectiveness of autologous blood predeposit in patients undergoing radical prostatectomy procedures. Urology 1994;44:226-31.

21. Sculco TP. Blood management in orthopedic surgery. Am J Surg 1995;170:(6A Suppl):60S-63S
22. Goodnough LT, Vizmeg A, Robecks R, et al. Prevalence and classification of anemia in elective orthopedic surgery patients: implications for blood conservation program. Vox Sang 1992;63:90-95.
23. Goodnough LT, Brittenham G. Limitations of the erythropoietic response to serial phlebotomy: implications for autologous blood donor programs. J Lab Clin Med 1990;115:28-35
24. Goodnough LT, Rudick S, Price TH, et al. Increased collection of autologous blood preoperatively with recombinant human erythropoietin therapy. N Engl J Med 1989;321:1163-67.
25. Beris P, Mermillod B, Levy G, et al. Recombinant human erythropoietin as an adjuvant treatment for autologous blood donation. Vox Sang 1993;65:2124-18.
26. Biesma DH, Marx JJ, Kraaijenhagen RJ, et al. Lower homologous blood requirement in autologous blood donors after treatment with recombinant human erythropoietin. Lancet 1994;344:367-70.
27. Mercuriali F, Zanella A, Barosi G, et al. Use of erythropoietin to increasae the volume of autologous blood donated by orthopedic patients. Transfusion 1993;33:55-59.
28. Price TH, Goodnough LT, Vogler WR, et al. Improving the efficacy of autologous blood donation with low hematocrit: a randomized, double-blind, controlled trial of recombinant human erythropoietin. Am J Med 1996;101(Suppl 2A):22S-27S.
29. Healy JC, Frankforter SA, Graves BK, Reddy RL, Beck JR. Preoperative autologous blood donation in total-hip arthroplasty. A cost-effectiveness analysis. Arch Pathol Lab Med 1994;118:465-70.
30. Britton L, Eastlund D, Dziuban S, et al. Predonated autologous blood use in elective cardiac surgery. Ann Thorac Surg 1989;47:529-32.
31. Spiess BD. Pro: autologous blood should be available for elective cardiac surgery. J Cardiothorac Vasc Anesth 1994;84:231-37
32. D'Ambra MN, Kaplan DK. Alternatives to allogeneic blood use in surgery: acute normovolemic hemodilution and preoperative autologous donation. Am J Surg 1995; 170:6A (Suppl):49S-52S.
33. Monk TG, Goodnough LT, Birkmeyer JD, et al. Acute normovolemic hemodilution is a cost-effective alternative to preoperative autologous donation in patients undergoing radical retropubic prostatectomy. Transfusion 1995;35:559-65.
34. Monk TG, Goodnough LT, Andriole GL, et al. Preoperative recombinant human erythropoietin therapy enhances ther efficacy of acute normovolemic hemodilution. Anesth Analg 1995;80:S230.
35. Stehling L, Zauder HL. Acute normovolemic hemodilution. Transfusion 1991;31: 857-68.
36. Williamson KR, Taswell HF. Intraoperative blood salvage: a review. Transfusion 1991;31:662-75.
37. Giordano GF, Giordano DM, Wallace BA, et al: An analysis of 9918 consecutive perioperative autotransfusions. Surg Gyn Obst 1993;176:103-10.
38. Makuuchi M, Kosuge T, Takayama T, et al. Surgery for small liver cancers. Semin Surg Oncol 1993;9:298-304.
39. Baer HU, Stain SC, Guastella T, Maddern GJ, Blumgart LH. Hepatic resection using a water jet dissector. HPB Surg 1993;60:189-96; discussion 196-8.
40. Wu CC, Yang MD, Liu TJ. Improvements in hepatocellular carcinoma resection by intraoperative ultrasonography and intermittent hepatic inflow blood occlusion. Jpn J Clin Oncol 1992;22:107-12.
41. Zhou XD, Tang ZY, Yu YQ, et al. Microwave surgery in the treatment of hepatocellular carcinoma. Semin Surg Oncol 1993;9:318-22.

42. Green MR, Christensen KP. Arthroscopic versus open Bankart procedures: a comparison of early morbidity and complications. Arthroscopy 1993;9:371-74.
43. Raut VV, Stone MH, Wroblewski BM. Reduction of postoperative blood loss after press-fit condylar knee arthroplasty with use of a femoral intramedullary plug. J Bone Joint Surg Am 1993;75:1356-57.
44. Levy AS, Marmar E. The role of cold compression dressings in the postoperative treatment of total knee arthroplasty. Clin Orthop 1993;297:174-78.
45. McCormick PA, Dick R, Burroughs AK. Review article: the transjugular intrahepatic portosystemic shunt (TIPS) in the treatment of portal hypertension. Aliment Pharmacol Ther 1994;80:273-82.
46. Orloff MJ, Bell RH Jr., Orloff MS, Hardison WG, Greenburg AG. Prospective randomized trial of emergency portacaval shunt and emergency medical therapy in unselected cirrhotic patients with bleeding varices [see comments]. Hepatology 1994; 20:863-72.
47. Parodi JC, Criado FJ, Barone HD, Schonholz C, Queral LA. Endoluminal aortic aneurysm repair using a balloon-expandable stent-graft device: a progress report. Ann Vasc Surg 1994;8:523-29.
48. Yusuf S, Baker D, Chuter T, Whitaker S, Wenham P, Hopkinson B. Transfemoral endoluminal repair of abdominal aortic aneurysm with bifurcated graft. Lancet 1994;344:650-51.
49. Senagore AJ, Luchtefeld MA, Mackeigan JM, Mazier WP. Open colectomy versus laparoscopic colectomy: are there differences? Am Surg 1993;59:549-53; discussion 553-54.
50. Go H, Takeda M, Takahashi H, et al. Laparoscopic adrenalectomy for primary aldosteronism: a new operative method. J Laparoendosc Surg 1993;30:455-59.
51. Suzuki K, Kageyama S, Ueda D, et al. Laparoscopic adrenalectomy: clinical experience with 12 cases [see comments]. J Urol 1993;150:1099-102.
52. Vietz PF, Ahn TS. A new approach to hysterectomy without colpotomy: pelviscopic intrafascial hysterectomy. Am J Obstet Gynecol 1994;170:609-13.
53. Arbogast JD, Welch RA, Riza ED, Ricaurte EL, Pieper DR. Laparoscopically assisted vaginal hysterectomy appears to be an alternative to total abdominal hysterectomy. J Laparoendosc Surg 1994;4:185-90.
54. Tan AK, Rothstein J, Tewfik TL. Ambulatory tonsillectomy and adenoidectomy: complications and associated factors. J Otolaryngol 1993;22:442-46.
55. Wyman A, Rogers K. Randomized trial of laser scalpel for modified radical mastectomy [see commentsj. Br J Surg 1993;80:871-73.
56. Tchabo JG, Thomure MF, Tomai TP. A comparison of laser and cold knife conization. Int Surg 1993;78:131-32.
57. Bhatta N, Isaacson K, Flotte T, Schiff I, Anderson RR. Injury and adhesion formation following ovarian wedge resection with different thermal surgical modalities. Lasers Surg Med 1993;13A:344-52.
58. Blackwell KE, Ross DA, Kapur P, Calcaterra TC. Propofol for maintenance of general anesthesia: a technique to limit blood loss during endoscopic sinus surgery. Am J Otolaryngol 1993;14:262-66.
59. Kram H, Nathan R, Stafford F, et al. Fibrin glue achieves hemostasis in patients with coagulation disorders. Arch Surg 1989;124:384-88.
60. Fremes S, Wong B, Lee E, et al. Metaanalysis of prophylactic drug treatment in the prevention of postoperative bleeding. Ann Thorac Surg 1994;58:1580-88.
61. Rupp RE, Ebraheim NA, Saddemi SR, et al. Management of a multiply injured Jehovah's Witness with severe acute anemia. Orthop Rev 1993;22:847-50.
62. Ford PA, Henry DH. Using r-HuEPO in patients unwilling to accept blood transfusions. Erythropoiesis. 1996;7:63-66.

63. Ravikumar TS, Mani S, Zamek R, et al. Preoperative erythropoietin (Procrit) in abdominal cancer surgery [abstract no. 74]. In: Perry MC (ed). Proceedings of the 32 nd Annual Meeting of the American Society of Clinical Oncology, 1996 May 18-2l; Philadelphia. Toronto: WB Saunders, 1996:276.
64. Canadian orthopedic perioperative erythropoietin study group. Effectiveness of perioperative recombinant human erythropoietin in elective hip replacement. Lancet 1993;34:1227-32.
65. Faris P. Use of recombinant human erythropoietin in the perioperative period of orthopedic surgery. Am J Med Suppl 1996;101:28-32.
66. D'Ambra MN, Lunch KE, Bocaggno J, et al. Effect of perioperative administration of recombinant human erythropoietin in CABG patients. Anesthesiology (Abstract) 1992;77:Al59.
67. Goldberg MA. Erythropoiesis, erythropoietin, and iron metabolism in elective surgery: preoperative strategies for avoiding allogeneic blood exposure. Amer J Surg. 1995;170(Suppl):37S-43S.
68. Breymann C, Bauer C, Major A, et al. Optimal timing of repeat rh-erythropoietin administration improves its effectiveness in stimulating erythropoiesis in healthy volunteers. Brit J Haematol 1996;92:295-301.

HOW TO SAVE BLOOD: ALTERNATIVE APPROACHES IN ANAESTHESIOLOGY AND SURGERY

A.W.M.M. Koopman-van Gemert

Introduction

Surgical patients often require peri-operative blood transfusions. In total in the Netherlands yearly about 1 million of cellular products are transfused. Transfusion of blood products may induce side effects, which may be toxic, infectious or immunological. The latter effects include antibody formation or a modulation of the immune response. Clinical studies showed an improved survival of transplantated organs after allogeneic blood transfusions. Immune suppression inducing Human Leukocyte Antigen (HLA)-antibodies are probably the underlying mechanism. It has been thought that prevention of the formation of HLA-antibodies may improve survival after cancer surgery. However prospective studies, comparing for instance the effect of transfusion of autologous or leukocyte filtered blood with that of normal allogeneic blood transfusions, showed no difference in survival or metastatic complications [1,2,3]. These studies have been done for colon tumours, which are weak immunogenic. At this moment the influence of different transfusion therapies on immunogenic tumours such as kidney tumours or haematological malignancies has not been investigated yet.

On the other hand it has been shown in some studies that after allogeneic blood transfusions the incidence of postoperative infections is higher than after autologous or leukocyte depleted blood transfusions [4]. Other studies however didn't confirm these results [4]. Probably more studies must be done to resolve this problem.

Interestingly the safety of blood transfusions is always considered as an important point. Since it became clear that Human Immunodeficiency Virus (HIV) can be transmitted through blood transfusions the rules to prevent blood transfusion related infections became more severe. In comparison with the risks for transmission of infectious diseases, the effects of blood transfusion on the immune system are less investigated and less regulated. The reason for this attitude is not clear. Although everybody agrees with the statement that a blood transfusion is a transplantation, the precautions taken for a tissue transplantation are not the same as for a blood transfusion.

The advocation of techniques to prevent a blood transfusion could be an important measurement.

Surgical and anaesthesiological blood saving techniques

The methods we are talking about include several surgical, anaesthesiological and specific transfusion techniques (Table 1) reducing patient's exposure to allogeneic blood transfusions [5]. Surgical techniques proved to be efficient are positioning of the patient, use of tourniquets, infiltration of the wound with local vasoconstrictors, direct control of bleeding and the use of electrosurgery. Posture influences intra-operative bleeding both by reducing the arterial blood pressure if the operation side is above the level of the heart (less bleeding) and by pooling of the blood in the venous vascular beds if the venous return is prevented for instance by compression of the caval vein (more bleeding).

Table 1. Methods to prevent donor blood transfusions

Surgical techniques
– Positioning
– Tourniquets
– Control of bleeding
– Electrosurgery
– Local vasoconstrictors
Anaesthesiological techniques
– Epidural or spinal anaesthesia
– Local anaesthesia
– Controlled hypotension
– Normothermia
Transfusion techniques
– Artificial plasma components
– Normo- and hypervolemic haemodilution
– Pre-operative autologous donation
– Cell saver techniques
– Artificial oxygen carriers
– Minimal peri-operative HCT

Several anaesthesiological techniques can be used to influence intra-operative bleeding. Spinal and epidural anaesthesia cause a pharmacological sympatectomy giving an arteriolar dilatation as well as a reduction of the venous tone. If the block extends to T1-4 the reflex tachycardia is prevented as well. These methods of anaesthesia effectively minimise peri-operative blood loss.

The same is true for controlled hypotension by means of volatile anaesthetics or short acting vasodilators such as sodium nitroprusside.

A different approach to reduce peri-operative blood loss is archived by optimalization of the coagulation system and reduction of the fibrinolysis. Keeping the patient warm is very important for an optimal function of the cooperation cascade. Medications such as aprotinin, tranexamin and epsilon aminocapronic acid (EACA) influence platelet and fibrinolytic function [6]. Our meta-analyses showed that aprotinin significantly reduces the use of allogeneic blood transfusions in cardiac surgery [7]. Tranexamin and epsilon aminocapronic acid also showed to be effective, but too few patients have been studied to definitively determine the benefit of these medications at this moment.

Stimulation the red blood cell production is another approach of blood saving techniques. Administration of erythropoietin caused a significant increase in red blood cells and as a consequence a significant reduction of the use of allogeneic blood transfusions as well [8-11]. This method also increases the number of preoperatively donated units of blood. There is no experience with the use of thromboplastin for this purpose.

During the operation the anaesthesiologist has to make a transfusion plan [12]. First of all he has to consider the minimum haematocrit (HCT) he will accept for this patient [13] and if he plans to give blood there are several alternative blood transfusion methods, such as artificial plasma products, normo- and hypervolemic haemodilution, preoperative autologous blood donation (PAD) and cell salvage techniques he can use [14-21].

Our ISPOT meta-analyses showed PAD to be an efficient method [22].

Haemodilution however, a method to deliberately decrease patient's HCT, has been shown to be less effective [23]. Our meta-analyses showed a too wide variation in results to be reliable. Normovolemic haemodilution is performed by withdrawing patient's blood and simultaneously replacing the collected blood by artificial plasma products. Hypervolemic haemodilution is done by infusion of fluid to overload.

Intra- and postoperative cell salvage however is more efficient [16,17,21]. The blood shed peri-operatively is aspirated and meanwhile anticoagulated, and then automatically centrifuged and washed in a cell saver. Only the red cell suspension is reinfused. This method can also be used for salvage of drain blood. Unwashed cell salvage techniques are also used for the salvage of drain blood.

Momentarily some machines offer a combination of techniques and make it possible to obtain platelet rich plasma and red blood cells pre-operatively (normovolemic haemodilution) and to perform cell salvage peri-operatively with the same machine. It has been shown that such an application of a combination of techniques is much more efficient.

A method still in clinical trial is the infusion of artificial blood products such as haemoglobin solutions or fluorocarbons. Maybe in the future these products will offer us the opportunity temporarily to allow a deeper fall in HCT without endangering patient's oxygen transport.

Discussion

Application of these alternative approaches to minimise the use of allogeneic blood is important. Internationally many differences exist in practice variation. Also in the field of blood bankers not all alternative techniques to minimise the need for donor blood are stimulated. Especially there is reluctance to predonation. The arguments include logistical, economical and emotional reasons, because of an increase of workload and fear for reduction of donor's motivation for voluntary blood donation. It should be clear however that such an attitude can be discussed because stimulation of blood saving techniques in fact shows respect for the blood donor, since his blood is used efficiently and only when really needed.

On the other hand it becomes more and more evident that it is not only the application of these techniques, but also the physician's attitude in transfusion therapy, that is important. The physician decides what to do.

Table 2. ASA classification

Class 1	Mild to moderate disease
Class 2	Systemic disease, limiting activity, but not incapacitating
Class 3	Severe incapacitating systemic disease: constant threat to life
Class 4	Moribund, not to expect to survive 24 hours without surgery
Class 5	Normal healthy patient with a localised process

Table 3. Transfusion concept

- Define expected blood loss
- Define type of surgery
- ASA class
- HCT
- Techniques possible:
  - evidence based
  - expected salvage of donor blood
- Available techniques in your hospital
- Acceptable costs
- Wish patient

Table 4. Example of a transfusion algorithm

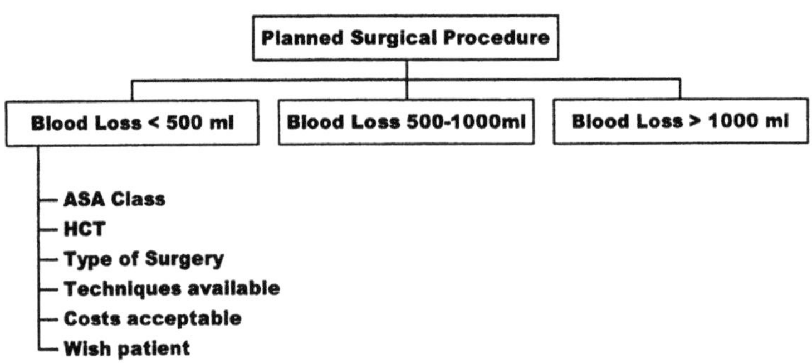

To stimulate the use of alternative methods and to optimise the rational use of allogeneic blood (in my view) one should develop a transfusion algorithm in each hospital. Before starting to make an algorithm it should be defined which techniques the hospital can offer the patient, at what expenses and for what type of surgery [21, 25-29]. These decisions should be evidence based on results of meta-analyses or scientific studies. Furthermore there must be consensus in the hospital about the minimal accepted HCT above which a blood transfusion is not necessary. Thereafter the anaesthesiologist can make a risk analysis (Tables 2, 3 and 4) for the individual patient and plan a transfusion strategy, depending on the procedure planned, on the expected blood loss, on Physical Status Classification of the American Society of Anesthesiology (ASA class) of the patient, on the pre-operative measured HCT and the wish of the patient [30,31]. Perioperative measurements of the HCT or the haemoglobin level and of coagulation values, can be helpful as guiding parameters. Integrated in a total concept of patient therapy this will make physicians more alert of the possibilities available to reduce patient's risks and to improve the quality of health care. Of course the costs of these techniques differ internationally. Therefore each hospital has to balance the transfusion related risks of the patient in his country against the health care budget available [21, 25-29]. Reduction in hospitalisation time and reduction of complications or medications are important factors to take into account as well [21].

The goal of our patient treatment should be trying to offer the best clinical treatment with the least number of complications, at an acceptable price and an acceptable risk. Meanwhile more studies must be performed to evaluate the importance and the efficiency of the different methods of blood transfusion therapy and their influence on patient's immune system and final outcome [4].

References

1. Wheatley T, Veitch PS. Editorial. Effect of blood transfusion on postoperative immunocompetence. Brit. J Anaesth 1997;78:489-92.
2. Vamvakas EC, Moore SB. Effect of autologous transfusion on length of survival. Vox Sang 1995;69:147-48.
3. Williamson I. Annotation. Homologous blood transfusion: the risks and alternatives. Brit J Haem 1994;88:451-58.
4. Blajchman MA. Allogeneic blood transfusion, immunomodulation, and postoperative bacterial infection: Do we have the answer yet? Transfusion 1997;37:121-25.
5. Simpson P. Perioperative blood loss and its reduction: the role of the anaesthetist. Review article. Brit J Anaesth 1992;69:498-507.
6. Verstraete M. Clinical application of inhibitors of fibrinolysis. Austral Drug Inform Serv 1985;29:236-61.
7. Laupacis A, Fergusson D, for the International Study of Peri-operative Transfusion (ISPOT) investigators. Drugs to minimize peri-operative blood loss in cardiac surgery. Mata-analyses using peri-operative blood transfusion as the outcome. Anesth Analg 1997;85:1258-67.
8. Laupacis A, Fergusson D, for the International Study of Peri-operative Transfusion (ISPOT). Erythropoietin to minimize peri-operative blood transfusion. Four meta-analyses of randomized trials. Transfus Med (under review).

9. Anonymous. Canadian Orthopedic Perioperative Erythropoietin Study Group. Effectiveness of perioperative recombinant human erythropoietin in elective hip replacement. Lancet 1993;341:1227-32.
10. Yuen K, Matthews JP. Recombinant human erythropoietin (R-HuEPO) and autologous donation. Document from Janssen Cilag Limited 1995.
11. EPREX (epoetin alpha) product monograph, Janssen-Ortho Inc. Canada, 1996.
12. Spiess BD. Anesthetic care and blood loss. In: Benumoff JL, Spiess BD, editors. Anesthesiology Clinics of North America. Philadelphia: WB Saunders Company, 1990;18:441-49.
13. Carson JL, Soence RK, Poses RM et al. Severity of anaemia and operative mortality and morbidity. Lancet 1988;i:727-29.
14. Kafer ER. Acute intraoperative hemodilution and perioperative blood salvage. In: benumof JL, Spiess BD (eds). Anesthesiology Clinics of North America: Hemorrhagic disorders. Philadelphia: WB Saunders Company 1990;8:543-67.
15. Messmer K. Preoperative hemodilution. In: Rossi EC, Simon TL, Moss GS, editors. Principles of Transfusion medicine. Baltimore: Williams and Wilkins 1991:405-9.
16. Williamson KR, Taswell HF. Intraoperative blood salvage: a review. Transfusion 1991;31:662-75.
17. Pineda AA, Valbonesi M. Intraoperative blood salvage. Baill Clin Haematology 1990;3:385-403.
18. Kruskall MS. Intraoperative autotransfusion. In: Rossi EC, Simon TL, Moss GS, editors. Principles of transfusion Medicine. Baltimore: Williams and Wilkins, 1991: 411-17.
19. AABB. Guidelines for blood salvage and reinfusion in surgery and trauma. American Association Blood Banks, Arlington, Virginia 1990:1-12.
20. NBREP Expert Panel. The use of autologous blood. JAMA 1990;263:414-17.
21. Koopman-van Gemert AWMM. Peri-operative autotransfusion by means of a blood cell separator. Academic thesis Nijmegen, Catholic University of Nijmegen 1993: 1-168.
22. Forgie M, Wells P, Laupacis A, Fergusson D. for the International Study of Perioperative Transfusion (ISPOT). Pre-operative autologous donation decreases allogeneic transfusion but increases exposure to all red cell transfusion - results of a meta-analysis. Arch Intern Med 1998;158:610-16.
23. Bryson GL, Laupacis A, Wells GA, for the International Study of perioperative transfusion (ISPOT). Does acute normovolemic hemodilution reduce perioperative allogeneic transfusion? A meta-analysis. Anesth Analg 1998;86:9-15.
24. Lubarsky DA, Hahn C, Bennett DH et al. The hospital cost (fiscal year 1991/1992) of a simple perioperative allogeneic red blood cell transfusion during elective surgery at Duke University. Anesth Analg 1994;79:629-37.
25. Etachson J, Petz L, Keeler et al. The cost effectiveness of preoperative autologous blood donations. N Engl J Med 1995;332:719-24.
26. Goldfinger D, Haimowitz M. Controversies in transfusion medicine. Is autologous blood transfusion worth the cost? Pro. Transfusion 1994;34:75-8.
27. AuBuchon JP, Bikmeyer JD. Controversies in transfusion medicine. Is autologous blood transfusion worth the cost? Con. Transfusion 1994;34:79-83.
28. Goodnough LT. Cost-effective strategies for autologous blood procurement before surgery. Vox Sang 1994;67:187-90.
29. Ferguson KJ, Strauss RG, Toy PTCY. Physician recommendation as the key factor in patient's decision to participate in preoperative autologous blood donation programs. Am J Surg 1994;168:2-5.
30. Domen RE, Ribicki LA, Hoeltge GA. An analysis of autologous blood donor motivational factors. Vox Sang 1995;69:110-13.

THE USE OF TECHNOLOGIES TO DECREASE PERIOPERATIVE ALLOGENEIC BLOOD TRANSFUSION: AN INTERNATIONAL SURVEY OF PRACTICE

D. Fergusson, I.D. Graham, A. Laupacis
International Study of Peri-operative Transfusion (ISPOT) Investigators[1]

Introduction

Since the discovery in the 1980's that blood transfusion can transmit HIV, there has been interest in technologies that reduce the amount of allogeneic blood used during and after surgery. This interest persists despite the fact that the probability of receiving HIV and hepatitis from allogeneic blood transfusion is now very rare.

The International Study of Peri-Operative Transfusion (ISPOT) investigators are evaluating the use of technologies to minimise peri-operative transfusion in ten countries (Australia, Canada, Denmark, France, Israel, Japan, Netherlands, Spain, United Kingdom, and the United States). The study consists of three phases: 1) systematic reviews to determine the efficacy, safety and cost-effectiveness of the technologies [1-4]; 2) surveys to determine the degree to which the technologies are used; and 3) interviews with clinicians, interest groups and policy makers to assess the factors contributing to the use (or lack of use) of the technologies. The technologies studied are drugs (aprotinin, desmopressin (DDAVP), tranexamic acid (TXA), epsilon aminocapronic acid (EACA), and erythropoietin (EPO)), pre-operative autologous donation (PAD), acute normovolemic haemodilution (ANH) and cell salvage (CS). In this paper we report preliminary results about the degree to which these technologies are currently used in nine of the ten countries (data are not available for Spain).

Method

In each country, either a census (i.e. all hospitals) or a random sample of hospitals with medical/surgical beds was surveyed between 1995 and 1997. (Table 1) The questionnaire, developed by the Canadian investigators served as a template which the other countries adopted and translated as needed to meet their own circumstances.

---

1. This work was carried out at the Clinical Epidemiology Unit, Loeb Research Institute, Ottawa Civic Hospital, University of Ottawa, Canada, supported by a Fellowship from the International Society of Technology Assessment in Health Care (ISTAHC) and funds from Janssen Ortho Inc.

Table 1. Survey of characteristics and response rates

	Type of hospitals surveyed	Survey	Recipients	Hospitals surveyed	Hospital response rate
Australia	Census	Mail	(1)	400	87%
Canada	Census (>50 medical/ surgical beds)	Mail	(2), (3), (4), (5), (6), (7)	269	95%
Denmark	Census	Mail	(2), (3), (4), (5), (6), (7)	62	98%
France	Random sample (surgical beds)	Mail and telephone	(8), (9)	241	93%
Isreael	Census (>50 beds)	Mail and telephone	(2), (3), (4), (5), (6), (7)	31	100%
Japan	Random sample (>100 beds)	Mail	(2), (3), (10)	724	70%
Netherlands	Census	Telephone	(9)	112	100%
Scotland	Census (>100 beds)	Mail and telephone	(11), (3), (2), (4), (5), (6), (7)	35	68%
United States	Random sample (>50 medical/ surgical beds)	Mail	(2), (3), (4), (6)	1000	54%

(1) Chief executive officer
(2) Chief of surgery
(3) Chief of anaesthesiology
(4) Chief of orthopaedics
(5) Chief of vascular surgery
(6) Chief of cardiac surgery
(7) Chief of urology
(8) Hospital pharmacy
(9) Operating room head nurse
(10) Directors of hospitals
(11) Head of pharmacy

The survey was administered by mail, telephone or both (Table 1). Mail surveys were in the form of a one page questionnaire, a postcard, or a more detailed questionnaire (United States). The most suitable recipients of the questionnaires were determined by the investigators of each country (Table 1). All surveys asked whether the technologies were currently being used or not being used in the hospital for orthopaedic, cardiac, urologic or vascular surgery to reduce perioperative allogeneic transfusion. Some countries included other specialties such as gynaecology and plastic surgery but those results are not presented in this paper. If the technology was used in that hospital, the amount of use was not elicited in the mail surveys. However, the telephone survey conducted in the Netherlands asked recipients to describe the amount of use in qualitative terms. If respondents stated that they "rarely" used a technology, this was interpreted as a "no". This assumption was only adopted for the Netherlands' survey. The surveys in Denmark and France did not include EACA because this technology was not available in either country. The Japanese survey did not ask about the use of technologies in vascular surgery. Countries in which the survey was administered by mail conducted one follow-up mailing of non-responders.

A majority of countries sent surveys to more than one recipient per hospital in order to maximise the likelihood of a response (Table 1). If there was a discrepancy among respondents at the same hospital as to whether a technology was used or not, it was assumed that the technology was used (e.g. if one individual indicated that aprotinin was being used and another stated that it was not used, we assumed that it was being used). Data were collected, entered, and analysed in each country (except the United States where data entry and analysis of data was done in Canada) and summary results were submitted to the Canadian co-ordinating centre on a standard data form.

Table 2. Hospital response rates by speciality

	Cardiac		Orthopaedic		Urology		Vascular	
	Surveyed	Re-sponded	Surveyed	Re-sponded	Surveyed	Re-sponded	Surveyed	Re-sponded
Australia*	59	–	323	–	287	–	185	–
Canada	36	92%	176	91%	149	93%	92	96
Denmark	5	80%	39	95%	6	100%	2	100
France*	27	–	172	–	132	–	138	–
Israel	13	100%	31	100%	31	100%	23	100
Japan	164	100%	581	75%	441	76%	ns	ns
Netherlands	13	100%	111	100%	104	100%	110	100%
Scotland	4	100%	26	62%	12	92%	17	53%

* Not know what proportion of hospitals have the various specialities;
ns = not surveyed.

Results

The number of hospitals surveyed and the response rates are given in Table 1. The response rate by surgical specialty is provided in Table 2. The results are presented according to the type of surgery and country. For most countries, the data are presented as the proportion of hospitals with a particular specialty that use the technology (e.g. 71% of Canadian hospitals that perform cardiac surgery used aprotinin). In the United States, the data are presented by hospital rather than specialty, and the same is true for France for PAD, CS, and ANH.

In order to standardise the descriptions of the use of the technologies, we have used the following definitions: "not used in any hospitals" – 0%; "used in a minority of hospitals" – 1-33%; "used in a moderate amount of hospitals" – 34-66%; "used in a majority of hospitals" – 67-99%; "used in all hospitals" – 100%. The Tables should be consulted for the exact percentages.

Table 3. Proportion of hospitals performing cardiac surgery using the technology

Country (number of hospitals)	Apro-tinin	TXA	EACA	DDAVP	EPO	CS	ANH	PAD
	%	%	%	%	%	%	%	%
Australia (59)	42	0	0	29	0	42	56	42
Canada (33)	71	70	72	78	24	72	43	ns
Denmark (4)	100	100	na	33	0	75	50	25
France (27)	52	44	na	38	12	ns	ns	ns
Israel (13)	92	69	0	8	0	50	69	39
Japan (164)	33	40	2	2	73	79	42	77
Netherlands (13)	39	31	39	8	0	31	0	0
Scotland (4)	100	50	50	0	25	75	100	50

na = technology not available in that country; ns = not surveyed

Type of surgery

a) Cardiac surgery: The proportion of hospitals using drugs to reduce allogeneic transfusion in cardiac surgery was considerably higher than that for the other three specialties (Table 3). This is especially evident for aprotinin and TXA. EACA was used in a moderate to majority of hospitals in three countries (Canada, Netherlands, Scotland) and it was not used in four countries (Australia, Denmark, France, and Israel). DDAVP was used in fewer hospitals than aprotinin in all countries except Canada. A moderate amount of Japanese hospitals performing cardiac surgery used EPO while it was rarely or not used in the other countries. As for the non-pharmaceutical technologies, the use of CS varied from 31% of hospitals in the Netherlands to 75% of Danish and Scottish hospi-

Table 4. Proportion of hospitals performing orthopaedic surgery using the technology

Country (number of hospitals)	Apro-tinin	TXA	EACA	DDAVP	EPO	CS	ANH	PAD
	%	%	%	%	%	%	%	%
Australia (323)	1	0	0	1	1	22	14	61
Canada (160)	6	4	6	20	13	19	43	ns
Denmark (37)	3	3	na	0	6	39	17	0
France (172)	9	9	na	18	6	ns	ns	ns
Israel (31)	0	3	0	0	3	13	16	23
Japan (434)	1	23	1	0	51	20	10	60
Netherlands (111)	1	2	1	1	0	25	19	9
Scotland (16)	0	0	0	0	6	25	6	13

na = technology not available in that country; ns = not surveyed tals. The proportion of hospitals using ANH and PAD varied from zero to 100% among countries.

b) Orthopaedic surgery: Pharmaceuticals were used in a smaller proportion of hospitals in orthopaedic than in cardiac surgery (Table 4). TXA was used in 23% of Japanese hospitals performing orthopaedic surgery, DDAVP in 20% of Canadian and 18% of French hospitals, and EPO in 51% of Japanese and 13% of Canadian hospitals. In the other countries these drugs were used in less than 10% of hospitals. Non-pharmacological technologies were used to a greater degree than drugs, although there was wide variation among technologies and countries.

Table 5. Proportion of hospitals performing urologic surgery using the technology

Country (number of hospitals)	**Apro-tinin**	**TXA**	**EACA**	**DDAVP**	**EPO**	**CS**	**ANH**	**PAD**
	%	%	%	%	%	%	%	%
Australia (287)	0	1	2	1	0	4	6	31
Canada (139)	9	3	35	25	10	8	29	ns
Denmark (6)	20	50	na	0	17	0	33	0
France (132))	4	19	na	14	3	ns	ns	ns
Israel (31)	0	16	0	7	0	7	16	16
Japan (336)	0	21	1	0	29	1	7	30
Netherlands (104)	0	8	3	0	0	0	7	0
Scotland (11)	9	18	18	0	0	0	0	0

na = technology not available in that country; ns = not surveyed

Table 6. Proportion of hospitals performing vascular surgery using the technology

Country (number of hospitals)	**Apro-tinin**	**TXA**	**EACA**	**DDAVP**	**EPO**	**CS**	**ANH**	**PAD**
	%	%	%	%	%	%	%	%
Australia (185)	1	1	1	3	1	28	19	41
Canada (88)	10	12	21	26	9	27	41	ns
Denmark (2)	50	50	na	0	0	100	50	0
France (138)	13	13	na	22	3	ns	ns	ns
Israel (23)	0	17	0	4	4	26	26	4
Japan (ns)	ns	ns	ns	ns	ns	ns	ns	ns
Netherlands (110)	0	0	0	0	0	20	11	3
Scotland (9)	11	0	0	0	0	22	22	0

na = technology not available in that country; ns = not surveyed

c) Urologic surgery: Technologies were used in fewer hospitals in urologic surgery than in cardiac surgery (Table 5), although TXA was used more frequently than in orthopaedic surgery. Cell salvage was rarely or not used in urologic surgery, and the use of ANH varied between 0% (Scotland) and 33% of hospitals (Denmark). PAD was not used in Denmark, Netherlands, and Scotland and was used in few Australian, Israeli and Japanese hospitals.

d) Vascular surgery: The use of pharmaceuticals in vascular surgery was similar to that in urologic surgery (Table 6). The use of CS ranged from 20% to 100% of hospitals, ANH from 11% to 50% and PAD from 0% to 41%.

Country

The pattern of technology use varied among the countries. Australia was a low user of pharmaceuticals in all four specialties except for aprotinin and DDAVP in cardiac surgery. Canada was a high user of all drugs in cardiac surgery, and tended to use EACA and DDAVP more frequently than the other countries in all four specialties. Denmark was a high user of aprotinin and TXA, except in orthopaedics. Denmark was also a high user of CS and ANH, except in urologic surgery, but used PAD rarely in cardiac surgery and not at all in the other surgeries. The use of technologies in France tended towards the average. Except for aprotinin and TXA in cardiac surgery, the pharmaceuticals were not used or were used in a minority of Israeli hospitals. Israel used CS, ANH, and PAD an average amount compared to the other countries. Japan had a high use of EPO but a relatively low use of the other drugs. Compared to the other countries, the Netherlands was a low user of all technologies. Similarly, Scotland was a low user of all technologies except in cardiac surgery.

Table 7. United States: proportion of hospitals using the technology

	Aprotinin	**TXA**	**EACA**	**DDAVP**	**EPO**	**CS**	**ANH**	**PAD**
Hospitals	413	401	407	404	214	420	411	206
% using technology	61	9	50	52	43	82	33	83

The proportion of hospitals using each technology in the United States is presented in Table 7. Data have not been broken down by specialty. A moderate proportion of hospitals use the drug technologies except TXA where it is used in a minority of hospitals. Use of CS and PAD is used in a majority of hospitals while ANH is used in a moderate proportion of hospitals.

Discussion

The results of this survey indicate that there is considerable practice variation in the use of technologies to minimise exposure to peri-operative allogeneic transfusion, both among technologies and among countries. Three limitations of this study must be acknowledged. First, we asked respondents to report what was done in their hospital, and did not perform actual audits of practice. Nonetheless, the degree of practice variation is so great that it is unlikely that this accounts for all of the variation observed. Second, in a minority of hospitals there was disagreement among respondents about whether or not the technology was used. A phone follow-up in Canada suggested that this usually occurred if the technology was used very infrequently (one responder indicating the technology was not used and the other indicating that it was). These hospitals were classified as users of the technology. Third, in order to maximise the response rate, we made the initial survey instrument extremely brief. We asked whether a hospital used a technology, but in those which did, we did not ask about the actual proportion of patients in whom the technology was used. Thus, it is possible that 100% of *hospitals* in one country reported using CS for vascular surgery, yet only a minority of *patients* undergoing vascular surgery would have received the technology. Most countries are now conducting a more detailed survey of the frequency of use in the hospitals that are using the technologies.

There are many possible reasons for the amount of variation in practice found in this survey. For instance, many of the technologies are effective at reducing the need for perioperative allogeneic transfusion [1-4] and clinicians and patients can therefore use a number of technologies to achieve the same goal. It is intriguing that some countries use desmopressin, which has been found to be ineffective in two meta-analyses [1,5]. It is possible that desmopressin is being used only for patients with von Willebrand's disease or uraemia. The frequent use of EPO in Japanese hospitals may be explained by the fact that many of the trials of peri-operative EPO were done in that country [6-9], and one of the manufacturers of EPO is located in Japan.

Although many of the technologies have been shown to be efficacious, some clinicians may be unaware of this information. Many physician specialties are involved in decisions about perioperative transfusion including surgeons, anaesthetists, transfusion specialists, haematologists, and internists. These physicians tend to read different journals, attend their own specialty meetings and conferences, and are thus exposed to different information about these technologies (e.g. anaesthetists are likely to be more aware about the issues related to aprotinin than transfusion specialists). Thus, it is not surprising that practice variation exists within and between specialties.

Each of the technologies is associated with side-effects, the frequency and seriousness of which is not always clear [1,2,4]. At the same time, the likelihood of receiving HIV or hepatitis from allogeneic blood transfusion has decreased considerably in the last decade [10,11], while the possibility of transmitting new agents such as prions exists [12]. Thus, patients and physicians in one centre may come to very different conclusions about the benefit:risk ratio of these technologies than individuals at other centres. Physicians training at one centre will be exposed to a different pattern of practice than physicians training at another centre. In some countries, the media and public may be much more aware and vocal about issues related to blood transfusion than in others. Finally, economic factors such as the type of health care system and the method of payment for blood and the technologies probably affects their use.

Future research from the ISPOT group will determine the actual degree to which these technologies are used in the ten countries, and examine the factors leading to these patterns of practice.

References:

1. Laupacis A, Fergusson D for the International Study of Peri-Operative Transfusion (ISPOT) Investigators. Drugs to minimize peri-operative blood loss in cardiac surgery – Meta analyses using peri-operative blood transfusion as the outcome. Anesth Analg 1997;85:1258-67.
2. Forgie M, Wells PS, Laupacis A, Fergusson D for the International Study of Peri-Operative Transfusion (ISPOT) Investigators. Pre-operative autologous donation decreases allogeneic transfusion but increases exposure to all blood products – Results of a meta analysis. Arch Intern Med 1998;158:610-16.
3. Bryson GL, Laupacis A, Wells GA, for the International Study of Peri-Operative Transfusion (ISPOT) Investigators. Does acute normovolemic hemodilution reduce perioperative allogeneic transfusion? A meta analysis. Anesth Analg 1998;86:9-15.
4. Laupacis A, Fergusson D, for the International Study of Peri-Operative Transfusion (ISPOT) Investigators. Erythropoietin to minimize peri-operative blood transfusion. Four meta-analyses of randomized trails. Transfus Med (under review).
5. Cattaneo M, Harris AS, Stroberg U, Mannucci PM. The effect of desmopressin on reducing blood loss in cardiac surgery – A meta analysis of double-blind, placebo-controlled trials. Tromb Haemost 1995;74:1064-70.
6. Watanabe Y, Fuse K, Naruse Y, et al. [Cardiac surgery without homologous blood transfusion--the effectiveness and the indication of recombinant human erythropoietin]. [Japanese]. *Nippon Kyobu Geka Gakkai Zasshi.* 1994;42:499-507.
7. Konishi T, Ohbayashi T, Kaneko T, Ohki T, Saitou Y, Yamato Y. Preoperative use of erythropoietin for cardiovascular operations in anemia. Ann Thorac Surg 1993; 56:101-3.
8. Kyo S, Omoto R, Hirashima K, Eguchi S, Fujita T. Effect of human recombinant erythropoietin on reduction of homologous blood transfusion in open-heart surgery. A Japanese Multicenter study. Circulation 1992;86(Suppl):II413-18.
9. Watanabe Y, Fuse K, Naruse Y, et al. Subcutaneous use of erythropoietin in heart surgery. Ann Thorac Surg 1992;54:479-83.
10. Lackritz EM, Satten GA, Aberle-Grasse J, et al. Estimated risk of transmission of the numan immunodeficiency virus by screened blood in the United States. N Engl J Med 1995;333:1721-25.
11. Schreiber GB, Busch MP, Kleinman SH, Korelitz JJ, for the Retrovirus Epidemiology Donor Study: The risk of transfusion-transmitted viral infections. N Engl J Med 1996; 334:1685-90.
12. Raymond GJ, Hope J, Kocisko DA, et al. Molecular assessment of the potential transmissibilities of BSE and scrapie to humans. Nature 1997 Jul 17;388: 285-88.

UMBILICAL CORD BLOOD AS AN ALTERNATIVE SOURCE OF HAEMATOPOIETIC STEM CELLS FOR TRANSPLANTATION

H.C.J.M. Jacobs, J.H.F. Falkenburg

Introduction

Transplantation of allogeneic haematopoietic stem cells plays an important role in the treatment of haematological diseases, including inherited immunologic or haematopoietic disorders, some metabolic diseases and haematologic malignant disorders, in particular leukaemia [1]. About 30% of the patients who need a haematopoietic stem cell transplantation do have an HLA-identical family donor.

For patients who do not have a family donor, it is possible to search for an HLA-identical unrelated donor [2,3]. Large international registries of potential bone marrow donors have been established. In spite of the enormous size of the registries, matched unrelated bone marrow transplantation is available for only half of the patients who lack an HLA-identical family donor. The probability of finding an HLA-identical unrelated donor for a patient who belongs to an ethnic minority group (15% of the search requests in The Netherlands) even smaller due to the relatively low numbers of volunteers from ethnic minority groups in the national and international registries [4]. As a result of the ethnic imbalances in the registries individuals belonging to an ethnical minority have a 75% lower chance of finding an identical unrelated donor.

Therefore additional sources of haematopoietic stem cells have been explored to be used for transplantation.

Umbilical cord blood as an alternative source of haematopoietic stem cells for bone marrow reconstitution

Recently it has been demonstrated that umbilical cord blood (UCB) contains a large number of stem and progenitor cells that can be used as an alternative source of bone marrow repopulating cells in allogeneic stem cell transplantation [5-12]. UCB is the blood which remains in the umbilical cord and placenta after a baby has been delivered and the umbilical cord has been clamped. A total amount of 50-200 ml blood can be harvested from a single umbilical cord containing sufficient stem cells to transplant both children and adults [13].

Gluckman, Broxmeyer and colleagues reported the first successful umbilical cord blood transplantation in 1988 in a patient with Fanconi anaemia [5,6].

Since the first transplantation, umbilical cord blood from a sibling has been used as a source of haematopoietic stem cells in more than 100 allogeneic transplantations. Wagner et al reported on umbilical cord blood transplantations from sibling donors in 44 children, with acquired or congenital lympho-haematopoietic disorders, neuroblastoma or metabolic diseases, between October 1988 and September 1994 [9]. Patients who had HLA-identical and HLA-1 antigen disparate grafts (n= 38), had a probability of engraftment at 50 days of 85%. No patient had late graft failure. The probability of grade HIV graft-versus-host disease (GvHD) at 100 days was 3% and the probability of chronic GvHD at one year was 6%. With a follow-up of 1-6 years, the probability of survival for recipients of HLA-identical or HLA-1 antigen disparate grafts was 72%.

In 1992 the New York Blood Center started to explore the feasibility of using cryopreserved umbilical cord blood from unrelated donors for the transplantation of haematopoietic stem cells [14]. Kurtzberg et al described in 1996 the results of 25 transplantations using umbilical cord blood from unrelated donors [7]. All transplants were performed with cryopreserved UCB from the umbilical cord blood bank of the New York Blood Center. Nearly all of the patients were children, with a variety of malignant and non-malignant disorders. Twenty-four of the 25 patients had HLA-1 to HLA-3 antigen disparate grafts. In 23 of the 25 patients the infused haematopoietic stem cells engrafted. Acute grade III GvHD occurred in 2 of the 21 patients who could be evaluated and 2 patients had chronic GvHD. With a follow-up of 12.5 months and a minimal follow-up of 100 days, the overall 100-day survival rate among these patients was 64% and the overall event-free survival was 48%.

These reports illustrate that allogeneic stem cell transplantation with UCB from both related and unrelated donors is feasible and may show advantages over allogeneic bone marrow transplantations. These advantages are:

- UCB transplants may show lower incidence of (severe) graft-versus-host disease.
- Viral contamination in UCB is substantially lower than in adult bone marrow.
- UCB is usually discarded with the placenta and can be harvested without any risk to mother or infant.
- The cryopreserved UCB can be made available on demand and eliminates the delay and uncertainties that may complicate the collection of bone marrow from unrelated donors.
- For non-caucasian patients UCB is often the only source of haematopoietic stem cells because ethnic minority groups are not well represented in registries of bone marrow donors.

However, a disadvantage of UCB transplantation is the limited number of nucleated cells in a UCB transplant which could delay the speed of engraftment. Moreover an important question is whether the absence of GvHD may be associated with a decreased graft versus leukaemia effect, which may influence the survival of patients with leukaemia.

The Eurocord Transplant Group registered cord blood transplantations performed in Europe. Analysis was performed on 143 transplantations at 45 centres, using cord blood from related and unrelated donors between October 1988 and December 1996 [12]. Of the 143 patients, 95 received transplants to treat haematological malignancies, 26 had a bone marrow failure syndrome, 8 had haemoglobinopathy and 14 had other types of genetic diseases. The median age of the patients was 6 years (0.2-45 years); 23 patients were older than 15 years. The overall survival at one year for all 143 patients was 49%. Variables associated with better survival were: younger age (<6 years), lower weight (<20 kg), HLA identical transplants, cytomegalovirus-negative status in recipient and infusion of at least 3.7×10^7 nucleated cells per kg body weight.

For patients receiving cord blood from related donors, one-year survival was 63%. Acute GvHD II-IV occurred in 5 of the 60 patients who received HLA matched cord blood and in 9 of the 18 recipients of HLA mismatched cord blood. 85% of the patients receiving $\geq3.7\times10^7$ nucleated cells/kg and 73% of the patients who received $<3.7\times10^7$ nucleated cells/kg had neutrophil engraftment within 60 days.

One-year survival for patients who received cord blood from unrelated donors, was 29%. The incidence of acute GvHD II-IV was not affected by the number of HLA mismatches. Neutrophil engraftment within 60 days occurred in 94% of the patients who received $\geq3.7\times10^7$ nucleated cells/kg and in 76% of the patients who received $<3.7\times10^7$ nucleated cells/kg.

Cord blood banks

Since successful umbilical cord blood transplantations have been reported, cord blood banks are being developed world-wide [15-18]. The first cord blood bank was initiated at the New York Blood Center in February 1993. More than 6000 umbilical cord blood transplants have been collected, processed, HLA antigen-typed, tested for transmissible infectious diseases, and cryopreserved. In The Netherlands, France, Germany, Italy, Belgium, Spain and the UK similar cord blood banks are being developed (European Cord Blood Banks). The ultimate goal of the New York Blood Center Placental Program as well as of the European Cord Blood Bank is the provision of umbilical cord blood stem cells for transplantation in recipients lacking suitably matched sibling donors.

Cord blood banking in The Netherlands

In The Netherlands, the EuroCord Nederland Foundation (ECN) was started in 1994 to co-ordinate the development of a national cord blood bank [19]. In this organisation the blood banks in Leiden, Groningen and Nijmegen, the Central Laboratory of the Blood Transfusion Service (CLB) in Amsterdam, Europdonor Foundation and the department of Hematology of the Leiden University Medical Centre collaborate in their effort to establish a national cord blood bank for unrelated transplants. The aim is to obtain a cord blood bank of at least 5000 transplants for patients who lack an HLA-identical related or unrelated bone marrow donor.

Regional obstetric units are contacted by the blood banks and CLB to organise the collection of UCB. After the collection, the UCB transplant is transported to the blood bank where it is processed and typed for HLA and blood groups, tested for viral and bacteriological contamination and cryopreserved. Each blood bank forms together with the obstetric units and diagnostic laboratories a regional cord blood bank. These regional cord blood banks are located in Amsterdam, Groningen, Leiden and Nijmegen. After a UCB transplant meets all quality requirements, it is reported to ECN. The HLA-typing and nucleated cell counts of the released transplants from the regional cord blood banks are entered into the network of the Bone Marrow Donors Worldwide (BMDW) by Europdonor, and made available to all participating Transplant Centres. Figure 1 shows the organisation structure of the EuroCord Nederland Foundation.

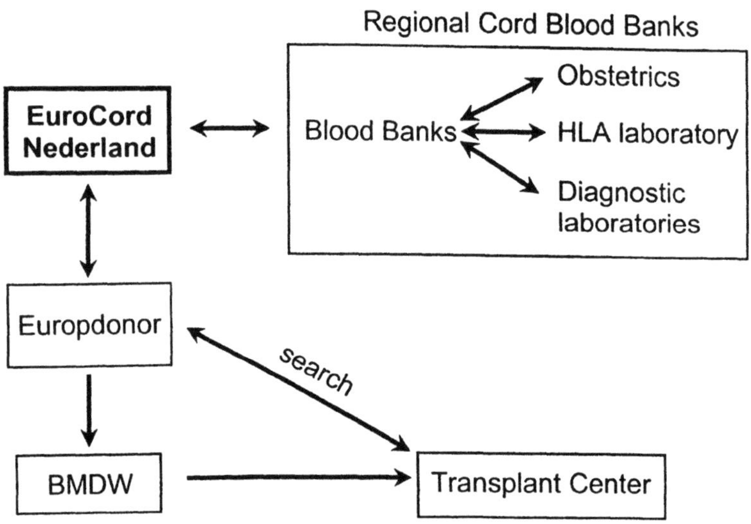

Figure 1. Organisation structure of the EuroCord Nederland Foudation.

Procedure in The Netherlands

At the participating obstetric units the mother is informed about the possibility to donate UCB after her child's birth. Prior to delivery informed consent is asked and the mother has to complete an information form concerning infectious disease history, genetic diseases and ethnic background of both parents. Knowledge of the ethnic background is important for optimal matching of UCB transplant and patient, and it will also help to identify certain genetic diseases like sickle cell anaemia and thalassemia.

UCB is collected by specially trained personnel either during the third stage of labour (placenta is still in utero) or after placental delivery (ex utero). A minimal collection volume of 50 ml is necessary to be used for banking. From this volume, 5-7 ml is used for diagnostic purposes, including nucleated cell counts, ABO/Rhesus blood group typing, HLA typing, infectious disease testing (hepatitis B, hepatitis C, HIV, HTLV, syphilis), bacteriological cultures and CD34 determination. Approximately 3 cm of the umbilical cord is cryopreserved for future DNA isolation and HLA class II oligonucleotide typing.

Within 48 hours before or after delivery, 10 ml of blood is taken from the mother and analysed for markers of infectious diseases, including Hepatitis B, Hepatitis C, HIV, HTLV and Syphilis. A volume of 20 ml of blood is taken from the mother for HLA-typing and future diagnostic procedures. At a regular control visit at 6-8 weeks after delivery the mother is questioned about her health and the health of her baby.

After cord blood collection, the UCB transplant is transported to the blood bank, where it is processed and cryopreserved using dimethylsulfoxide (DMSO) as cryoprotectant. UCB transplants are cryopreserved either as whole blood transplants or after volume reduction. Different methods for volume reduction are being used, including hydroxyethyl starch (HES) sedimentation and density cell separation. Cryopreservation of UCB is performed within 24 hours after collection. Vials for future diagnostic purposes and at least two reference vials are separately cryopreserved. Reference vials contain the final suspension that is cryopreserved and are used for control haematopoietic progenitor cell cultures after cryopreservation and determination of the identity of the transplant when it will be actually used.

The UCB transplants and vials are kept at the regional cord blood banks. UCB transplants which fulfil all criteria necessary for the release of the transplant are reported to ECN. Information concerning the UCB transplants, including volume, nucleated cell counts, HLA typing, blood group, viral status, sex and race is transferred to Europdonor. Europdonor enters the HLA-typing and nucleated cell counts of transplants into the network of the Bone Marrow Donors Worldwide (BMDW) to make them available to all participating transplant centres. If a request is made for a specific transplant, the medical advisory team of ECN will consider the use of the UCB transplant and the use of cryopreserved control vials for additional testing.

Table 1. Characteristics of the regional cord blood banks.

	Leiden	Nijmegen	Amsterdam	Groningen
Started	1995	1996	1997	experimental phase
Collection method	ex utero	ex utero	in utero/ex utero	in utero
Processing method	whole blood / HES	density gradient	density gradient	HES
Total units stored (Nov. '97)	418	150	152	0
Units available (Nov. '97)	143	109	0	0

Results

A total amount of 720 cord blood units has been cryopreserved in the Dutch cord blood bank from March 1995 to November 1997 (Table I). The data of 250 units are entered in the registry of the BMDW and are available to patients from all over the world.

Thusfar two umbilical cord blood transplantations have been performed in The Netherlands, and one cord blood unit has been used for a patient in Switzerland.

References

1. Armitage JO. Bone marrow transplantation. N Engl J Med 1995; 330: 827-38.
2. Downie TR, Hows JM, Gore SM, Bradley BA, Howard MR. A survey of use of unrelated volunteer donor bone marrow transplantation at 46 centres worldwide, 1989-93. Bone Marrow Transplant 1995;15:499-503.
3. Kernan NA, Bartsch G, Ash RC, et al. Analysis of 462 transplantations from unrelated donors facilitated by the National Marrow Donor Program. N Engl J Med 1993; 328:598-602.
4. Howard MR, Gore SM, Hows JM, Downie TR, Bradley BA. A prospective study of factor determining the outcome of unrelated marrow donor searches: report from the International Marrow Unrelated Search and Transplant Study Working Group on behalf of collaboration centres. Bone Marrow Transplant 1994;13:389-96.
5. Broxmeyer HE, Douglas GW, Hangoc G, et al. Human umbilical cord blood as a potential source of transplantable haematopoietic stem/progenitor cells. Proc Natl Acad Sci USA 1989;86:3828-32.
6. Gluckman E, Broxmeyer HA, Auerbach AD, et al. Haematopoietic reconstitution in a patient with Fanconi's anemia by means of umbilical cord blood from an HLA-identical sibling. N Engl J Med 1989;321:1174-8.
7. Kurtzberg J, Laughlin M, Graham ML, et al. Placental blood as a source of haematopoietic stem cells for transplantation into unrelated recipients. N Engl J Med 1996; 335:157-66.
8. Kurtzberg J, Graham M, Casey J, Olson J, Stevens CE, Rubinstein, P. The use of umbilical cord blood in mismatched related and unrelated haematopoietic stem cell transplantation. Blood Cells 1994;20:275-83.
9. Wagner JE, Keman NA, Steinbuch M, Broxmeyer HE, Gluckman E. Allogeneic sibling umbilical-cord-blood transplantation in children with malignant and non-malignant disease. Lancet 1995;346:214-19.
10. Wagner, JE. Umbilical cord blood transplantation. Transfusion 1995;35:619-21.
11. Wagner JE, Rosenthal J, Sweetman R, et al. Successful transplantation of HLA-matched and HLA mismatched umbilical cord blood from unrelated donors: analysis of engraftment and acute graft-versus-host disease. Blood 1996;88:795-802.
12. Gluckman E, Rocha V, Boyer-Chammard A, et al. Outcome of cord blood transplants from related and unrelated donors. N Engl J Med 1997;337:373-81.
13. Broxmeyer HE, Hangoc G, Cooper S, et al. Growth characteristics and expansion of human umbilical cord blood and estimation of its potential for transplantation in adults. Proc Natl Acad Sci USA 1992;89:4109-13.
14. Rubinstein P, Rosenfield RE, Adamson JW, Stevens CE. Stored placental blood for unrelated bone marrow reconstitution. Blood 1993;81:1679-90.

15. Silberstein LE, Jefferies LC. Placental-blood banking - a new frontier in transfusion medicine. N Engl J Med 1996;335:199-201.
16. Gluckman E, Wagner J, Hows J, Kernan N, Bradley B, Broxmeyer HE. Special Report: Cord blood banking for haematopoietic stem cell transplantation: an international cord blood transplant registry. Bone Marrow Transpl 1993;11:199-200.
17. Newton I, Charbord P, Schaal JP, Herve P. Toward cord blood banking: density-separation and cryopreservation of cord blood progenitors. Exp Hematol 1993; 21:671-74.
18. Rubinstein P, Dobrila L, Rosenfield RE, et al. Processing and cryopreservation of placental/umbilical cord blood for unrelated bone marrow transplantation. Proc Natl Acad Sci USA 1995;92:10119-22.
19. Falkenburg JHF, Lim FTH. Navelstrengbloed ter vervanging van beenmerg voor allogene transplantatie van hematopoëtische stamcellen. Ned Tijdschr Geneeskd 1995;139:1319-22.

CORD BLOOD BANKING AND TRANSPLANT IN EUROPE

E. Gluckman, V. Rocha, C. Chastang, on behalf of Eurocord[1]

Introduction

Allogeneic haematopoietic stem cell transplantation (HSCT) has been used to treat thousands of patients, adults and children, with life-threatening haematological diseases. The principal limitations of allogeneic bone marrow transplantation are the lack of suitable HLA-matched donors and the complications of graft-versus-host disease associated with HLA disparities. In the absence of a suitable HLA identical sibling donor, alternative donors such as mismatched related or matched unrelated donors are searched. In these transplants, major and minor histocompatibility differences are often unrecognised by current matching tests, explaining the relatively high frequency of post transplant complications, graft failure, graft-versus-host disease and delayed immune reconstitution. The description of new more sensitive techniques of typing by molecular biology and has decreased the probability of finding a fully matched donor. Despite a bone marrow donor registry which contains more than 4 millions bone marrow donors world-wide, some patients cannot be transplanted because of the lack of an HLA identical donor.

Since the first cord blood transplant performed in 1988 [1], cord blood transplantation is increasingly used as a new source of haematopoietic stem cells and more than 500 cases have been reported. In order to develop and evaluate cord blood transplant results, the European Blood and Marrow Transplantation group (EBMT) has organised a concerted action the Eurocord Group.

The objectives of Eurocord are:

- to standardise the methods of collection, testing and cryopreservation of cord blood;
- to study the properties of haematopoietic progenitors and gene transfer in cord blood;
- to study the immune function of cord blood lymphocytes;
- to co-ordinate and facilitate the exchange of sera and cells from donor and recipients of cord blood transplants;

1. Eurocord is supported by a European concerted action BIOMED II BMHA-CT96-0833.

- to establish a European Registry of patients treated by cord blood transplants and design protocols comparing cord blood transplants with alternative conventional blood and bone marrow haematopoietic stem cell transplants.

Cord blood banking

In Europe, cord blood banking has been developed in several countries including Germany, France, UK, Italy , Belgium, the Netherlands and Spain. Other local banks have been collecting cord blood mostly for related transplants, the New York Cord Blood directed by P. Rubinstein being the most active [2,3].

Issues of standardisation of methods quantification of haematopoietic stem cells, development, of techniques for cell concentration and enrichment without substantial loss of haematopoietic progenitors, detection of transmissible infectious and genetic diseases, detection of maternal cell contamination and, legal and ethical aspects of cord blood banking and transplant have been discussed extensively.

Collection and cell processing

Two techniques are used, one is to collect cord blood in the delivery room, while the placenta is still in utero, the other is to collect cord blood after delivery in an adjacent room.

Because of the small volume of cord blood ranging from 40 to 150 ml, there is some concern that any attempt at cell manipulation and concentration might result in a considerable cell loss which might impair engraftment [2]. Many banks freeze in a programmed cell freezer whole cord blood in 20% DMSO. Thawing technique is well established, it aims at removing red cells and DMSO [3].

Evaluation of stem cell content is a very important issue since several studies have shown that there is a correlation between the number of mononucleated cells infused and engraftment. There is a correlation between placental weight, time of clamping, speed of processing, volume collected and stem cell content. There is a lot of variation between laboratories which explain why quantification has been a problem and why, in the European study, a correlation was found between the number of mononucleated cells and engraftment, this correlation was not found, anymore, when looking at the number of CD34+ cells and CFU-GM.

Infectious diseases screening

Syphilis and viral tests including HIV, hepatitis B and hepatitis C, CMV are performed on maternal blood. In some countries, HTLV-I and toxoplasmosis are also tested. Most of the time, virology tests are not performed directly on cord blood but a separate aliquot is kept to perform these tests before transplantation. When possible, cord blood is quarantined until a confirmatory test is performed on the mother 3 to 6 months after delivery. In the other cases, performance of very sensitive tests, including viral antigen or nucleic acid screening tests, before delivering the transplant, should considerably decrease the risk of viral transmission [4].

Bacterial infection is also a major issue but it seems that the frequency of bacterial contamination diminishes with the expertise of the staff in charge of the collection.

Genetic diseases

This should be directed by the familial history, the ethnic background and the follow-up of the donor. Tests on cord blood are expensive and there is no real consensus on the type and number of tests which should be performed.

HLA and red cell typing

HLA typing is performed on an aliquot of cord blood. Usually, HLA-A and HLA-B antigens are identified by serology and HLA-DRB1 by DNA amplification methods. In addition, Eurocord is collecting DNA from donor and recipient to perform molecular typing for HLA-C, -DQB 1, -DPB 1, some HLA-A and -B antigens and other markers.

Ethical and legal aspects [5]

It is generally agreed that cord and placental blood is a discarded product and can be used without asking permission but, informed consent must be asked for doing tests on mother and cord blood. In some countries, mother's informed consent is asked after delivery and, if it is obtained, a full medical history is taken, blood sample is drawn from the mother to test for infectious disease markers. In other countries, information on cord blood donation for allogeneic use is given long before delivery and the informed consent process engaged in advance. This gives the opportunity of excluding donors with high risk of transmitting any infectious or genetic disease through careful collection of the family and mother history.

There has been some concerns about the process of information of the family on the results of infectious and genetic disease screening. Another issue is the follow-up of the donor and, in case of need, the possibility for the family to retrieve the autologous cord blood.

Clinical outcome in recipients of cord blood transplant from related and unrelated donors: Eurocord registry [6]

Using the data bases of the European Blood and Marrow Transplantation Group (EBMT) and of the French Society of Bone Marrow Transplantation, centres who had reported cord blood transplants were invited to join Eurocord. In addition non European centres volunteered to enter into the study. Overall 45 centres reported between 1 and 22 cases, verified for data accuracy by a clinical co-ordinator. Of 148 cases reported before December 31, 1996, 5 were excluded because the patients had received bone marrow in addition to CB. Seventy eight patients had received a related and 65 an unrelated CBT. These 2 groups were analysed separately for all endpoints.

Conditioning regimens varied according to diagnosis, previous treatment and disease status. Patients who received a CBT from an HLA identical sibling CBT had been given the conditioning for a bone marrow transplant. Total body irradiation (TBI) combined with cyclophosphamide or other chemotherapy was used in 60 patients, Busulfan was used instead of TBI in 40 patients who received a related CBT (mean age 4 years, range 0.2 to 11 years) and in 24 patients who received an unrelated CBT (mean age 8 years, range 0.3 to 28 years). In 49 patients receiving a mismatched CBT, antithymocyte globulin (ATG) or a monoclonal anti-T cell antibody were given before transplantation. GvHD prophylaxis consisted of cyclosporine (CSA) either alone or combined with prednisone or methotrexate. Established GvHD was usually treated with prednisone. Haematopoietic growth factors G-CSF (granulocyte colony stimulating factor) or GM-CSF (granulocyte macrophage colony stimulating factor) were given after the transplantation in 104 patients (73%) at various dates and doses.

CB was provided from cord blood banks (CBB) in New-York (47 cases), Milan (14 cases), Paris (11 cases), Dusseldorf (6 cases) and local cord blood banks (65 cases). The median volume collected was 99 ml (range 37 to 360), the total median number of NC was 10.8×10^8 (range 1.3 to 58), the median number of CD34+ cells was 3.8×10^6 (range 0.02 to 38) (n=31) and the median number of CFU-GM (colony forming unit granulocyte and macrophage) was 4.4×10^5 (range, 0.01 to 298) (n=83). Collections from related and unrelated donors had similar properties. The median number of nucleated cells infused after thawing was 3.7×10^7 (range, 0.7 to 30), the median number of CD34+ cells was 2×10^5/kg (range 0 to 45) (n=67) and the median number of CFU-GM infused was 2.4×10^4/kg (range 0 to 222) (n=104). HLA typing was performed by serology for class I HLA-A and HLA-B antigens and by low resolution generic oligotyping for DRB1. In related cord blood transplants, 60 patients were transplanted with an HLA genoidentical sibling, 3 had 1 antigen, 5 had 2 antigens, 9 had 3 antigens and 1 had 4 HLA antigens differences. In unrelated cord blood transplants, 9 patients were HLA identical, 43 had 1 HLA difference, 11 had 2 differences and 2 had 3 HLA antigens differences.

Surrogates for engraftment were the time to recover neutrophil and platelet counts after transplantation. Neutrophil recovery was defined as the time to reach an absolute neutrophil count (ANC) $\geq$ 500/µl for 3 consecutive days, no engraftment was defined as no sign of engraftment after day 60 or patients who had another transplant or patients with autologous reconstitution defined as the reappearance of cells with recipient markers such as sex, ABO or HLA markers. Platelet engraftment was defined as the time to reach a sustained platelet count $\geq$20,000/µl in the absence of platelet transfusions. Graft rejection has defined as engraftment followed by pancytopenia or GvHD without signs of myeloid engraftment. Patients, in whom there was no engraftment, were excluded if they died before day 60. Acute GvHD was scored according to standard criteria. Grade 0 and 1 were not counted as significant acute GvHD. For patients surviving more than 100 days, GvHD was defined as chronic and coded as limited or extensive. Relapse, complications and causes of death were also reported.

Patient characteristics

In the total population donor sex was male in 81 and female in 62 cases. In 78 related CBT, 76 donors were siblings, 1 was a cousin and 1 was a child to mother CBT. Of the 143 patients, 95 received a transplant for treatment of a haematological malignancy, 26 had a bone marrow failure syndrome (BMFS), 8 had an haemoglobinopathy and 14 had another type of genetic diseases. Of 62 patients with acute leukaemia, 37 were transplanted in first or second complete remission and 35 were in a more advanced stage, and 10 patients had previously received a bone marrow transplantation (9 autologous and 1 allogeneic).

Overall results

Overall one-year survival was 49±5%, for the entire group of 143 patients. For recipients of CB from related donors, overall one-year survival was 63±6% (Table 1) and for recipients of CB from unrelated donors 29±7% ($p=0.0001$ by the log-rank test, Table 2). In the group of 143 patients, factors associated with prolonged one-year survival were age <6 years ($p=0.0001$), weight <20 kg ($p=0.0001$), infusion of $\geq 3.7\times10^7$/kg NC ($p=0.04$), HLA identity ($p=0.0001$), and recipient negative CMV serology ($p=0.0001$). As the outcome in recipients of CB from related or unrelated donors differed considerably, we decided to analyse related and unrelated CBT separately.

Survival (Table 1, 2)

Among recipients of CBT from related donors, one-year overall survival was 63%±6% with a median follow-up of 29 months (range 1 month to 8 years). It was 73% in HLA matched and 33% in HLA mismatched CBT ($p=0.006$). Variables associated with improved survival were age <6 years, weight <20 kg, negative recipient CMV serology and HLA identity. By using the Cox's model, the most favourable factors were weight <20 kg with a relative risk (RR) of 4.2, 95% confidence interval (CI): 1.9-9.4, $p= 0.0004$ and, negative recipient CMV serology with a RR of 2.4, 95% CI: 1.1-5.5, $p=0.02$.

In recipients of CBT unrelated donors, one-year survival was 29±7% with a median follow-up time of 10 months (1 to 30 months). The number of HLA differences between donor and recipient did not influence survival, probably because we did not use high resolution molecular typing for class I and class II antigens. Negative recipient CMV serology was associated with better survival ($p=0.03$). Patients who received $<3.7\times10^7$ nucleated cells/kg had a one-year survival of 22%, whereas among those with $>3.7\times10^7$ nucleated cells/kg, one-year survival was 41% ($p= 0.07$).

Engraftment

In the entire group of 143 patients, the median time to reach an ANC >500/μl was 30 days (8 to 56) and >20,000/μl platelets (PLTS) was 56 days (9 to 180 days). The probability of an ANC ≥500/μl by day 60 after the transplantation was 79% in recipients of related CB and 87% in recipients of unrelated CB. For platelets, the corresponding probabilities were 62% and 39%.

Table 1. Factors associated with one year survival after cord blood transplantation: related donors (n=78)

	n	Death	%	P
Overall diagnosis	78	30	63	
Leukaemia	46	22	55	0.15
BMFS	17	6	65	
Haemoglobinopathy	8	0	100	
Inborn error	7	2	69	
Age (median):				
– <6 years	45	9	83	0.0001
– 6-15 years	30	19	36	
– ≥15 years	3	2	33	
Weight (median):				
– <20 kg	40	7	82	0.0002
– 20-45 kg	35	21	87	
– ≥45 kg	3	2	33	
Number of nucleated cells infused/kg:				
– $<3.7\times10^7$	48	16	57	0.29
– $\geq3.7\times10^7$	40	14	68	
CMV serology:				
– Negative	40	9	74	0.002
– Positive	36	20	42	
ABO compatibility:				
– Matched	55	26	55	0.04
– Minor mismatched	8	2	75	
– Major mismatched	15	2	85	
– Matched	55	26	55	0.01
– Mismatced	23	4	82	
Number of HLA disparities:				
– 0	60	18	73	
– 1	3	1	67	
– 2	5	2	60	
– 3	9	8	10	
– 4	1	1	0	
– 0	60	18	73	0.006
– ≥1	18	12	33	

Table 1 (continued)

	n	Death	%	P
Gender (recipient/donor):				
– Identical	41	12	73	0.07
– Non identical	36	17	53	
TBI:				
– No	50	14	74	0.02
– Yes	28	16	46	
Serotherapy (ATG + Mac):				
– No	57	22	65	0.93
– Yes	21	8	62	
Prednisone:				
– No	66	22	69	
– Yes	12	8	31	
Growth factors (G-CSF and/or GM-CSF):				
– No	25	10	61	0.72
– Yes	53	20	64	
Day of onset:				
– 0-5 days	24	10	58	0.38
– 6-21 days	13	3	84	
– ≥22 days	11	4	64	
MTX:				
– No	50	15	70	0.03
– Yes	28	15	51	
Serotherapy (in GvH prophylaxis):				
– No	74	28	64	0.67
– Yes	4	2	50	

Considering the group of 78 patients who received CB from a related donor, among 46 patients with malignant diseases, 4 were excluded, 7 did not engraft, (3 received later an autologous bone marrow transplantation, 1 had a reconstitution with his own pretransplant cells and 3 died with an aplastic bone marrow). Of the 17 patients with BMFS, in this group of 78 patients, 3 were excluded, 3 did not engraft, (2 had a second transplant and 1 was aplastic at time of death). Five of 8 patients with Fanconi anaemia are alive with signs of engraftment of the transplanted cord blood. In 8 patients with haemoglobinopathies, 4 did not engraft, (2 received a second BMT) and 2 patients had a reconstitution with their own pretransplant cells. In 7 patients with inborn errors, 5 engrafted, 1 was excluded and 1 did not engraft.

Table 2. Factors associated with one year survival after cord blood transplantation: related donors (n=65)

	n	Death	%	P
Overall diagnosis	65	38	29	
Leukaemia	49	27	31	0.0001
BMFS	9	8	0	
Inborn error	7	3	57	
Age (median):				
– <6 years	27	16	35	0.13
– 6-15 years	18	9	40	
– ≥15 years	20	13	16	
Weight (median):				
– <20 kg	24	13	38	0.18
– 20-45 kg	21	13	29	
– ≥45 kg	20	12	28	
Number of nucleated cells infused/kg:				
– $<3.7\times10^7$	36	23	22	0.07
– $\geq3.7\times10^7$	29	15	41	
CMV serology:				
– Negative	26	11	42	0.03
– Positive	39	27	20	
ABO compatibility:				
– Matched	20	3	57	0.12
– Minor mismatched	20	13	21	
– Major mismatched	4	16	21	
– Matched	20	8	57	0.05
– Mismatced	44	29	21	
Number of HLA disparities:				
– 0	9	5	0	
– 1	43	25	36	
– 2	11	6	34	
– 3	2	2	0	
– 0	9	5	0	
– ≥1	56	33	33	0.077

Table 2 (continued)

	n	Death	%	P
Gender (recipient/donor):				
– Identical	30	17	29	0.99
– Non identical	32	18	37	
TBI:				
– No	30	21	26	0.04
– Yes	35	17	34	
Serotherapy (ATG + Mac):				
– No	13	9	37	0.97
– Yes	52	29	32	
Prednisone:				
– No	18	15	17	0.01
– Yes	47	23	34	
Growth factors (G-CSF and/or GM-CSF):				
– No	14	8	36	0.61
– Yes	51	30	29	
Day of onset:				
– 0-5 days	32	17	30	0.72
– 6-21 days	12	9	22	
– ≥22 days	7	4	43	
MTX:				
– No	56	32	29	0.80
– Yes	9	6	30	
Serotherapy (in GvH prophylaxis):				
– No	62	36	30	0.67
– Yes	3	2	0	

Among 65 recipients of CB from unrelated donors, of the 49 malignant diseases, 7 were excluded, 5 did not engraft. Of 9 patients with BMFS, 8 had Fanconi anaemia, 4 were excluded, 11 did not engraft and died after a second CBT and 1 patient is alive. In 7 patients with inborn errors, 2 were excluded and 1 did not engraft.

Factors associated with engraftment were judged by ANC and platelet counts 60 days after the CBT. In the entire group, 60 days ANC ≥500/μl was associated with $\geq 3.7\times10^7$ nucleated cells /kg (p=0.001) and, platelet ≥20.000/μl, with recipient weight >20 kg (p=0.02) and HLA identity compared to any HLA difference (p=0.0001).

Among recipients of CS from related donors, engraftment was influenced by age (p=0.02), weight (p=0.02) and number of nucleated cells/kg infused (p=0.06). By Cox's analysis, age < 6 years was associated with a higher chance of reaching > 500/µl ANC before day 60 (RR: 0.5, 95%, CI: 0.2-0.9, p: 0.008). For platelets, the most important factor was HLA identity (p=0.0009). Similarly, in the recipients of CB from unrelated donors, ANC and platelet engraftment were associated with a higher number of nucleated cells/kg infused and HLA identity.

Graft-versus-host disease

In recipients of CB from a related donor, acute GvHD ≥ grade II was observed in 14 cases (grade II in 10 cases, grade III in 3 cases and grade IV in 1 case). Chronic GvHD was observed in 8 of 56 patients surviving more than 100 days. In 65 recipients of CB from an unrelated donor, acute GvHD ≥ grade II was observed in 21 cases (grade II in 8 cases, grade III in 9 cases and grade IV in 4 cases). Chronic GvHD was absent in 23 patients surviving more than 100 days.

In related CBT, the number of HLA differences was the most important factor, the incidence of acute GvHD ≥ grade II was 9% in HLA identical related CBT and 50% in HLA mismatched related CBT (p=0.0001). In Cox's analysis, HLA difference was the only factor associated with increased risk of GvHD (RR: 7.7, 95% CI: 2.5-23, p=0.0003).

In unrelated CBT, the incidence of acute GvHD was not modified by the number of HLA differences. CMV negative serology was associated with a decreased risk of acute GvHD (p=0.04).

Other complications, leukaemic relapse and cause of death

Malignant relapse was observed in 22 out of 95 cases. Of the 46 patients transplanted for malignancies with related CBT, 15 patients relapsed, (4 with AML, 5 with ALL, 1 with CML). 5 patients (2 with neuroblastoma and 3 with myelodisplastic syndrome MDS) died of resistant disease. Of 49 patients transplanted for malignancies with an unrelated CBT, 7 patients relapsed.

In 30 out of 78 related CBT, the primary cause of death was relapse in 11 cases, rejection in 8 cases, infection in 6 cases, liver veno-occlusive disease in 2 cases, GvHD in 1 case, cardiac toxicity in 1 case, haemorrhage or other cause in 2 cases. In 38 out of 65 patients who died after unrelated CBT, the primary cause of death was relapse in 6 cases, interstitial pneumonitis in 7 cases, acute respiratory distress syndrome in 2 cases, liver veno-occlusive disease in 3 cases, cardiac toxicity in 2 cases, GVH in 4 cases, rejection in 4 cases, infection in 10 cases, haemorrhage and other cause in 2 cases .

Other results

J. Kurtzberg et al [7] reported a series of 25 patients who received an unrelated cord blood transplant provided by the New York cord blood bank. All except one were children, 23 had a malignancy, 12 were in first or second complete remission (standard risk), 7 were in relapse or in advanced stage of the disease, 2 had leukaemia complicating Fanconi anaemia and Kostmann's syndrome, 1 neuroblastoma and 1 common variable immunodeficiency disease, myelodisplastic syndrome. There were various degrees of HLA incompatibilities. The number of nucleated cells infused correlated with the rate of myeloid engraftment (p:0.002). GVH was observed but it was mild. Twenty-two of these patients engrafted with a median time to reach >500/μl ANC of 22 days. However, all patients received G-CSF to accelerate engraftment. Twelve of the 25 patients had an event free survival rate of 48%. Seven of the 19 patients undergoing transplantation for malignant conditions survived, 6 of 12 patients transplanted in first or second CR survived but most have a short follow-up of less than one year only, 1 of 8 patients who underwent CBT while in remission and survived for more than 100 days had a leukaemic relapse.

J. Wagner et al [8] reported 18 patients who received an unrelated CBT from the New York cord blood bank. Most were children, 13 had a malignant disease, 5 patients only were in 1st or 2nd remission, the other had more advanced disease. Among 5 good risk patients, all were alive with a very short follow-up ranging from 317 to 170 days. The median number of NC/kg was 4.1×10^7/kg (range 1.4 to 40) and of 13 patients surviving for more than 30 days, all engrafted with a median time to reach 500 ANC of 24 days.

More recently, Duke and Minneapolis University pooled there observations of 111 patients transplanted with an unrelated cord blood donor from August 1993 to August 1997. In 51 cases, the donor was HLA identical or with 1 HLA difference, in 58 cases, there were 2 or 3 HLA differences and in 2 cases 4 HLA differences. The mean volume collected was 84 ml (range 40-214) and the median number of nucleated cells infused was 3.5×10^7/kg (range 0.7-33.8). The probability of engraftment was 79%, there was no difference according to HLA differences. The median time to reach more than 500 PMN/mm^3 was 23 days (12-59) and more than 50,000 platelets was 2.4 months [1-8]. in univariate analysis, the speed of engraftment was associated with the number of cells, the number of CD34+ and the number of CFU-GM infused. The probability of grade II-IV GvHD was 35% without differences according to HLA disparities. The frequency of chronic GVH was very low. With a median follow-up time of 1 year, the probability of 2 years survival was 45%. The only factor predictive of survival was the number of cells infused.

Discussion

Possible clinical advantages of CB as a source of allogeneic haematopoietic stem cells for transplantation may be related to differences between fetal and adult haematopoietic stem cells [9,10].Compared to adults HSC, CB HSC have distinctive proliferative advantages including higher number of colonies in culture, increased cell cycle rate, autocrine production of growth factors and longer telomeres [11,12]. All these properties should favour engraftment and growth of CB HSC. Moreover, relative immaturity of CB lymphocytes might reduce the risk and severity of GvHD which, in turn, could permit a greater HLA disparity between donor and recipient than is usually accepted with adult blood or marrow HSC transplants. CBBs have developed world-wide and there has been a considerable effort to standardise banking procedures [6,7]. CBBs have several advantages including availability of this source of cells, low viral infection rate at birth, and possibility to collect cord blood in ethnic groups not represented in BM donor registries. There are potential problems related to legal and ethical issues concerning patents on CB cells and issues on informed consent and follow-up of the donor for detection of possible transmission of genetic or infectious diseases.

This report indicates that CB is an alternative source of HSC for use in patients with malignant and non malignant haematological diseases. With this new source of HSC and other technical developments in haematopoietic stem cell transplantation, we may be able to identify a donor for any given patient who needs a transplant. This new situation calls for carefully planned prospective studies of the clinical efficacy of different strategies of selecting donors.

References

1. Gluckman E, Broxmeyer HE, Auerbach AD, et al. Hematopoietic reconstitution in a patient with Fanconi's anemia by means of umbilical cord blood from an HLA-identical sibling. New Engl J Med 1989;321:1174-8.
2. Rubinstein P, Rosenfield RD, Adamson JW, Stevens CE. Stored placental blood for unrelated bone marrow reconstitution. Blood 1993;81:1679-90.
3. Rubinstein P, Dobrila L, Rosenfield RE, et al. Processing and cryopreservation of placental/umbilical cord blood for unrelated bone marrow reconstitution. Proc Natl Acad Sci USA 1995;92:10119-22.
4. Silberstein LE. Jeffreys LC. Placental blood banking: a new frontier in transfusion medicine. N Engl J Med 1996;335:199-201.
5. Sugarman J, Reisner EG, Kurtzberg J. Ethical aspects of banking placental blood for transplantation. JAMA 1995;21;:783-5.
6. Gluckman E. The therapeutic potential of foetal and neonatal hematopoietic stem cells. N Engl J Med 1996; 335:1839-40.
7. Kurtzberg J, Laughlin M, Graham L, et al. Placental blood as a source of hematopoietic stem cells for transplantation into unrelated recipients. N Engl J Med 1996; 335:157-66.
8. Wagner JE, Rosenthal J, Sweetman R, et al. Successful transplantation of HLA. Matched and HLA mismatched umbilical cord blood from unrelated donors: analysis of engraftment and acute graft versus host disease. Blood 1996;88:795-802.
9. Morrison SJ, Wandycz AM, Akashi K, et al. The aging of hematopoietic stem cells. Nature Med 1996;2:1011-6.
10. Morrison SJ, Prowse KR, Ho P, et al. Telomerase activity in hematopoietic cells is associated with self-renewal potential. Immunity 1996;5:207-16.
11. Mayani H, Lansdorp PM. Thy-1 expression is linked to functional properties of primitive hematopoietic progenitors cells from human umbilical cord blood. Blood 1994;83:2410-7.
12. Vaziri H, Dragowska W, Allsop RC, et al. Evidence for a mitotic clock in human hematopoietic stem cells: loss of telomeric DNA with age. Proc Natl Acad Sci USA 1994;91:9857-60.

Appendix

Eurocord centers:

- ABECASIS M, BMT Unit, Inst. Portugues Oncologia, Lisboa, Portugal.
- ARCESE W, Institute of Hematology, degli Studi « La Sapienza », Roma, Italy.
- BADELL SERRA I, Department of pediatrics, Hospitai Santa Creu i Santa Pau, Barcelona, Spain.
- BEKSAC M, Department of Hematology/Oncology, Ibni Sina Hospital, Ankara, Turkey.
- BERNAUDIN F, Service d'Hématologie, Hôpital Henri-Mondor, Créteil. France.
- BOGDANIC V, Division of Haematology/BMT Unit, University Hospital Center-Rebro, Zagreb, Croatia.
- BOSI A, BMT Unit, Department of Hematology, Ospedale di Carregi, Firenze, Italy.
- CAHN JY, Service d'Hématologie, Hôpital Jean Minjoz, Besançon, France.
- CORNU G, Department of Pediatrics, University of Louvain, Brussels, Belgium.
- DELLIERS LG, Instituto Scienze Mediche, University of Milano, Italy.
- DOKAL I, Department of Hematology, Hammersmith Hopital, London, UK.
- FAVRE C, BMT Unit Pediatric Department, University of Pisa, Pisa, Italy.
- FERNANDEZ MN, Servicio de Hematologia y Hemoterapia, Clinica Puerta de Hierro, Madrid, Spain.
- FERREIRA E, Serviço de Transplante de Medula Ossea, Hospital Israelita Albert Einstein, Sao Paulo, Brazil.
- FISHER A, Unité d'Immunologie et d'Hématologie, Hôpital Necker, Paris, France.
- GIBSON BES, Royal Hospital for Sick Children, Glasgow, UK.
- GLUCKMAN E, Service d'Hématologie Greffe de Moelle, Hôpital Saint-Louis, Paris, France.
- JOUET JP, Service des maladies du Sang, Hôpital Claude Huriez, Lille, France.
- KINOSHITA A, Kelo Bone Marrow Transplant Program, Department of Pediatrics, Keio University School of Medicine, Tokyo, Japan.
- KOBYLKA P, Institute of Hematology and Blood Transfusion, Praha, Czech Republic.
- LAPORTE JP, Department of Hematology, Hôpital Saint-Antoine, Paris, France.
- LOCATELLI F, Pediatric Clinic, University of Pavia, Pavia, Italy.
- LUTZ P, Unité d'Hématologie-Oncologie, Hôpital Civil, Strasbourg, France.
- MASSZI T, Department of Hematology BMT Unit, St. Laszlo Hospital, Budapest, Hungary.
- MILLONE J, Instituto de Transplante de Medula Ossea, Fundacion Mainetti, Cronnet, Argentina.
- MILOVIC V, Instituto de criopreservacion y transplante de medula ossea. Antartida Hospital Privado, Buenos Aires, Argentina.
- MINIERO R, Department of Pediatrics, University of Torino Ospedale Regina Margherita, Torino, Italy.
- NAGLER A, Department of BMT, Hadassah University Hospital, Jerusalem, Israel.
- ORTEGA JJ, Hospital M. Infantil Vall d'Hebron, Barcelona, Spain.
- PASQUINI R, Serviço de Transplante de Medula Ossea, Hospital de Clinicas, Curitiba, Brazil.
- PENSION A, BMT Unit Clinica Pediatrica III, Policlinico S, Orsola Malphighi, Bologna, Italy.

- PEREZ-OYTEZA J, Servicio de Hematologia, Hospital Ramon y Cajal, Madrid, Spain.
- PETERS C, St Anna Kinderspital, Vienna, Austria.
- PLOUVIER E, Service d'Oncologie-Hématologie Pédiatrique, Hôpital Saint-Jacques, Besançon, France.
- REIFFERS J, Hôpital du Haut Levêque, Pessac, France.
- ROBERTS I, Department of Hematology, Hammersmith Hospital, London, UK.
- ROITTMAN S, Serviço de Hematologia e Transplante de Medula Ossea, Hospital de Clinicas, Porto Alegre, Brazil.
- SAARINEN U, Children's Hospital, University of Helsinki, Helsinki, Finland.
- SOUILLET G, Immuno-Hématologie Pédiatrique et Transplantation de moelle osseuse, Hôpital Debrousse, Lyon, France.
- STARY J, Pediatric Department Oncology, University Hospital Motol, Praha, Czech Republic.
- TAKAUE Y, University of Tokushima, Japan.
- URBAN C, Division of Pediatrics Hematology/Oncology, University Children's Hospital, Graz, Austria.
- VEYS P, Great Ormond Street Hospital for Children NHS Trust, London, UK.
- VILMER E, Hôpital Robert Debré, Paris, France.
- VOSSEN JM, BMT Unit and Department of Hematology, University Hospital Leiden, The Netherlands.
- WIKTOR-JEDRZEJCZACK, Department of Immunology, Warsaw, Poland.
- YANIV I, Bone Marrow Transplantation Unit, Children's Medical Center of Israel, Tel Aviv University, Tel Aviv, Israel.
- ZINTL F, Department of Pediatrics, University of Jena, Jena, Germany.

Cord Blood Banks:
- BENBUNAN M, Hôpital Saint Louis, Paris, France.
- BROSSARD Y, CHP Hôpital Saint Vincent de Paul, Paris, France.
- RUBINSTEIN P, New-York Cord Blood Bank, New-York, USA.
- WERNET P, Bone Marrow Donor Center, Dusseldorf, Germany.
- SIRCHIA G, Milano Cord Blood Bank, Milano, Italy.
- RAFFOUX C. MD France Greffe de Moelle Hôpital Saint Louis, Paris for reviewing HLA typing.

DISCUSSION

L.T. Goodnough, H.J.C. de Wit

J.C. Fratantoni, Rockville, MD, USA: It was interesting that you got some response from the 1990 SANGUIS report when you looked at the results in 1995. In the United States there was a conference on fresh frozen plasma in 1984[1] and they spelled out very few logical indications of fresh frozen plasma. They then looked at the results of that conference several years later and it had no effect on physicians' use of fresh frozen plasma at all. There was no change in the reimbursement policies for fresh frozen plasma in the States. Regarding aid to the SANGUIS study, was there any change in the financial policies towards fresh frozen plasma that may have led to some changes that you saw?

Ph. Baele, Brussels, B: It is difficult to answer this question because there were several concomitant changes including new rules asking the clinicians to sign a new paper before transfusion of plasma, telling that it was one of 5 or 6 admitted indications. Even so I am not confident that the results I showed you in my hospital can be extended to other hospitals, especially recollecting the wide variations found in Belgium. We extend from both sides further than the variation found for the SANGUIS study; we go higher on one side and lower on the other. So, I am not sure that feeding back those results to the medical community as a whole has changed dramatically the behaviour of people who were not concerned. Those are the feed-back data. We went back to our teams, we discussed with each team their own results comparing them with the array of the results of the rest of Europe and then they understood how they were different from the others and they tried to add up or to correct or to whatever they wanted to add up or correct. I think personalising feed-back is the trick.

L.T. Goodnough, St. Louis, MO, USA: Do you think that the availability of solvent detergent plasma is a roadblock to educating physicians to use less plasma?

Ph. Baele: I do not think so, because the switch to viral inactivated plasma was made about four years ago in Belgium.

1. National Institute of Health Consensus Conference. Fresh frozen plasma: indications and risks. JAMA 1985;253:551-53.

H.J.C. de Wit, Leeuwarden, NL: If I may comment; the introduction of viral safe plasma at least in our region where we use quarantined plasma, was used to discuss again the use of plasma with all clinicians. While introducing viral safe plasma usage dropped by 50%; so you can use it as a moment to discuss again about indications and proper use.

If I may ask a question; you added two drugs to the list of pharmacological methods to limit blood loss. To limit blood use which is very good, α_2 agonists might be the easiest to use and it might be broader used than only in large surgical procedures. Would it be worthwhile to have a broader look in normal surgical procedures?

Ph. Baele: This has been done for maxillofacial procedures for example also for wisdom teeth removal, but is different. Only bowel manipulation gives you that tremendous increase in prostaglandines. Of course you have also other benefits in using anti-inflammatory drugs to reduce swelling for example; reduced bleeding then becomes a minor side-benefit.

L.T. Goodnough: Dr. Rocha, do you have a minimum dose of cord cells that you require for transplantation in terms of nucleated cells or CD34.

V. Rocha, Paris, F: The Eurocord protocol has established a minimum of $1x10^7$ nucleated cells infused (after thawing) per kg of recipient. We have to calculate a median loss of 20% of nucleated cells after thawing. The number of CD34 cells infused was not analysed in consequence of different ways of counting CD34+ cells by different centres.

L.T. Goodnough: So it is 1×10^7 nucleated cells infused per kg.

V. Rocha: We have been looking at the outcome of patients who received between 1.0 and 2.0 x 10^7 nucleated cells infused/kg and we found that there was in the 143 patients a 69% probability of neutrophil engraftment (ANC>500/μl) and 49% of reaching 20,000 platelets on day 62. Also the delay of engraftment was longer.

L.T. Goodnough: These children or the recipients are they given growth factors during the transplantation.

V. Rocha: Yes, this was a multicentre and retrospective study, so each centre has its own protocol to begin haematopoietic growth factors. This is the reason we have not analysed the influence of G-CSF. Our goal in Eurocord group is to begin a randomised protocol to study the influence of growth factors for engraftment.

L.T. Goodnough: Your survival data for the CMV positive recipients especially in the unrelated patients, it looks as if there is a free fall in survival within several months after transplantation; that looks just like it is continuously going down. Does that surprise you?

V. Rocha: Indeed, this is a very striking factor but not unexpected, since CMV serology prior to transplant is an adverse factor for survival in unrelated bone marrow transplant setting.

M.K. Elias, Groningen, NL: Dr. Rocha, you mentioned that the survival in the unrelated setting is 20%. There is a great discrepancy between your results and those of the recent American study in which they found 50% survival with similar criteria[2]. How would you explain this; would the significance in outcome be attributable to the method of HLA typing?

V. Rocha: We cannot compare the results between these two analyses since indications, HLA typing, disease status and choice of donor are not the same and, we know the influence of all these factors in the outcome of transplantation.

M.K. Elias: Using high resolution DNA typing in the American study and serological HLA typing in the European one means that there are more HLA discrepancies in the population of Gluckman?

V. Rocha: For this analysis we have only studied low resolution HLA typing since approximately 85% of the unrelated cord blood units delivered had high resolution HLA typing. Cord Blood Banks have a depository of DNA of these units and our goal is to check out all units.

F. Falkenburg, Leiden, NL: Well I think it also is very important to realise that there are centres and in particular centres in the United States like Duke university where umbilical cord blood transplantation is performed almost up front, a first choice. Whereas in Europe in many centres all the other possibilities are first excluded before someone does an umbilical cord blood transplantation, which results in a selection of very unfavourable patients. Even the ones that look on paper as low risk patients in fact are frequently patients that are relatively at a high risk because of long term search for an unrelated donor. So, I think there are really two different populations.

M.K. Elias: Dr. Falkenburg, you mentioned in the characteristics of the UCB grafts that the HLA typing comes in the first place.

F. Falkenburg: The order of characteristics was not based on preference.

M.K. Elias: But would you give now the priority of the number of nucleated cells in view of the analysis of the phase I trial presented by Wagner, recently[2].

---

2. Fourth International Cord Blood Congress, Italy, September 1997.

It came to light that the only factor affecting survival is the dozen of nucleated cells. So in view of this knowledge my question would be if Eurocord would chose between two grafts, one perfect match with low number of progenitors and the other one or two antigen disparity and a high number of progenitors; for which of the two variables would the choice be made?

F. Falkenburg: It is impossible to answer this question from a scientific point of view. It would depend for instance on the age of the patient and the disease. If you have a 20 years old patient, there are too few patients transplanted to make any judgements. My bet is that HLA typing is important in those cases. Now I think that if you look at the kinetics of stem cell transplantation in animals but also in humans and you think about doubling the number of progenitor cells gives you at most two to three days of reduction of time between the transplantation and the recovery of the first cells. So, I think in an elderly patient where the risk of graft versus host disease is higher and the risk of infections is also higher, like in unrelated bone marrow transplantations, the better the match the better the outcome. So, in that situation I would chose for an HLA match. Of course you need a certain minimal number of cells to do the transplantation. If you have a very young patient of about one year old, the likelihood of engraftment is high anyway, but in those patients the risk of graft versus host disease is also relatively low. So, for very young patients my choice is not relevant. In the elderly patient I think HLA typing is extremely important, but of course, you need as many cells as you can get.

J.C. Fratantoni: Dr. Spence you ended up by talking about transfusion medicine people educating their surgical colleagues. It has been my impression that that often is not very effective. I will put it bluntly; some wise man told me a long time ago that surgeons have to teach surgeons and to educate them. What do you think about that and what might be the best way for surgeons in the US and in Europe.

R.K. Spence, Staten Island, NY, USA: Maybe we should start with a big hammer to get their attention. I think we have come a long way in educating surgeons by drawing their attention to the issue. One of the primary elements of education is you have to identify the problem first and you have somehow to be aware of it; I think we have done that to a great extent, for example with orthopaedic surgeons it is now acceptable to consider autologous predonation as an alternative in orthopaedic surgery; it is almost a standard of care and standard of care in the US is really a legal terminology so that most orthopaedic surgeons that were taken to court by a patient and had not offered autologous predonation there is a chance he can loose a lawsuit, because of that he could be held liable. So we have got at least to that point. We can get surgeons' attention through liability as we started the conference in the beginning talking about it is one of the areas of concern. Moreover we have to stop arguing back and forth amongst ourselves as to how good is this technology compared to another technology. Let us take a look at everything, put it on the table and bring it into the medical schools. Start teaching the students there; bring it into the residencies and make it part of the curricula. That is where I think we will see the best impact: teach people early as part of their clinical practices in the training. If you go after the grey hairs like me it is a lot tougher to get to change ways.

A.W.M.M. Koopman-van Gemert, Blaricum, NL: As an anaesthesiologist I can only watch the sutures. There are different techniques if I see surgeons working for the same procedure. I think some of them have learned techniques to lose little or very little blood and others are trained different. I know in the United States they have bloodless hospitals and they operate in a certain way. I think that can be developed more because for me as an anaesthesiologist it is incredible that for the same procedure for instance an aneurysm of the aorta some can do with 500 ml blood loss and the other for the same procedure 2,000 ml. I can imagine sometimes it is more difficult but that is not always the case. I think techniques are also important to train and to try to find out what makes the difference for a surgeon, is it the surgical field, the tissue layer he uses. I know from the bloodless hospitals that they can do much more and that we often are in too much hurry and want to make production. Maybe when we do it somewhat easier and take more time it could be very important.

R.K. Spence: One thing what will work is to get you guys out of the blood bank and get us out of the operating room and meet in the transfusion committee. I found that that worked when I was in my former institution, getting the surgeons and anaesthesiologists involved in the transfusion committee and establish some of the practices. Set the rule, set the guidelines and let everybody play by those rules, I think that can make a difference.

C.Th. Smit Sibinga, Groningen, NL: Could I also make a comment and contribute. It is not only the surgeon but it is also the response of the anaesthesiologist to what the surgeon really does. I have observed both of them and seen differences in responses of anaesthesiologists to certain blood losses. That varies from immediate action with transfusion to more expectative type of approaches looking at what happens, what was the cause of the bleed at that point in time and could we cover the period in an other way rather than transfusing immediately. I think we should not only have the surgeons and the blood bankers together at the table but include the anaesthesiologists and get all three of us together.

A.W.M.M. Koopman-van Gemert: Yes, I agree. It is more important as a hospital to decide what to offer, how we shall do it and what will be the haematocrit and then make the guidelines. Everyone should not only follow but use the guideline. I think that is the better way because then you have direct interaction between everybody and you can talk about why do you use that kind of technique and why do you respond in that way.

C.Th. Smit Sibinga: That is correct. I am glad you mentioned to practise guidelines, because dr. Fergusson if I may turn the question to you at the very last part of your presentation you mentioned the practised guideline and you said perhaps I would suggest that would be a top priority to start with a practised guideline and then follow the rest of the things; am I correct?

D. Fergusson, Ottawa, C: Yes, it was not a major point to mention practised guidelines, I do not know if they really work or not; that has not been fully evaluated and practised guidelines can change, can vary from province to province in Canada, from institute to institute so I think the jury is still open on practised guidelines.

C.Th. Smit Sibinga: The guide as such will not work if those who have to work with the guideline are not informed and are not educated.

D. Fergusson: Absolutely, it cannot happen in a vacuum and develop by surgery.

C.Th. Smit Sibinga: There should be something as a reference to support the guideline to follow and only if you do so you can create a reference to which you could evaluate the ultimate practice.

D. Fergusson: I agree with that, yes.

R.K. Spence: Let me just comment if I may. Practised guidelines are the first step but they are a very needed step. I was fortunate to work with a group that published the practised guidelines and issues in surgery that was published in 1995. The editors of the American Journal of Surgery just loved us, because that is the most successful supplement they ever printed[3]. They have printed it twice now; 50,000 copies of that for distribution so in addition to the initial mailing they put in over a 100,000 copies of that. People ask for that because there is no basic information put together in that format. I think this group has a great opportunity to get this information together and distribute it, but then just what dr. Fergusson said you need as a number one to put it in use and as you say also dr. Smit Sibinga that you have to put it in use and then look at the educational tools for evaluating, how long it has been used. But the first steps creating information creating educational tools and resources, proceedings of this kind of meeting to be distributed well beyond the Netherlands that would be wonderful.

D.B.L. McClelland, Edinburgh, UK: Dr. Rocha, you showed this remarkable fact of recipients CMV status and survival; have you analysed that in terms of the age of the recipients.

---

3. Spence RK. Consensus Conference: blood management surgical practice guidelines. Am J Surg 1995;170:6A(suppl).

V. Rocha: Indeed, if we analyse the related group, there is a correlation between CMV status and age. In a multivariate analysis, a positive CMV serology is the most important factor. In the unrelated group this correlation is not significant and CMV positivity probably reflects a multifactorial consequence as the status of disease.

D.B.L. McClelland: The other thing that worries me about the CMV observation is just the virus that you are looking for. Could it be that it is an indicator for susceptibility or exposure to other agents which might in fact be the critical factor or at least a co-factor in the way the recipient handles the graft. Earlier in your presentation you mentioned a much lower level of virus infection in the cord data.

V. Rocha: Dusseldorf cord blood bank has performed CMV-PCR of all units and only 0.12% of the units were positive. It probably means that the donor/recipient rate of infection is negligible. The problem of CMV status is a well known factor affecting the outcome of transplants mainly unrelated and mismatched transplants, correlated with acute GvHD and non engraftment. CMV disease was not an important cause of death in this group of patients. As it is a retrospective and multicentre study we do not know which kind of prophylaxis and treatment for CMV was used. Transplant centres are afraid of using Gancyclovir as a prophylaxis due to the myelosuppression. Another hypothesis is the non-exposure of cord blood lymphocytes to CMV antigens. Prospective studies on immunological reconstitution might help us to understand this phenomenon.

F. Falkenburg: I think the problem with this is that there is now one variable that comes out but still it is a very small group of patients. If you look at unrelated bone marrow transplantation, there is a correlation between the risk of infection and mismatch. Apparently, it is easier to cope with the infection if the match is better. It looks like an overall immune reaction that causes certain complications. In CMV disease after transplantation for instance, you may have a pulmonary disease and then an overall immune response which also activates the CMV or the CMV infection may be the primary trigger. In that case it induces both graft versus host disease and pneumonitis and other infections after cord blood transplantation, because normally foetal or child T-cells will see the CMV in a primary infection in contrast to BMT. So it could be that the type of infection is different if you come with naive cells, than in a situation where T-cells are already developed in an individual.

C.Th. Smit Sibinga: Another aspect which was touched upon in the cord cell presentations which intrigue us all is the fact that indeed the cord cells are less mature and show a much more intense cell renewal capacity than those which you generally collect from the peripheral blood. The point, however, is that with the seemingly long recovery of a certain amount of countable cells in the peripheral blood following the transplantation so far all the presentations here as well as in other meetings mention the amount of complications in terms of infections and bleeding to be extremely low. You did not mention it at all; you only mentioned the engraftment failures and the HLA problems, the graft versus host. But the other point is the bleeding occasions.

F. Falkenburg: I think it is very important to distinguish between overall engraftment and speed of engraftment. The major difference that has been presented is the speed of engraftment; the speed of engraftment is slower when the number of cells infused per kg bodyweight is lower. But that does not entirely predict overall engraftment. So, those are in fact two different things. From a hypothetical point of view you need only one real good stem cell for long term engraftment. But you need a lot of little more mature cells for short term engraftment. So the total number of CD34 positive cells like in mobilised peripheral blood is probably very relevant for the short term engraftment. But it may not be that relevant for overall engraftment if you live long enough to get good engraftment and to survive infection.

C.Th. Smit Sibinga: An other facet of the diamond is the repopulation of the marrow space as such and the maturation with the recovery of the peripheral blood. Seemingly there is a difference between these also. So, what seems to happen is a repopulation of the marrow to a certain stage. It does not come to full maturation and lineaging, reason why we do not see for a long a time a recovery of mature cells in peripheral blood where there is already a substantial degree of repopulation of marrow.

F. Falkenburg: You probably refer to the studies for instance of Wagner[4] where he found three or four weeks after transplantation there are hardly any cells in the periphery whereas when he performed bone marrow aspirates he saw very high numbers of cells in the marrow. But the problem is that the major infections are not as far as I understand within the first four weeks, but they are the opportunistic infections that come later. It is not the classical bacterial infection which is probably the main course of death of infections within the first four weeks but after that it is the combination of a T-cell immunity, B-cell immunity and granulocytopenia. So, in that situation the immaturity of the T-cells that you infuse may in fact be a disadvantage for the first month after the transplantation as far as the likelihood of coping with opportunistic infections is involved.

L.T. Goodnough: Dr. Fergusson I have a question for you and maybe the drs. Murphy and McClelland can help. The consensus conference of the Royal College of Physicians of Edinburgh on autologous blood[5] if I remember was fairly definite about the idea that autologous blood donation is not a standard of care in the European Union and there was a fairly long list of pretty exclusive exclusions for cardiac surgical patients. But I was intrigued to see that 50% of the Scottish hospitals in cardiac surgery indicated that they do offer autologous

---

4. Wagner JE. Umbilical cord blood transplantation. Transfusion 1995;35:619-21.
5. Consensus Conference on Autologous Transfusion. Royal College of Physicians of Edinburgh, Edinburgh, Soctland 1995.

blood donation at their hospital; it did exceed urologic surgery and orthopaedic surgery in Scotland. I was wondering if you had an opinion on that.

D. Fergusson: That is four centres, four centres performing cardiac surgery and it was used in two of them.

J.P. AuBuchon, Lebanon, NH, USA: I find the idea of cord blood stem cell transplantation very exciting and very intriguing but also in some aspects very troubling. The issues that are not resolved for me or that I have difficulty coming to a conclusion now are the ethical issues. For example, children have been conceived for the purpose of providing a bone marrow donor. If the intended recipient is large how quickly should the cord be clamped? What type of informed consent is appropriate and should a parent be offered the opportunity to have this frozen cord blood sample reserved for the child for autologous transplantation for thirty years later possibly rather than have it been used for allogeneic purposes? There are no easy answers to all these questions.

F. Falkenburg: Many of those issues are debating issues in particular keeping the cord blood for autologous transplantation. One simple problem is costs. It may be very nice to have your own cord blood if you have breast cancer in 60, 70 years and use it for autologous transplantation. I think it is not very likely at this moment that we can predict what the type of treatment will be by then. But there are also diseases where an autologous transplantation is probably not the best choice and leukaemia maybe one of those. But of course you can endlessly discuss that situation. About clamping or any type of those arguments about conceiving a donor. I think there is an overall difference between a family donor and an unrelated donor, a directed donation and a non-directed donation, because that situation is not very much different in allogeneic transplantation. There is of course also already a long discussion whether for instance the donor in a HLA-identical sibling situation benefits from a transplantation or not and there have been many ethical discussion about that. As far as the unrelated transplants are involved I think there is consensus that for harvesting for unrelated cord blood transplantation those who are collecting the material and are banking the material should not be involved in any decisions made in the delivery room. The related situation is of course different because that is a directed donation, and there is in a certain way a benefit of the family for a large transplant.

IV. THE BALANCE OF RISKS, BENEFITS AND COSTS

INDICATIONS FOR RED BLOOD CELL TRANSFUSION

C.R. Valeri, P. Crowley, J. Loscalzo

Introduction

Since 1983 when it became apparent that the human immunodeficiency virus (HIV) could be transmitted through blood transfusions, the number of blood transfusions administered in the United States has decreased significantly [1-7]. Before the potential risk of HIV infection from donor blood became known, a haematocrit value of 30% and a haemoglobin concentration of 10 g/dl served as the clinical indication for a red blood cell transfusion [8]. Currently, a more restrictive transfusion practice is employed, where haematocrit values must reach much less than 30% even, though much of the reported data in support of this practice have been obtained from retrospective studies [9-22].

Red blood cell transfusion: risks vs benefits

The potential risks of a transfusion include haemolytic transfusion reactions, transfusion-related graft-versus-host disease, non-haemolytic febrile transfusion reactions, transmission of disease, immune suppression, and posttransfusion infection [5-7,23-28].

The benefits of red blood cell transfusion are increases in oxygen carriage and delivery to tissues; increased carbon dioxide carriage and delivery to the lungs; regulation of acid-base balance; and increased red blood cell volume, plasma volume, and total blood volume [23,24].

When to transfuse red blood cells

Decisions on when or whether to transfuse red blood cells must take the following into consideration:

Patient condition

Whether or not to transfuse a patient depends upon the patient's pathophysiology; the clinical situation, whether for elective, urgent or emergency reasons; the disease for which the patient is being transfused; and whether the transfusion is required before, during, or after surgery. In addition, the physician must also consider the patient's cerebrovascular, cardiovascular, haemodynamic, pulmonary, and haematologic status. Most anaemic patients increase blood flow to compensate for a decrease in oxygen carriage. However, decreases in haematocrit and haemoglobin concentrations in patients with impaired blood flow as a result of cardiac dysfunction, coronary artery or cerebrovascular disease, and failure of pulmonary function to properly oxygenate the blood may result in increased morbidity and mortality [22].

Red cell volume status

The decision to transfuse or not is usually based on measurements of haematocrit value and haemoglobin concentration in the patient's peripheral venous blood. However, these measurements do not give a true indication of the red blood cell deficit because they yield inaccurate estimates of red blood cell volume, plasma volume, and total blood volume [23,24]. Anaemic patients are usually hypovolemic [29]. In the hypovolemic anaemic patient, there may be decreases in both plasma volume and red blood cell volume but not in the peripheral venous haematocrit and haemoglobin concentration [23,24,30-32]. Thus, it is necessary to measure more than the peripheral venous haematocrit value and haemoglobin concentration to accurately estimate the therapeutic effectiveness of a red blood cell transfusion. Accurate measurements of red blood cell volume, plasma volume and total blood volume are difficult to obtain because testing requires the use of radioactive labelling of autologous red blood cells with chromium-51 (51-Cr) or technetium-99m (99mTc) [29,33].

Assessment of central vs peripheral volume restoration

Clinicians usually assess the restoration of blood volume from measurements of mean arterial pressure; heart rate; pulmonary artery wedge pressure; cardiac output; arterial pO_2, pCO_2, pH; and urine output [30,34,35]. These measurements assess the central blood volume but not the peripheral blood volume or the total blood volume. The peripheral blood volume refers to the volume of blood in the muscles, bones, skin, and, importantly, the gastrointestinal tract.

In anaemic patients, mortality is usually associated with a failure to restore perfusion and oxygen delivery to vital organs, and morbidity with a failure to restore perfusion and oxygen delivery to both vital organs and non-vital organs such as the gastrointestinal tract and the extremities. In hypovolemic anaemic patients, a reduction in perfusion to the gastrointestinal tract may produce intestinal ischaemia with entry of bacteria from the gut into the circulation producing endotoxin-mediated multiple organ dysfunction [36-38].

Changes in the haematocrit and haemoglobin values as indicators of red cell transfusion effectiveness

With the current practice of relying solely on measurements of peripheral haematocrit level and haemoglobin concentration to identify the red blood cell transfusion trigger, many patients might be deprived of transfusion therapy that would be beneficial to their well being.

Extensive studies in patients with traumatic injuries exhibiting hypovolemic anaemia with significant reductions in red cell, plasma and total blood volumes have shown that although transfusions of red blood cells increased both red blood cell and plasma volumes, only minimal increases in the haematocrit value and haemoglobin concentration were observed [30,31]. The increased plasma volume seen in these hypovolemic anaemic patients following a red blood cell transfusion was a consequence of recruitment of extravascular proteins via the lymphatic circulation into the systemic circulation [23,24,30-32].

The traumatised hypovolemic anaemic patients had normal central red blood cell volumes and significantly reduced peripheral red blood cell and total red blood cell volumes [30]. The transfusion of washed red blood cells to these patients resulted in a significant increase in peripheral red blood cell volume, but there was no increase in the central red blood cell volume during the 24-hour posttransfusion period [30].

The role of the red blood cell

The role of red blood cells in the carriage and delivery of oxygen to tissues, carriage and delivery of carbon dioxide to the lungs, and regulation of acid-base balance is well established. However, the role of red blood cells in the regulation of plasma volume has only recently been recognised [30-32]. The red blood cell volume plays a role in the regulation of the plasma volume; in most patients without renal insufficiency, a reduction in red blood cell volume usually is associated with a reduction in plasma volume and total blood volume [23,24,30,32].

Alternatives to red blood cell transfusion

In recent years, the clinical use of erythropoietin to treat normovolemic anaemic patients with renal disease has resulted in a considerable improvement in their well-being [39]. Erythropoietin is usually administered to normovolemic anaemic patients with renal disease to achieve a haematocrit value of 30 to 35% and haemoglobin concentration of 10 to 12 g/dl. Human recombinant erythropoietin also has been recommended in the hope of reducing allogeneic blood transfusions in surgical patients. Human recombinant erythropoietin has been recommended for anaemic patients with haemoglobin concentrates of greater than 10 g/dl and less than 13 g/dl undergoing elective surgery and patients at high risk for significant perioperative blood loss.

Summary

Because of the limited value of the haematologic and haemodynamic measurements in assessing the need for a red blood cell transfusion, clinical judgement is especially important. Symptoms of red cell volume deficit such as tachycardia, shortness of breath, pallor, decreased tissue turgor, postural hypotension, light-headedness-dizziness, decreased appetite, weakness, and fatigue must be taken into account. A patient should be properly apprised of the potential risks and benefits of a transfusion and in some cases even allowed to play a role in this important decision.

The benefits of an haematocrit range of 30 to 35% include improved oxygen delivery and enhanced haemostasis, which will help minimise complications in patients at high risk for ischaemia and perioperative non-surgical bleeding. In these settings, the conservative transfusion practice using a lower haematocrit range should be replaced with a more aggressive approach. The known risks of blood transfusion would appear to be sufficiently low and the benefits sufficiently high to justify maintaining a haematocrit value of at least 30%. An even higher haematocrit value of 35% may be desirable in patients who have overt cardiopulmonary disease or who are at high risk for myocardial ischaemia. Retrospective studies conducted to persuade us that a conservative approach to red cell transfusion is a safe and prudent practice are not what we need. What is needed is a series of well-designed, prospective, randomised trials to evaluate the impact of a more aggressive transfusion policy on perioperative mortality, morbidity, and non-surgical bleeding in patients with known cardiopulmonary disease or who are at high risk for myocardial and cerebrovascular ischaemia.

Acknowledgements

The authors acknowledge the editorial assistance of Ms. Cynthia A. Valeri and Ms. Gina Ragno and the secreterial assistance of Ms. Marilyn Leavy.

References

1. Surgenor DM, Wallace EL, Hale SG, Gilpatrick MW. Changing patterns of blood transfusion in four sets of United States Hospitals, 1980 to 1985. Transfusion 1988;28:513-8.
2. Surgenor DM, Wallace EL, Hao SHS, Chapman RH. Collection and transfusion of blood in the United States, 1982-1988. N Engl J Med 1990:322:1646-51.
3. Wallace EL, Churchill WH, Surgenor DM, et al. Collection and transfusion of blood and blood components in the United States, 1992. Transfusion 1995;35:802-12.
4. Consensus Conference. Perioperative red blood cell transfusion. JAMA 1988;260: 2700-3.
5. Dodd RY. The risk of transfusion-transmitted infections. N Engl J Med 192;322:419-21.
6. Schreiber GB, Busch MP, Kleinman SH, Korelitz JJ. The risk of transfusion-transmitted viral infections. N Engl J Med 1996;344:1685-90.
7. Holland PV. Viral infections and the blood supply. N Engl J Med 1996;334:1734-5.
8. Finch CA, Lenfant C. Oxygen transport in man. N Engl J Med 1972;286:407-15.
9. Kitchens CS. Are transfusions overrated: surgical outcome of Jehova's Witnessess. Am J Med 1993;94:117-9.
10. Viele MK, Weiskopf RB. What can we learn about the need for transfusion from patients who refuse blood? The experience with Jehova's Witnesses. Transfusion 1994; 34:396-401.
11. Lunn JN, Elwood PC. Anaemia and surgery. Brit Med J 1970;3:71-3.
12. Doldman L, Caldera DL, Nussbaum, et al. Multifactorial index of cardiac risk in noncardiac surgical procedures. N Engl J Med 1977;297:845-50.
13. Czer LSC, Shoemaker WC. Optimal hematorcrit value in critically ill postoperative patients. Surg Gynecol Obstet 1978;147:363-68.
14. Rawstron RE. Anaemia and surgery: a retrospective clinical study. Aust NZ J Surg 1980;39:425-32.
15. Friedman BA, Burns TL, Schork MA. An analysis of blood transfusion of surgical patients by sex: a quest for the transfusion trigger. Transfusion 1980;20:179-88.
16. Carson JL, Poses RM, Spence RK, Bonavita G. Severity of anaemia and operative mortality and morbidity. Lancet 1988;i:727-9.

17. Salem-Schatz SR, Avorn J, Soumerai SB. Influence of clinical knowledge, organizational context and practice style on transfusion decision making: implications for practice change strategies. JAMA 1990;264:476-83.
18. Mangano DT, Browner WS, Hollenberg M, et al. Association of perioperative myocardial ischemia with cardiac morbidity and mortality in men undergoing noncardiac surgery. N Engl J Med 1990:323:1781-8.
19. Carson JL, Willet LR. Is a hemoglobin of 10 g/dL required for surgery? Med Clin North AM 1993;77:335-47.
20. Nelson AH, Fleisher LA, Rosenbaum SH. Relationship between postoperative anemia and cardiac morbidity in high risk vascular patients in the intensive care unit. Crit Care Med 1993;21:860-6.
21. Hebert PC, Wells G, Marshall J, et al. Transfusion requirements in critical care. A pilot study. JAMA 1995:273:1439-44.
22. Carson JL, Duff A, Poses RM, et al. Effect of anaemia and cardiovascular disease on surgical mortality and morbidity. Lancet 1996;348:1055-60.
23. Valeri CR. Physiology of blood transfusion. Little, Brown & Co. In: Barie PS, Shires GT (eds). Surgical intensive care. 1993:681-721.
24. Valeri CR. Transfusion medicine and surgical practice. In: Bulletin of the American College of Surgeons 1993;78:20-24.
25. Triulzi DJ, Vanek K, Ryan DH, Blumberg N. A clinical and immunologic study of blood transfusion and postoperative bacterial infection in spinal surgery. Transfusion 1992;32:517-24.
26. Vamvakas EC, Carven JH, Hibberd PL. Blood transfusion and infection after colorectal cancer surgery. Transfusion 1996;36:1000-8.
27. Jeter ECK, Spivey MA. Noninfectious complications of blood transfusion. Hem/Onc Clin of N Am 1995;9:187-204.
28. Klein HG. New insights into the management of anemia in the surgical patient. Am J Med 1996;101(suppl 2A):12S-15S.
29. Valeri CR, Cooper AG, Pivacek LE. Limitations of measuring blood volume with iodinated I125 serum albumin. Arch Int Med 1973;132:534-43.
30. Valeri CR, Altschule MD. Hypovolemic anemia of trauma: the missing blood syndrome. Chemical Rubber Company, Boca Raton, FL, 1981.
31. Biron PE, Howard J, Altschule MD, Valeri CR. Chronic deficits in red-cell mass in patients with orthopaedic injuries (stress anemia). J Bone Joint Surg 1972;54-A:101-14.
32. Valeri CR, Donahue K, Feingold HM, Cassidy GP, Altschule MD. Increase in plasma volume after the transfusion of washed erythrocytes. Surg Gynecol Obstet 1986;162:30-6.
33. Jones J, Mollison PL. A simple and efficient method of labelling red cells with ^{99m}Tc for determination of red cell volume. Br J Haematol 1978;38:141-8.
34. Fisher JB, Dennis RC, Valeri CR, et al. Effect of graft material on loss of erythrocytes after aortic operations. Surg Gynecol Obstet 1991;171:131-6.
35. Cordts PR, LaMorte WW, Fisher JB, et al. Poor predictive value of hematocrit and hemodynamic parameters for erythrocyte deficits after extensive elective vascular operations. Surg Gynecol Obstet 1992;175:243-8.
36. Deitch EA, Berg RD. Bacterial translocation from the gut: a mechanism of infection. J Burn Care Rehab 1987:8:475-82.
37. Marik P. Gastric intramucosal pH. A better predictor of multiorgan dysfuntion and death than oxygen derived variables in patients with sepsis. Chest 1993;104:225-9.
38. Ivatury R, Simon J, Islam S, et al. A prospective randomized study of end points of resuscitation after major trauma: global oxygen transport indices versus organ specific gastric mucosal pH. J Am Coll Surg 1996;183:145-54.

39. McMahon LP, Dawborn JK. Subjective quality of life assessment in hemodialysis patients at different levels of hemoglobin following use of recombinant human erythropoietin. Am J Nephrol 1992;12:162-9.
40. Cazzola M, Mercuriali F, Brugnara C. Use of recombinant human erythropoietin outside the setting of uremia. Blood 1997;89:4248-67.

COST-EFFECTIVENESS OF CONVENTIONAL AND ALTERNATIVE APPROACHES IN TRANSFUSION PRACTICE: THE VALUE OF DECISION ANALYSIS

J.P. AuBuchon

Introduction

The allogeneic blood supply currently provides haemotherapy support with an unprecedented degree of safety: the risk of morbidity or mortality after transfusion has never been lower. This starting point is a difficult one on which to build improvement. Although the public is always looking for improvements in safety, the public is also looking for careful management of resources allocated to healthcare. What is the best way to improve the safety of transfusion?

This situation is not unique in healthcare where improvement is always sought but resources are not unlimited. In choosing between competing interventions, choices must be made in resource allocation that affect the total health gain received by the population, since resources directed toward one opportunity often detract from those available for others. As the health benefits from different interventions are different, and since the marginal return on healthcare investments may be asymptotic, there are important implications of resource allocation decisions.

Decision analysis

The situation described above is one in which decision analysis techniques may provide useful insights. Cost-effectiveness analysis, a mathematical method of projecting the effects of a health-related decision in a way that allows comparative quantification of net benefit in comparison to the resources consumed, may provide particularly helpful insights [1].

Goals

The goals of decision analysis can be framed in two contexts. In the first, the technique can be applied to an individual patient's situation, quantifying, for example, the potential outcomes for a patient choosing between two therapeutic options [2]. In this application, the chances of better health with each can be compared to the risks of a side-effect. Another use of decision analysis is with a macroeconomic focus, determining the effect of applying two different interventions to a population or a group of patients. In this use, the impact of resource consumption takes on meaning as well so that the relative benefit achieved for resources expended can be calculated and compared for the competing interventions.

Outcomes

The outcome of an intervention in a decision analysis model is usually stated as years of life extended (either average extension or an aggregate total for a population), adjusted for the quality of life. This quality adjustment recognises that people value not only the length of life but also the quality of health experienced. A quality adjustment factor (from 1.0 for perfect health to 0 for death) is multiplied by longevity to yield quality-adjusted life years (QALYs), a commonly used outcome metric. As this measurement is independent of the actual illness or intervention under study, models using it as an outcome measure can be compared directly with each other.

The determination of the quality of life perceived in different states of health is a science in itself and beyond the scope of this presentation [1]. There are several ways by which this quality factor can be determined, but different perspectives (that of the patient versus that of an unaffected person, for example) can have a large impact. In addition, imminence of death can dramatically alter one's perspective and quality ratings [3,4]. Furthermore, allowing a visible segment of the population to avoid certain, premature death may lead to assignment of higher utility for an intervention than one that provides a more distributed but less dramatic (albeit even larger) health gain for the population [5]. These vagaries must be considered when comparing outcomes of interventions.

Cost-effectiveness analysis

Cost-effectiveness analysis (CEA), a commonly used form of decision analysis, is a methodology that compares the net health effects for a population through application of an intervention as compared to the change in resource consumption the intervention requires [1]. The outcome of a model is usually expressed as a marginal *cost-effectiveness ratio*: the difference in resource consumption between two interventions divided by the difference in (quality-adjusted) life years their application provides. A multitude of these analyses has shown that most generally accepted interventions in medicine have a cost-effectiveness below USD 50,000/QALY [see references 6 and 7].

The construction of a CEA can be a simple or complex task but generally can be divided into three phases. First, a decision tree is usually constructed to represent all the various possibilities that might occur once a particular intervention had been chosen. Then, the literature is consulted or experiments are performed to determine the probability that each of these chance events may occur. Finally, the total cost of the path to each outcome is determined along with a quantitation of the health state and longevity of each outcome. The mathematical calculations required can then be performed readily through a variety of software packages, on a spreadsheet, or manually.

Decision analysis techniques provide a means to compare objectively the health interventions to be applied to a particular situation or that are competing for the same resources. These models do not provide a complete decision making tool, however, as they cannot capture all aspects of a situation, particularly those costs and outcomes that have an intangible element [6,7]. Care must also be taken in analysing the report of an analysis to ensure that the model has not included assumptions that unduly bias the result and that future costs and future benefits have been discounted to represent appropriate time preferences.

Applications of decision analysis in transfusion medicine

There are many options available in blood banking and transfusion medicine that offer the potential for improved safety for the recipient. As healthcare resources remain limited, decision analysis techniques may be applied to help determine the relative benefits and cost-effectiveness of each. These analytic techniques can also serve to illustrate where attention should be focused. For example, the greatest risk of death due to transfusion is not related to HIV or hepatitis transmission; *several-fold more people die each year in the United States due to receiving a unit of blood intended for another patient through an entirely preventable chain of events!* [8]. In addition, because the risk of infectious disease transmission is already so low, any unintended side-effects of an "improvement" in blood safety have the real potential to overwhelm the intended benefit and yield a net *decrement* of safety to the blood supply and of health to the population.

Preoperative autologous donation

Although preoperative autologous donation (PAD) before elective surgery is very popular among patients, its application must be carefully guided to ensure that a reasonable health return is achieved for the commitment of resources and that, indeed, the intervention produces more good than harm for the patient.

In coronary artery bypass grafting (CABG) surgery, the cost-effectiveness of PAD is approximately USD 500,000/QALY; PAD in this situation is far less cost-effective than most health interventions [9]. Cost-effectiveness is improved if PAD occurs in situations where transfusion is more likely and/or the patient has a greater expected longevity [9,10]. Thus PAD can offer more benefit if directed toward younger patients undergoing surgeries with considerable blood loss.

Most models of PAD cost-effectiveness in CABG have assumed that delaying surgery to collect the necessary units and the donation process itself would have no untoward impacts on the patient. However, patients awaiting bypass surgery have a definite mortality (about 0.5%/month), and serious reactions occur once every 17,000 autologous donations, usually without a definable predisposition [11,12]. Removing the assumption of lack of negative effect of the donation process, the PAD CEA model indicated that only one peridonation mortality amongst patients awaiting CABG *negates all the health benefits* of having autologous blood available [9]. It is unlikely that the procedure can be conducted with that level of safety in this patient population! Of course, its use in other settings, such as orthopaedic surgery and a healthier population of patients, would not include such a harsh warning, but the importance of contrasting the potential benefits with the potential risks for every patient being considered for PAD is clear.

PAD is best applied to patients predicted to have significant postoperative longevity, who are scheduled to undergo a procedure in which there is a significant likelihood of transfusion, and for whom the donation process is likely to be well tolerated. Care must be taken that the donation not just leads to an increased likelihood of transfusion to make up for what has been previously collected! [13,14].

Infectious disease testing

The allogeneic blood supply has achieved a very high degree of safety through a variety of measures, including donor screening and laboratory testing. Improvements in and additions to these protocols over the last decade have yielded a very low probability of infection – but also a low potential yield from additional interventions [15,16].

This limitation for future improvements can be seen in analysing the cost-effectiveness of laboratory testing to reduce the risk of HIV transmission. HIV *antibody* testing, in aggregate, costs approximately the same amount as taking care of the transfusion recipients who would otherwise have contracted HIV; thus this intervention not only prevented the vast majority of transfusion-transmitted cases that were occurring when it was introduced but was also very cost-effective at USD 3,600/QALY [17]. Because the number of cases transmitted through transfusion was reduced to approximately one per half million units in Europe and the US through continued improvements in donor questioning and testing by the mid-1990's, even the relatively low per-unit cost of HIV p24 antigen testing still yielded a cost-effectiveness estimate of USD 2.3 million/QALY [17].

The actual cost-effectiveness of p24 antigen testing has been much poorer than anticipated. This additional testing was projected to detect approximately 8 infectious units each year in the US that would not have otherwise been detected. However, in the first year and a half after its implementation, only one donation out of approximately 18 million was interdicted solely because of this test. This disparity has been attributed to a longer interdonation interval amongst seroconverters, possibly related to the acute HIV viral syndrome. If this experience of using the HIV antigen test continues, the cost-effectiveness of its use will exceed USD 20 *million*/QALY!

More recently, attention has been focused on the potential application of genetic amplification technologies to blood donor testing. Because of cost and throughput considerations, these are currently being considered in a pooled testing format. As a result, the increased sensitivity for early infections is potentially diminished, and the reduction in the infectious window period has been estimated to be 1-3 d (as compared to 6 d for HIV antigen testing). The low potential yield and poor cost-effectiveness of this testing is compounded by its application to plasma intended for manufacture to products that currently undergo one or more viral inactivation techniques that effectively produce a non-infectious final component. Obviously, the yield (benefit) of applying genetic amplification testing to these plasma units will be unmeasureable and its cost-effectiveness abysmally poor.

This analysis highlights that there is more to a decision than a CEA. As the public remains panicky about HIV transmission, almost any expenditure that reduces HIV risk through transfusion becomes absolutely necessary. Cost was clearly excluded from the regulatory decision process regarding HIV p24 antigen testing in the United States, and further decisions with similar underpinnings may be anticipated.

However, adding a new test may make the blood supply less safe, paradoxically. First, the blood collecting agency's systems must be able to accommodate the increase in units quarantined and discarded; past increases due to new testing protocols have sometimes resulted in erroneous releases (although at a time when there was less emphasis on good manufacturing practices). Also to consider is the "magnet effect", the potential that persons at risk for HIV infection might be attracted to donate blood in order to have access to the latest detection technology in a socially acceptable venue. As 15-25% of HIV positive donors admit that obtaining test results was primary reason in their donation [18], a modest increase in the number of "test seekers" could lead to an actual increase in the number of undetected infectious (window period) donations [19].

Viral inactivation of plasma

Several techniques are approaching approval for viral inactivation of plasma. The solvent-detergent (SD) treatment for frozen plasma (FP) is already in use in several European countries. However, a CEA has raised both economic and safety concerns [20].

Because the blood supply already is of low infectivity and since many recipients of FP do not survive long enough to reap the benefits of having avoided a viral transmission, the cost-effectiveness of SD FP is predictably poor, approximately USD 300,000/QALY. As with PAD, this cost-effectiveness estimate improves if the intervention is directed toward patients with improved chances for survival, such as those undergoing plasma exchange for thrombotic thrombocytopenic purpura as opposed to plasma transfusion during surgery for a ruptured abdominal aortic aneurysm. Similarly, if SD FP is in short supply, the greatest benefit would be achieved by directing it toward patients with the greatest (expected) longevity.

However, the SD process involves pooling many units together in order to inactivate lipid enveloped viruses, including HIV, HBV and HCV. The pooling process provides an inadvertent means to distribute non-enveloped viruses even further, since these would escape inactivation and be transfused from one donor to a large number of recipients. Although the blood-borne non-enveloped viruses known today cause little morbidity for most of those infected, viral evolution could lead to the appearance of a new, non-enveloped virus that could have a devastating impact: a non-enveloped virus causing HIV-like consequences would have to be present only at an undetectable low frequency (1 in 71 million) before all the benefits of avoiding HIV, HCV and HBV were negated!

Other techniques of viral inactivation in plasma are under investigation or are already implemented. For example, methylene blue treatment inactivates some but not all blood-borne viruses and does so in a process that can be applied to units individually. Attention must also be focused, however, on the chemical residuals in units and their removal [21] in order to ensure that risks of viral transmission are not being replaced with those of chemical exposure.

Concluding comments

The current level of safety afforded by the allogeneic blood supply leaves little room for improvement and even less an opportunity for "cost-effective" improvement in most developed countries. There remain opportunities to reduce the risk of viral transmission, but their yields will be small and will undoubtedly provide less health benefit than other uses of limited healthcare resources.

It is the responsibility of knowledgeable professionals to attempt to direct attention toward those risks that can be ameliorated and, by virtue of their frequency or severity, will yield the greatest health benefit if reduced. The largest risks faced by a transfusion recipient at present are probably not those on which the public and regulatory agencies have most recently focused [22]. The risk of fatality from receiving the wrong unit of blood or from bacterial contamination of a component (especially platelets) far exceeds the likelihood of viral transmission [8]. While the clinical consequences of immunomodulation induced by allogeneic leukocyte exposure remain to be definitively defined, the potential for these effects to have a substantial impact on morbidity, mortality and healthcare costs demands further investigation and, possibly, action. By allowing transfusion safety discussions to be focused primarily on to vanishingly small residual risks of viral transmission (e.g., HIV and hepatitis), we are detracting from our efforts that could potentially save many more lives.

It is ultimately society's decision how its resources should be allocated, but it remains the responsibility of medical professionals to highlight for the public just how much "bang for the buck" they are getting when further improvements in blood safety are sought.

References

1. Gold MR, Siegel JE, Russel LB, Weinstein MC (eds). Cost-effectiveness in health and medicine. New York, Oxford, 1996.
2. Sox HC, Blatt MA, Higgins MC, Marton KI. Medical decision making. Boston, Buterworth-Heinemann, 1988.
3. Fowler FJ, Cleary PD, Massagli MP, Weissman J, Epstein A. The role of reluctance to give up life in the measurement of the value of health states. Med Decis Making 1995;15:195-200.
4. Schneiderman LJ, Kaplan RM. Fear of dying and HIV infection vs hepatitis B infection. Am J Publ Health 1992;82:584-6.
5. Hadorn DC. Setting health care priorities in Oregon. Cost-effectiveness meets the rule of rescue. JAMA 1991;265:2218-25.
6. AuBuchon JP. Lessons learned from decision analysis. Transfusion 1996;36:755-60.
7. AuBuchon JP. The role of decision analysis in transfusion medicine. Vox Sang 1996;71:1-5.

8. Linden JV, Paul B, Dressler KP. A report of 104 transfusion errors in New York State. Transfusion 1992;32:601-6.
9. Brirkmeyer JD, AuBuchon JP, Littenberg B, et al. The cost-effectiveness of preoperative autologous donation in coronary bypass surgery. Ann Thoracic Surg 1994;57:161-9.
10. Etchason J, Petz L, Keeler E, et al. The cost-effectiveness of preoperative autologous blood donations. N Engl J Med 1995;332:719-24.
11. Popovsky MA, Whitaker B, Arnold NL. Severe outcomes of allogeneic and autologous blood donation: frequency and characterization. Transfusion 1995;35:734-7.
12. AuBuchon JP, Popovsky MA. The safety of preoperative autologous blood donation in the non-hospital setting. Transfusion 1991;31:513-7.
13. Kanter MH, van Maanen D, Anders KH, Castro F, Mya WW, Clark K. Preoperative autologous blood donations before elective hysterectomy. JAMA 1996;276:798-801.
14. Goodnough LT, Monk TG, Brecher ME. Autologous blood procurement in the surgical setting: lessons learned in the last 10 years. Vox Sang 1996;71:133-41.
15. Busch MP, Korelitz JJ, Kleinman SH, Lee SR, AuBuchon JP, Schreiber GB. Declining value of alanine aminotransferase in screening of blood donors to prevent posttransfusion hepatitis B and C virus infection. The Retrovirus Epidemiology Donor Study. Transfusion 1995:35:903-10.
16. AuBuchon JP, Birkmeyer JD, Busch MP, Dodd RY, Lackritz EM, Peterson LR and HIV Blood Donor Study Group. Cost-effectiveness of anti-HBc testing to reduce HIV transmission risk. Transfusion 1996;36(abstract):43S.
17. AuBuchon JP, Birkmeyer JD, Busch MP. Cost-effectiveness of expanded human immunodeficiency virus-testing protocols for donated blood. Transfusion 1997;37: 45-51.
18. Leitman SF, Klein HG, Melpolder JJ, et al. Clinical implications of positive tests for antibodies to human immunodeficiency virus type 1 in asymptomatic blood donors. N Engl J Med 1989:321:917-24.
19. Korelitz JJ, Busch MP, Williams AE for the Retrovirus Epidemiology Donor Study. Antigen testing for human immunodeficiency virus (HIV) and the magnet effect: will the benefit of a new HIV test be offset by the numbers of higher-risk, test-seeking donors attracted to blood centers. Transfusion 1996;36:203-8.
20. AuBuchon JP, Birkmeyer JD. Safety and cost-effectiveness of solvent-detergent treated plasma. In search of a zero-risk blood supply. JAMA 1994;272:1210-4.
21. AuBuchon JP, Pickard C, Herschel L, O'Connor JL, Williams S. Preparation of methylene blue (MB) plasma with reduction in residual MB content by adsorption filtration. Transfusion 1996:36(abstract):65S.
22. AuBuchon JP, Kruskall MS. Transfusion safety: realigning efforts with risk. Transfusion 1998;(in press).

THE DESIGN OF TRANSFUSION IN RANDOMISED CONTROLLED TRIALS IN CRITICALLY ILL PATIENTS

P.C. Hébert[1]

Introduction

Anaemia is common in the critically ill and results in the frequent use of red cell transfusions [1,2]. For decades, an arbitrary transfusion threshold of 100 g/L has been employed widely in clinical medicine including the management of critically ill patients [3]. Recently, a re-evaluation of this practice was prompted both by the fear of transfusion-related infections such as AIDS and the prospect of an ever decreasing blood supply [4-6]. These concerns also resulted in the formulation of red cell transfusion guidelines by a number of organisations for the use of red cells [7-10]. However, published guidelines, for the most part, have not addressed how red cells should be administered in critically ill patients.

Despite the intense scrutiny of transfusion practice in the recent past, there remain very few well controlled clinical trials evaluating transfusion practice in various settings. In a recent systematic review of transfusion practice, we only identified randomised controlled trials (RCTs) contrasting two transfusion strategies in a total of 813 patients [11-16]. Only one study conducted in patients with sickle cell disease, was large enough to rule out clinically important differences in its primary outcome [15]. Four of the six studies were relevant to the care of critically ill patients. Two of these studies were undertaken in patients undergoing coronary revascularisation [11,12], one study [14] randomly allocated a general population of critically ill patients and the remaining study was conducted in trauma victims. In summary, five of the six studies enrolled too few patients to make significant inferences regarding important outcomes from red cell transfusions and the one remaining large RCT only documented the effects of transfusions using a disease-specific outcome in sickle cell disease.

Transfusion decisions in critically ill patients are therefore based on inferior levels of clinical evidence such as observational studies, poorly controlled clinical trials or laboratory studies. One of the explanations for the relative deficiency of clinical trials in critical care and transfusion medicine may be the methodologic challenges hampering the development and execution of RCTs in these settings. In this article, the controversies that form the basis for a more restrictive as opposed to a more liberal use of allogeneic red cells in critical care

---

1. Career scientist of the Ontario Ministry of Health.

will be described. Also some of the methodologic issues central to the development and conduct of transfusion studies in critical care settings will be outlined. An attempt has been made to present the many facets of contentious issues and where possible to make recommendations.

Critical care transfusion practice

While consensus statements and clinical practice guidelines have recommended moving away from the use of perioperative transfusion triggers, practitioners appear to be slow in modifying their approach to allogeneic transfusions. Several self-administered surveys conducted over the years have examined the use of triggers [17-21]. A 1992 Canadian survey of critical care practitioners [19] observed that 35% of respondents identified 90 g/L as minimum concentration and an additional 40% selected 100 g/L. These authors also noted significant difference among the four clinical scenarios and a number of potential risk factors. In a 4,470 patient cohort, we also documented a significant variation in nadir haemoglobin levels prior to transfusion amongst six academic intensive care units using multivariate techniques adjusting for the influence of diagnosis, disease severity, patient age and transfusion status ($p<0.0001$) [22]. The lack of direction emanating from guidelines as well as compelling evidence of individual and institutional practice variation indicates uncertainty regarding optimal haemoglobin levels and a need for further study.

Critically ill patients are affected by complex metabolic, respiratory and cardiovascular pathophysiological processes which predispose this patient population to the adverse consequences of anaemia (e.g. death and myocardial infarction). Physiological responses to anaemia, and possibly outcomes may be modulated through factors including advanced age, severity of illness, cardiac disease, haemodynamic instability as well diagnoses such as severe sepsis and adult respiratory distress syndrome (ARDS). Two large cohort studies have documented that increasing degrees of anaemia were associated with a disproportionate increase in mortality rates in the subgroup of patients with cardiac disease. Critically ill patients [l] with cardiac disease had a trend towards an increased mortality when haemoglobin values were <95 g/L (55% versus 42%, $p=0.09$) as compared to anaemic patients with other diagnoses. Patients with anaemia, a high APACHE II score (>20) and a cardiac diagnosis had a significantly lower mortality rate when given 1 to 3 or 4 to 6 units of allogeneic red cells [55% (no transfusions) versus 35%(1 to 3 units) or 32%(4 to 6 units) respectively, $p=0.0l$)]. In Jehovah's Witness patients undergoing surgical interventions [23], the adjusted odds of death increased from 2.3 (95%CI of 1.4 to 4.0) to 12. 3 (95%CI of 2.5 to 62.1) as preoperative haemoglobin values declined from a range of 100-109 g/L to 60-69 g/L in patients with cardiac disease. In non-cardiac patients with comparable levels of anaemia, there was no impact of anaemia on mortality. Even though both cohort studies were retrospective in nature and may not have been controlled for a number of important confounders, it appears that anaemia increases the risk of death in patients with cardiac disease.

In our multicentre cohort of critically ill patients, a disproportionate increase in mortality rates was observed in the most severely ill patients with anaemia as opposed to non-anaemic patients with comparable levels of illness severity [1]. Similar observations were made in a separate case-control study [24]. At present, there are no studies examining the independent contribution of age, cerebrovascular disease, respiratory disease and diseases such as sepsis and ARDS. However, alone or in combination, these factors may independently increase the mortality risk in anaemic critically ill patients. Therefore, critically ill patients appear to be at increased risk of complications from anaemia. In addition, some disease processes and patient characteristics may adversely affect certain anaemic patients more than others.

Critically ill patients may not only be at risk of complications from anaemia, but may also be at increased risks of adverse consequences from allogeneic red cell transfusions, particularly the immunosuppressive and microcirculatory effects of red cells. In a bibliographic search of the literature, we identified 6 randomized controlled clinical trials examining the role of transfused red cells in immunomodulation [25-30]. There were mixed results from these studies. Only three studies, comparing either leukodepleted red cells [27,28] or autologous transfusions [30], to allogeneic transfusions demonstrated decreased rates of postoperative infections. If allogeneic red cells result in clinically important immunosuppression, this may result in significant increases in the rates of nosocomial infections, multisystem organ dysfunction and death, given that infections are a major cause of morbidity and mortality in the ICU.

While the effect of haemoglobin levels (haematocrit) on systemic O_2 transport in the central circulation have been well studied, it remains unclear how raising haematocrit levels might impact on O_2 delivery in the microcirculation [31-33]. There are many storage-related changes in red cells [5,34-43] and changes caused by diseases such as sepsis [44-48] that decreases red cell deformability and the ability to off-load O_2 in the microcirculation. In conjunction with significant systemic microcirculatory dysfunction observed in many critically ill patients, the decrease in red cell deformability may dramatically affect tissue oxygen delivery in many critically ill patients [44-47]. Therefore, there is evidence to suggest that red cell transfusions increase systemic O_2 delivery but may have adverse effects on microcirculatory O_2 delivery to the tissues.

As described above, we only identified 6 RCTs attempting to contrast all of these benefits, risks, harms and costs of red cell transfusion in a total of 813 patients. The only level I RCT was conducted in patients with sickle cell disease [15]. One of the studies enrolled otherwise healthy patients with a gastrointestinal haemorrhage. The study documented an increase in coagulation abnormalities following the use of a more liberal transfusion strategy. Patients undergoing coronary revascularisation were included in two studies [11,12]. Johnson et al [12] randomized 39 patients to receive either a liberal transfusion strategy (maintaining haematocrit levels of 32% or haemoglobin concentrations of 105 g/L) or a conservative approach (maintaining haematocrit levels of 25% or haemoglobin concentrations of 82 g/L). There was not any difference in postoperative complication rates in the two groups even though the conservative group experienced a significant decrease in total postoperative blood use. A second

RCT, carried out by Weisel et al [11], assessed day five exercise tolerance as well as haemodynamic and myocardial metabolic response following normovolemic haemodilution in 27 patients. Patients received either red cells if their haemoglobin concentrations fell below 120g/L in addition to colloids in one group (n=13) versus crystalloids and allogeneic red cells only if haemoglobins fell below 70g/L (n=14). Though patients in the low haemoglobin trigger group received significantly less red cell transfusions than the other group, there were no differences in morbidity, mortality or exercise tolerance. In a small subset of patients (n=6), there were differences in the rate of myocardial lactate recovery in the low haemoglobin trigger group suggesting increased myocardial ischaemia from anaemia. Hébert et al [14] randomly allocated 69 critically ill patients to a restrictive red cell transfusion strategy (haemoglobin concentrations between 70 g/L-90 g/L) or a liberal strategy (haemoglobin concentrations between 100 g/L-120 g/L) in order to evaluate the impact of the treatments on mortality rates, organ dysfunction scores and other markers of morbidity.

The results showed that neither mortality nor the development of organ dysfunction were affected by the transfusion strategy. However, the maintenance haemoglobin concentrations between 70 and 90 g/L decreased the average number of units transfused from 4.8 to 2.5 units (a 48% reduction, $p<0.001$). Finally, a clinical trial in critically ill trauma victims randomly allocated 25 patients to allogeneic red cell transfusions once haematocrit levels reached either 30% or 40%. The authors concluded that there were no discernable differences in O_2 transport variables between both transfusion strategies [13]. In summary, five of the six studies enrolled too few patients to make significant inferences regarding important outcomes from red cell transfusions and the one remaining large RCT only documented the effects of transfusions using a disease-specific outcome in sickle cell disease.

From this review, it should be apparent that an optimal and safe lower limit to the transfusion threshold has not been established in critically ill patient populations [49]. There is therefore a need for further randomized controlled clinical trials. The remainder of the article will describe many difficulties inherent in performing transfusion trials in the critical care setting. The Transfusion Requirements in Critical Care trial, a randomized controlled clinical trial comparing a restrictive to a more liberal use of red cells in normovolemic critically ill patients will be presented as an example of such a trial and used to highlight some of the difficulties.

What is unique about critical care RCTs?

Critically ill patients have a number of features that have a profound influence on the study design. Specifically, the diverse study population and ill-defined diseases, the complex nature of critical care interventions and the choice of outcomes all pose unique difficulties. In terms of a critical care population, one of its unique aspects is that participating patients must be admitted to an ICU in order to be considered critically ill (this may also include a recovery room or a step-down unit in some studies). Therefore, eligibility is primarily predicated on location rather than specific diseases alone. Second, selection is also based on disease definitions, comprised of a constellation of physiologic and other biologic abnormalities as opposed to a single well defined disease entity such as a malignancy. Third, the diseases and pathologic processes, resulting in these severe homeostatic disturbances, are often in their late stages at the time of ICU admission. Co-morbid illnesses unrelated to the primary disease process may also have similar consequences.

In critical care, as in surgical disciplines, study interventions are administered in conjunction with other treatment modalitied by skilled multidisciplinary teams [50,51]. The large number of potential interventions as well as the complexity of care in the critically ill also create unique difficulties when performing clinical studies in this field. Investigators must therefore contend with involved treatment protocols. The degree of control or constraints imposed on experimental and non-experimental interventions should be considered early in the planning of an RCT [52]. Experimental constraints on study interventions can generally be implemented by using treatment protocols and by the selection of study centres. Thus, a number of difficult choices face the clinical investigator.

The selection of outcomes for RCTs evaluating transfusion practice in the critical care setting also poses unique challenges. Investigators might consider selecting a transfusion specific outcome such as a change in allogeneic exposure or total red cell transfusions as opposed to a more general outcome such as a 30 day all cause mortality rate. Transfusion specific outcomes such as a decrease in allogeneic exposure will be better able to detect differences between treatment groups and may be seen as beneficial to patients. However, the assumptions underlying such specific outcomes are that there are few significant complications from anaemia. From the previous discussion, it should be apparent that this assumption may not be valid. Given that red cell transfusions and decreased O_2 delivery caused by anaemia may have significant consequences in this patient population, an outcome such as mortality and multiple organ dysfunction scores may be considered more relevant. Even though outcomes such as mortality as a consequence of critical illness, is common, easily ascertained and important in this patient population, a mortality rate may nonetheless not easily discriminate amongst interventions. That is, as a primary outcome in an RCT, mortality might not detect differences in interventions when differences truly exist. An investigator must therefore either choose an outcome that is apt to discriminate or an outcome that encompasses that is better able to describe the overall risks and benefits of treatment interventions. This decision largely rests on the approach chosen in the study.

Overall design approaches

The ideal RCT establishes if therapeutic interventions work, as well as determines the overall benefits and risks of each alternative in pre-defined patient populations. This is accomplished by minimising the influence of chance, bias and confounding through appropriate choices in the design. In addition, the ideal

RCT should attempt to fulfil its objectives in the fewest patients possible (often termed *statistical efficiency*) [53]. Unfortunately, these objectives are often in direct conflict rather than complementary. For instance, by maximising the efficiency of a study, investigators might sacrifice their ability to draw conclusions in clinically important subgroups because confidence intervals around estimates of the outcome may be too wide.

The most important consequence of these conflicting objectives are that choices made in the design of RCTs must either focus on whether an intervention works or whether the intervention results in more good than harm for patients [53,54]. Trials which attempt to determine therapeutic *efficacy* address the *"Will the therapy work under optimal conditions?"* question, while trials attempting to determine therapeutic *effectiveness* address the *"Will the therapy do more good than harm under usual practice conditions in all patients who are offered the intervention?"* question. Clearly, both questions yield clinically useful information. Efficacy is often first established then the intervention is evaluated for its effectiveness.

Table 1. Theoretical reasons supporting the restrictive or the liberal use of allogeneic red cells in normovolemic critically ill patients

Rationale supporting the liberal use of red cells:
– Augmenting O_2 delivery may improve survival
– Increased risk of coronary ischaemia due to increased demand
– Age, disease severity and drugs may interfere with adaptation to anaemia
– Improved safety margin if further blood loss
Rationale supporting the restrictive use of red cells:
– Red cell transfusions impair microcirculatory flow
– Pathologic supply dependency is rare
– Risks of viral infections
– Immunodepression causing increased infections following transfusion
– Cardiac consequences of red cells less important

Study characteristics are frequently quite dissimilar between efficacy and effectiveness trials (Table l). As examples, efficacy trials would opt for restricted eligibility, rigorous treatment protocols and disease-specific outcomes responsive to the potential benefits of the experimental intervention. A similar study attempting to determine effectiveness would implement liberal eligibility criteria, loosely defined treatment protocols and outcomes which represent patients' overall response to an intervention. This approach is possible in very large trials because randomisation should provide an equal distribution of known and unknown risk factors among study groups. However, group comparability is not assured in smaller clinical trials. Unrestricted patient eligibility will improve the generalisability and ease of implementation of larger trials but potentially lead to significant imbalances in randomisation in smaller RCTs. Thus, one of the first steps in planning an RCT is to determine which of these two design approaches will best reflect the primary study question.

Table 2. Randomised clinical trials of transfusion practices

Authors/year published	Level of evidence	No. of patients	Study population	Interventions	Outcomes	Comments
Weisel, et al. [11] (1984)	II	27	CABG)**	Crystalloid alone (n=14) vs blood or colloid solutions (n=13)	[Hb]* lower in crystalloid group 20 h postoperation (p=0.01) Reduction in blood utilisation in the crystalloid group No difference in pulmonary edema and haemodynamic parameters (cardiac index and filling pressures)	Small sample size No difference in mortality or myocardial infarction rates Delayed recovery of myocardial extraction in a small number of patients in the crystalloid group
Johnson, et al. [12] (1992)	II	38	CABG**	Conservative group Hct maintained at 25% (n=20) vs liberal group Hct maintained at 32% (n=18)	Conservative group transfused with fewer units than the liberal group (p=0.012) Mean cardiac index same for both groups in the OR and 1 day postoperative Mean postoperative LOS: 7.6±1.9 days (liberal), 7.9±4.3 days (conservative) No difference in fluid requirement, haemodynamic parameters or hospital complications No relation between exercise tolerance on the 5th and 6th days and Hct	Small sample size No postoperative deaths reported No difference in ischaemic event
Blair, et al. [16] (1986)	II	50	GL*** haemorrhage	At least 2 units of PRCs (immediate) (n=24) vs no transfusion unless [Hb] <80g/L (delayed) (n=26)	Decrease transfusions in delayed group (2.6 vs 4.6 units/patient, p<0.05) The number of re-bled patients was greater in the immediate transfusion group 9 vs 1, p<0.01)	Small sample size Study design included a pilot study Laboratory and clinical measurements available No detailed data related to operative interventions and mortality rate

Authors/year published	Level of evidence	No. of patients	Study population	Interventions	Outcomes	Comments
						Prolonged clotting time and higher re-bleeding rate due to blood transfusions in the first 24 hours
Fortune, et al. [13] (1987)	II	25	Adult trauma	Hct = 30% (n=12) vs Hct = 40% (n=13)	5 units of PRC more in Hct = 40% groups No difference in haemodynamic parameters Higher intrapulmonary shunt in Hct = 40% group	Small sample size Physiologic outcome measurements only No data on mechanisms and type of traumatic injury No data on clinical outcomes
Hébert, et al. [14] (1995)	II	69	ICU	Restrictive group: [Hb] = 70-90 g/L (n=33) vs liberal group: [Hb] = 100-120 g/L (n=36)	Average daily [Hb] = 90 g/L vs 109 g/L ($p<0.001$) Number of units transfused 48% less in restrictive group (2.5 vs 4.8 units/patient) No difference in mortality and organ failures ($p>0.05$) No difference in ICU and hospital LOS ($p>0.05$)	Small sample size Pilot unable to detect difference in clinically important outcomes
Vichinsky, et al. [15] (1995)	I	604	Sickle cell disease in surgery	Aggressive (n=303) vs conservative (n=301) regimens	No difference in life-threatening complication rates but more transfusion-associated complications, i.e. haemolytic reactions and alloantibodies in the aggressive group	Total of 551 patients undergoing 604 operations Randomised procedures not patients Study in a specific population Only 1 patient died in all procedures

* Hb = haemoglobin concentration; ** CABG = coronary artery bypass grafting; *** GI = gastro intestinal

Table 3. Comparison of study characteristics using either an efficacy or an effectiveness approach when designing a study

Study characteristics	Efficacy trial	Effectiveness trial
Reseach question	Does the intervention work under ideal conditions?	Will the intervention result in more good than harm under usual practice conditions?
Setting	Restricted to centres of excellence	Open to all institutions
Patient selection	Specific diseases in well-defined patients	Wide range of patients identified using broad eligibility criteria
Study design	Small single or multicentre study	Very large multicentre clinical trial
Baseline assessment	Elaborate and detailed	Simple and clinician friendly
Intervention	Thightly controlled Optimal therapy under opimal study conditions	Less controlled Therapy administered According to ususal care
Treatment protocols	Rigorous and detailed Compliance essential	Very general Non compliance tolerated
Endpoints	Disease-related Related to biologic effect "surrogate"endpoints (e.g. allogeneic exposure)	Patient-related (e.g. all-cause mortality or quality of life)
Analysis	By treatment received Non-compliers excluded	Intention-to-treat All patients included
Data management:		
Data collection	Elaborate	Minimal and simple
Data monitoring*	Detailed and rigorous	Minimal

* Data monitoring refers to the review of source documents and adjudication/verification of outcomes.

The patient population in critical care RCTs

In choosing an efficacy approach, investigators would usually perform the study in a well-defined patient population where the intervention has the highest probability of demonstrating an effect. This may be done by narrowly defining the patient population through the use of restrictive eligibility criteria and disease definitions as well as selecting specialised centres with clinical expertise in the field. For instance, an investigator wanting to evaluate the effects of a restrictive versus a more liberal transfusion strategy might enrol trauma victims from a specialised trauma centre with a specified injury severity score and free of neurologic injury. The choosing to study some diseases in critical care, for instance severe sepsis or sepsis syndrome, may be further compounded by the lack of well established definitions that readily separate patients into diseased and non-diseased groups. A number of criteria must usually be met in order to fulfil these disease definitions. Investigators may also decide to use a more stringent disease definition as opposed to a broader definition. Choosing a narrowly defined study population through these different approaches will decrease overall variability attributed to patient selection but may have adverse consequences such as hampering patient recruitment and jeopardising the generalisability of the study results [55]. When defining the eligibility criteria for an effectiveness trial, investigators should consider utilising more liberal criteria in a wide range of clinical settings. Thus, as the study is being designed, medical or surgical critically ill patients with a broad range of primary diagnoses (or underlying conditions) from a range of tertiary care centres might be considered for enrolment in the study.

Using the Transfusion Requirements in Critical Care (TRICC) trial example, a study evaluating two transfusion strategies, the investigator might enrol a more generic population of critically ill patients or a very restricted sub-population such as trauma victims or patients undergoing coronary bypass grafting. Patients may also be enrolled from a greater number of sites including both community and tertiary level intensive care units. We opted for a hybrid approach by adopting permissive eligibility criteria. The study question is therefore being asked in a diverse group of ICU patients. When the study was being planned, we thought that the study question would be relevant to all critically ill patients. Also, the published evidence made it difficult to identify a specific subgroup in which the study question was the most controversial. We also believed that a study limited to such a subgroup would both jeopardise the feasibility of the study and compromise the generalisability of the results. We therefore elected to include a larger case mix and perform a detailed analysis of primary and secondary outcomes in clinically important subgroups. In practice, however, the eligibility criteria selected a very ill cohort of post-surgical patients or aggressively volume resuscitated medical patients in whom, we believe, the question is very relevant.

Given the inherent complexity of critically ill patients, we would generally recommend a hybrid approach. Thus, on the spectrum between an efficacy trial that focuses on highly selected patients and a large effectiveness trial that might enrol all potential patients with few exclusions, we would suggest that, whenever possible, critical care investigators should opt for the more restrictive end of the patient eligibility spectrum. We would further recommend that either extreme should be avoided in larger studies comparing clinical outcomes. Even though the use of more restrictive eligibility criteria and disease definitions in studies undertaken in tertiary care institutions may be preferred, choices should not jeopardise the feasibility of the study through their negative effects on patient recruitment. In practice, other considerations such as funding and resource constraints, the prevalence of the specific condition or disease process, the frequency of the primary outcome as well as the scientific or clinical interest of the investigative team will very likely impact on choice made in the selection of patients.

Critical care transfusion interventions

As one designs an RCT, decisions regarding the level of control should be imposed on the study intervention as well as all other aspects of the patient's care. This is a major concern in critical care given the complexity of patients and the enormous potential for confounding from any number of interventions. Experimental constraints on study interventions can generally be implemented through the modification of treatment protocols or by the selection of study centres. Thus, a number of choices face the clinical investigator. For example, should the administration of fluids and inotropic agents be standardised in a trial evaluating transfusion strategies? Or, should the use of antibiotics be tightly controlled in an RCT comparing the immunosuppressive effects of allogeneic versus autologous red cells? Similar questions regarding the selection of participating centres will also arise. The selection of Intensive Care Units may impact on many aspects of patient care within the trial given that most centres adopt various approaches to the care of the critically ill. Investigators must therefore consider whether the trial will be conducted exclusively in centres of excellence or in all ICUs that agree to participate?

Answers to these questions will in part depend on whether investigators wish to test therapeutic efficacy or effectiveness. Elaborate study protocols detailing the use of experimental and non-experimental therapies characterise efficacy evaluations. It is expected that the development and implementation of explicit and elaborate study protocols will decrease overall variability attributed to the confounding influence of co-interventions [56]. Decreased variation in the study may enable the detection of smaller clinically important treatment differences, if truly present. The development process itself may increase the uniformity of administering care among the investigators and participating centres. Because of the diversity of referral patterns and patients in different ICUs, selecting specific ICUs to participate may be a worthwhile method of ensuring compliance with the protocol and minimising patient heterogeneity. However, detailed protocols add complexity to the study and potentially provoke disagreements among investigators especially in multicentre RCTs. In a multidisciplinary setting, the clinical team(s) might also object to various aspects of the research protocol. Thus, non-compliance with the study protocol becomes a greater concern, both to minimise and to measure. In effectiveness trials, one attempts to understand whether an intervention will do more good than harm in the real world. In order to ascertain effectiveness, an investigator will develop extremely simple therapeutic protocols with minimal controls imposed on usual clinical care. In critical care, this may result in tremendous variability in the type and number of co-interventions performed in the study population. As a consequence, the benefits from the experimental therapy may be lost.

Opting for a compromise between rigorous experimental controls and usual care without any controls may often be the best solution. In the TRICC trial, physicians were asked to either maintain haemoglobin concentrations between 70 and 90 g/L or between 100 and 120 g/L. In addition to these simple target ranges, physicians were asked to administer red cells according to the American College of Physician guidelines. A number of policies were also used to minimise crossovers from one transfusion strategy to the other. When selecting potential study sites, tertiary level ICUs who had experience in implementing multicentre RCTs were identified and chosen as participating centres. There were, however, few experimental controls imposed on non-experimental therapies. We agreed that documentation of significant co-interventions would also be important given the inability to rigorously control many aspects of the patient's care.

Outcome in critical care transfusion trials

In most clinical trials, a number of potential outcomes, both fatal and non-fatal, will be considered by the clinical investigative team. If all were given equal consideration, there will be concerns arising from multiple comparisons and the interpretation of a study with heterogeneous findings. Thus, it is important to choose a primary outcome that will determine an intervention's therapeutic success or failure as well as secondary outcomes that will provide supportive secondary analyses. As a corollary, a predefined hierarchy implies that the investigators believe that clinically or statistically important differences in secondary outcomes, in the absence of important changes in the primary outcome, will not be interpreted as strong evidence of therapeutic benefit. The primary outcome is also essential in determining the sample size requirements in a clinical trial. Thus, once a decision has been made to determine either therapeutic efficacy or effectiveness (or possibly a hybrid approach), the second task facing investigators is ranking outcomes as primary and secondary.

In order to demonstrate efficacy, outcomes are generally chosen to evaluate the biological and disease-related effects of the interventions. It is also presumed that these outcomes are better able to detect clinically meaningful changes (responsiveness). For instance, decreasing the rate of allogeneic exposure in a study of evaluating a new alternative will be much easier to detect than an improvement in overall mortality. An assessment of oxygen kinetics including measures indicating the resolution of global or tissue specific ischaemia (e.g. lactate concentrations or mixed venous saturations) may also be considered as disease-related outcomes. However, the gains in responsiveness made by adopting such outcomes may be offset by the decrease in relevance to the patient.

Patient-related as opposed to disease-related or biological outcomes are usually assessed when attempting to establish the effectiveness of an intervention. In the TRICC trial, the primary outcome is overall 30 day mortality rates rather than cause-specific mortality rates (e.g. death due to myocardial infarction) or organ failure in a specific organ. The information derived from effectiveness trials and patient-related outcomes may be applicable to a broad range of patients but usually requires much larger sample sizes to demonstrate clinically important differences in outcomes.

The use of mortality as an outcome has been widely advocated by critical care researchers, the pharmaceutical industry and government agencies such as the Food and Drug Administration (FDA). A mortality rate, ascertained at a fixed time point (usually 28 or 30 days), was considered to be a frequent and clinically important event as well as objective and easily determined. However, in the past several years, a large number of negative clinical trials have led investigators to suggest that the choice of mortality as an outcome may have significant limitations. Indeed, in a recent Lancet article [57], Petros et al argued that mortality may not be able to distinguish the potential benefits of interventions in critically ill patients because of small studies being conducted in complex heterogeneous patients. Some of the possible solutions to this dilemma include developing new or re-evaluating existing alternative outcomes to ensure they are both clinically important as well as discriminate between treatment groups, the incorporation of mortality in outcomes such as organ failure scores and ensuring that mortality is, at a minimum, considered as a secondary endpoint in critical care RCTS.

Conclusions

In this article the divergent theoretical paradigms supporting a more restrictive and a liberal approach to the administration of red cell transfusions are described. From this review, it is very apparent that there is a need for larger randomized controlled clinical trials to evaluate existing and new therapeutic initiatives in transfusion medicine. A recent systematic review of the literature revealed very few well conducted larger RCTs evaluating various transfusion interventions [58]. Even newer pharmacological agents have only been subjected to smaller efficacy evaluations. Therefore, potential investigators are strongly urged to undertake larger clinical trials, able to ascertain clinically important benefits an risks of therapeutic interventions.

In designing RCTs in critical care, the investigator should be aware of different design approaches. Large effectiveness trials such as the very large ISIS trials in acute myocardial infarction [59,60] opt for very simple study designs accompanied by minimal data collection, monitoring of source documents and verification/adjudication of outcomes.

Using this approach, the ability to comment on biologic mechanisms, cointerventions and confounding factors may be severely limited [61]. In critical care, there are few examples of such large trials [62]. Indeed, the largest trials have only enrolled a few thousand patients. Therefore, it is suggested that RCTs evaluating various transfusion interventions consider using a hybrid approach [63-65]. Thus, many of the design characteristics adopted would be considered a compromise between a small RCT evaluating efficacy and a very large RCT evaluating the effectiveness of a therapy.

Acknowledgements

The author wishes to thank the Transfusion Requirements in Critical Care (TRICC) trial Executive Committee members for their wisdom and ongoing support, the TRICC investigators for their commitment to the study and its ideals and Drs George Wells and Andreas Laupacis for their mentorship.

References

1. Hébert PC, Wells G, Tweeddale M, et al. Does transfusion practice affect mortality in critically ill patients? Am J Crit Care 1997;155:1618-23.
2. Corwin HL, Parsonnet KC, Gettinger A. RBC transfusion in the ICU. Is there a reason? Chest 1995;108:767-61.
3. Cane RD. Hemoglobin: how much is enough? Crit Care Med 1990;18:1046-47.
4. Phillips TF, Soulier G, Wilson RF. Outcome of massive transfusion exceeding two blood volumes in trauma and emergency surgery. J Trauma 1987;27:903-10.
5. Welch HG, Meehan KR, Goodnough LT. Prudent strategies for elective red blood cell transfusion. Ann Intern Med 1992;116:393-402.
6. Surgenor DM, Wallace EL, Hale SG, Gilpatrick MW. Changing patterns of blood transfusions in four sets of United States hospitals, 1980 to 1985. Transfusion 1988;28:513-18.
7. American College of Physicians. Practice strategies for elective red blood cell transfusion. Ann Intern Med 1992;116:403- 6.
8. Petz LD, Tomasulo PA. Red cell transfusion. In: Kolins J, McCarthy LJ (eds). Contemporary transfusion practice. Arlington, VA: American Association of Blood Banks, 1987:1-26.
9. Consensus Conference (National Institutes of Health). Perioperative red blood cell transfusion. JAMA 1988;260:2700-3.
10. Expert Working Group. Guidelines for red blood cells and plasma transfusion for adults and children. Can Med Assoc J 1997;156:Sl-S24.
11. Weisel RD, Charlesworth DC, Mickleborough LL, et al. Limitations of blood conservation. J Thorac Cardiovasc Surg 1984;88:26-38.
12. Johnson RG, Thurer RL, Kruskall MS, et al. Comparison of two transfusion strategies after elective operations for myocardial revascularization. J Thorac Cardiovasc Surg 1992;104:307-14.
13. Fortune JB, Feustel PJ, Saifi J, Stratton HH, Neweil JC, Shah DM. Influence of hematocrit on cardiopulmonary function after acute hemorrhage. J Trauma 1987;27: 2434-49.
14. Hébert PC, Wells GA, Marshall JC, et al. Transfusion requirements in critical care. A pilot study. JAMA 1995;273:1439-44.
15. Vichinsky EP, Haberkern CM, Neumayr L, et al. A comparison of conservative and aggressive transfusion regimens in the perioperative management of sickle cell disease. N Engl J Med 1995;333:206-13.
16. Blair SD, Janvrin SB, McCollum CN, Greenhaigh RM. Effect of early blood transfusion on gastrointestinal haemorrhage. Br J Surg 1986;73:783-85.
17. Kowalyshyn TJ, Prager D, Young J. Preoperative hemoglobin requirements. Anesth Analg 1972;51:75-79.
18. Stehling LC, Ellison N, Faust RJ, Grotta AW, Moyers JR. A survey of transfusion practices among anesthesiologists. Vox Sang 1987;52:60-62.
19. Hébert PC, Schweitzer 1, Wells GA, et al. A survey of red cell transfusion practices in Canadian critical care practitioners. Clin Invest Med 1994;17(abstract):B22.
20. Nicholis MD, Whyte G. Red cell, plasma and albumin transfusion decision triggers. Anaesth Intensive Care 1993;21:156-62.
21. Price FV, Kelley JL, Edwards RP, Hasley PB, Amin RM. A survey of blood transfusion practices of gynecologic oncologists. Gynecol Oncol 1995;59:45-50.
22. Hébert PC, Wells G, Schweitzer I, et al. Red cell transfusion practices in the critically ill: the Canadian experience. Clin Invest Med 1995;18(abstract):B29.
23. Carson JL, Duff A, Poses RM, et al. Effect of anaemia and cardiovascular disease on surgical mortality and morbidity. Lancet 1996;348:1055-60.

24. Carson JL, Spence RK, Poses RM, Bonavita G. Severity of anaemia and operative mortality and morbidity. Lancet 1988;i:727-29.
25. Houbiers JGA, Brand A, van de Watering LMG, et al. Randomised controlled trial comparing transfusion of leucocyte-depleted or buffy-coat-depleted blood in surgery for colorectal cancer. Lancet 1996;344:573-78.
26. Van de Watering LMG, Houbiers JGA, Hermans J, et al. Leukocyte depletion reduces postoperative mortality in patients undergoing cardiac surgery. Br J Haematol 1996;93:312(abstract).
27. Jensen LS, Andersen AJ, Christiansen PM, et al. Postoperative infection and natural killer cell function following blood transfusion in patients undergoing elective colorectal surgery. Br J Surg 1992;79:513-16.
28. Jensen LS, Kissmeyer-Nielsen P, Wolff B, Qvist N. Randomised comparison of leucocyte-depleted versus buffy-coat-poor blood transfusion and complications after colorectal surgery. Lancet 1996;348:841-45.
29. Busch ORC, Hop WCJ, Hoynck van Papendrecht MAW, Marquet RL, Jeekel J. Blood transfusions and prognosis in colorectal cancer. N Engl J Med 1993;328:1372-76.
30. Heiss MM, Memple W, Jauch K, et al. Beneficial effects of autologous blood transfusion on infectious complications after colorectal cancer surgery. Lancet 1993;342: 1328-33.
31. Messmer KFW. Acceptable hematocrit levels in surgical patients. World J Surg 1987;11:41-46.
32. Messmer K, Kreimeier U, Intaglietta M. Present state of intentional hemodilution. Eur Surg Res 1986;18:254-63.
33. Messmer K, Sunder-Plassmann L, Klovekorn WP, Holper K. Circulatory significance of hemodilution: rheological changes and limitations. Adv Microcirc 1972;4:1-77.
34. Kennedy AC, Valtis DJ. The oxygen dissociation curve in anemia of various types. J Clin Invest 1954;33:1372-81.
35. Sugerman HJ, Davidson DT, Vibul S, Delivoria-Papadopoulos M, Miller LD, Oski FA. The basis of defective oxygen delivery from stored blood. Surg Gynecol Obstet 1970;137:733-41.
36. Race D, Dedichen H, Schenk WGJ. Regional blood flow during dextran-induced normovolemic hemodilution in the dog. J Thorac Cardiovasc Surg 1967;53:578-86.
37. Collins JA. Massive blood transfusion. Clinics Hematol. 1976;5:201-22.
38. Sohmer PR, Dawson RB. Transfusion therapy in trauma: a review of the principles and techniques used in the M.I.E.M.S. program. Ann Surg 1979;45:109-25.
39. McConn R, Derrick JB. The respiratory function of blood: transfusion and blood storage. Anesthesiology 1972;36:119-27.
40. Jesch F, Webber LM, Dalton JW, Carey JS. Oxygen dissociation after transfusion of blood stored in ACD or CPD solution. J Thorac Cardiovasc Surg 1975;70:35-39.
41. Haradin AR, Weed RI, Reed CF. Changes in physical properties of stored erythrocytes: relationship to survival in vivo. Transfusion 1969;9:229-37.
42. LaCelle PL. Alteration of deformability of the erythrocyte membrane in stored blood. Transfusion 1969;9:238-45.
43. Longster GH, Buckley T, Sikorsky J, Touey LAD. Scanning electron microscope studies of red cell morphology: changes occurring in red cell shape during storage and post transfusion. Vox Sang 1972;22:161-70.
44. Hurd TC, Dasmahapatra KS, Rush BF, Machiedo GW. Red blood cell deformability in human and experimental sepsis. Arch Surg 1988;123:217-20.
45. Langenfeld JE, Livingston DH, Machiedo GW. Red cell deformability is an early indicator of infection. Surgery 1991;110:398-404.

46. Baker CH, Wilmoth FR, Sutton ET. Reduced RBC versus plasma microvascular flow due to endotoxin. Circ Shock 1986;20:127-39.
47. Mollitt DL, Poulos ND. The role of pentoxyfilline in endotoxin-induced alterations of red cell deformability and whole blood viscosity in the neonate. J Pediatr Surg 1991;26:572-74.
48. Poweil RJ, Machiedo GW, Rush BFJ, Dikdan G. Oxygen free radicals: effect on red blood cell deformability in sepsis. Crit Care Med 1991;19:732-35.
49. Crosby ET. Perioperative haemotherapy: II. Risks and complications of blood transfusion. Can J Anesth 1992;39:822,-37.
50. Fielding LP, Stewart-Brown S, Dudley HAF. Surgeon-related variables and the clinical trial. Lancet 1978;778-79.
51. Van der Linden W. Pitfalls in randomized surgical trials. Surgery 1980;87:258-62.
52. Ratain JS, Hochberg MC. Clinical trials: a guide to understanding methodology and interpreting results. Arthritis Rheum 1990;33:131-39.
53. Sackett DL. The competing objectives of randomized trials. N Engl J Med 1980; 303:1059-60.
54. Sackett DL, Gent M. Controversy in counting and attributing events in clinical trials. N Engl J Med 1979;301:1410-12.
55. Fletcher RH, Fletcher SW, Wagner EH. Clinical epidemiology: the essentials. 2nd ed. Baltimore:Williams & Wilkins, 1988.
56. Kubinski JA, Rudy TE, Boston JR. Research design and analysis: the many faces of validity. J Crit Care 1991;6:1431-51.
57. Petros AJ, Marshall JC, van Saene HKF. Should morbidity replace mortality as an endpoint for clinical trials in intensive care? Lancet 1995;345:369-71.
58. Hébert PC, Schweitzer I, Calder L, Blajchman M, Giulivi A. Review of the clinical practice literature on allogeneic red blood cell transfusion. Can Med Assoc J 1997; 156:S9-S26.
59. ISIS-4 (Fourth International Study of Infarct Survival) Collaborative Group. ISIS-4: a randomised factorial trial assessing early oral captopril, oral mononitrate, and intravenous magnesium sulphate in 58,050 patients with suspected acute myocardial infarction. Lancet 1995;345:669-85.
60. ISIS-2 (Second International Study of Infarct Survival) Collaborative Group. Randomised trial of intravenous streptokinase, oral aspirin, both, or neither among 17,187 cases of suspected acute myocardial infarction: ISIS-2. Lancet 1988;349-60.
61. Lubsen J, Tijssen JGP. Large trials with simple protocols: indications and contraindications. Control Clin Trials 1989;10:151s-60s.
62. McCloskey RV, Straube RC, Sanders C, Smith SM, Smith CR, The CHESS Trial Study Group. Treatment of septic shock with human monoclonal antibody HA-1A. A randomized double-blind, placebo-controlled trial. Ann Intern Med 1994;121:1-5.
63. Ziegler EJ, Fisher CJJ, Sprung CL, et al. Treatment of gram-negative bacteremia and septic shock with HA-1A human monoclonal antibody against endotoxin. A randomized, double-blind, placebo-controlled trial. N Engl J Med 1991;324:429-36.
64. Fisher CJ, Dhainault JF, Opal SM. Recombinant human interleukin-1 receptor antagonist in the treatment of patients with sepsis syndrome: results from a randomized double-blind, placebo controlled trial. JAMA 1994;271:1836-43.
65. Abraham E, Raffin TA. Sepsis therapy trials. Continued disappointment or reason for hope? JAMA 1994;271:1876-78.

THE FUTURE OF HUMAN BLOOD RESOURCES

J.C. Fratantoni

Alternatives to transfusion

This Twente-Second International Symposium on Blood Transfusion has concentrated on alternative approaches to blood transfusion. That is really quite remarkable – a symposium on blood transfusion, organised and run by experts on blood transfusion is discussing alternatives to that very discipline. Perhaps remarkable, but a sign of intellectual health and vitality.

The place of blood transfusion in the medical armamentarium has changed radically in the past fifteen years. The state of mind that has led to discussion such as held at this symposium is well summarised in the advice that came from the American College of Physicians in 1992: "An allogeneic transfusion is an outcome to be avoided". This attitude is shared by the public, which has developed serious concerns about the safety of the blood supply. This is in sharp contrast to the situation that prevailed as recently as the late 1970s, when the transfusion community was proud of their achievements and the public gave them full confidence.

The past

At times it helps our thinking to step back a little and seek a better view of how we got to our present situation. If we think about the past, the relatively recent past, it is interesting to compare public attitudes toward other complex disciplines. In the cold war era, roughly from the late 19940s to 1990, public reaction to the military (or, at least, to the military-industrial complex) was mixed at best. Certainly, at times within the cold war era, there were strong negative feelings regarding defence spending and the ever present danger of nuclear war. This was in contrast to the unqualified public support enjoyed by the military during World War II and the immediate aftermath. During the war, while the public was in danger, and while the Allies were winning, there was confidence and trust in the military.

In the early 1980s, a different type of enemy appeared – AIDS. Most scientific authorities who have examined the record of those who were making decisions during those years have stated that the situation was handled as well as one could expect. Nonetheless, there were civilian casualties and, for some time, the enemy was winning. Public trust in the transfusion community was lost.

Reactions to AIDS

For purposes of our analysis, we will separate the reactions of the transfusion community to the events of the AIDS and post-AIDS eras into three categories:

- Immediate reactions: those that are sufficient to permit continued operations;
- Intermediate reactions: these are solutions that will partially address the problems at hand;
- Ultimate reactions: solutions based on sound science that satisfy all aspects of the problem.

Immediate actions

Situations requiring immediate action include those that have resulted from the increased regulatory, political and media attention to blood systems that has characterised the post-AIDS era. Recent examples include:

- A lengthy investigation in Canada resulting in a mandated change in directing authority of the nations' blood system;
- Extensive enforcement actions by the FDA resulting in imposition of judicial consent decrees on major blood systems including the American Red Cross, the New York Blood Center and United Blood Services. In effect, this meant that greater than 70% of the US blood supply was being managed by the federal government;
- Media and public scrutiny of all phases of blood operations in Ireland after a report in 1994 revealed that a production problem with anti-Rh immune globulin in the 1970s had led to transmission of hepatitis. The immune globulin manufacturing problem had been definitively resolved.

The immediate reactions taken by industry and the regulators have been designed to allay public fear, but they do not necessarily solve the underlying public health problem. Increased screening of blood and plasma donors, by questions and blood testing, has progressed to a point that may represent a loss of economic perspective. Some public health experts feel that the recent imposition of HIV antigen (p24) testing consumes resources that could be used more effectively.

The regulatory authorities have reacted with increased and more visible enforcement of the regulatory details, as illustrated above. There have also been situations in which policy has been made in the absence of clear data. An example is the FDA requirement that blood and plasma products be recalled if a donor is subsequently found to have been affected with, or at high risk for the spongiform encephalopathy, Creutzfeldt-Jakob Disease (CJD). To date, the transmission of CJD via transfusion is a theoretical possibility, not demonstrated with experimental or epidemiologic evidence. Nonetheless, the FDA has reacted to public concern and has made policy that is quite different from that put into effect by European authorities. The publication of the Institute of Medicine

(IOM) report on HIV and the Blood Supply was a crucial factor in the development of this policy.

Intermediate actions

The term "intermediate actions" is used to refer to responses to the type of problems discussed above that have the following properties:

- They alleviate, at least to some extent, the public fear;
- They provide some measure of improvement in the public health; but,
- They will not completely solve the underlying problem and, as a result, they will not fully address the economic challenges.

Dr. Lewis Thomas, one of the great biochemical thinkers of our time, referred to such approaches as "half-way technologies". Perhaps the most frequently cited example of a half-way technology is the respiratory assist devices used to treat patients with respiratory paralysis due to polio – these were called "iron lungs". Obviously, the definitive technology for that problem was the polio vaccine. Other examples of half-way technologies, examples that unfortunately are still with us, are renal dialysis and coronary artery bypass surgery. These procedures are accepted (in fact, they are demanded) by the public, are very expensive, but do not affect the basic cause of the medical problems involved.

We can find examples of half-way technologies within transfusion medicine. I believe that testing blood donors for infectious diseases qualifies as a half-way technology – it ameliorates public concern, is quite costly, but does not affect basic problems. The use of nucleic acid amplification techniques, such as the polymerase chain reaction (PCR), for donor testing adds sensitivity to the method, but still seems short of an ultimate solution.

A more fundamental question, and one that will be more contentious, relates to transfusion itself: is the transfusion of blood products derived from human donors a half-way technology? I will not try to answer that question, but will proceed to a discussion of ultimate responses and allow each of you to reach your own conclusions.

Ultimate actions

An increased understanding of the relevant basic science has led to complete solutions to some of the diseases discussed above in conjunction with half-way technologies. The paralytic complications of polio have been eliminated by controlling the disease with polio vaccine, the development of which was dependent upon fundamental research on growing viruses in tissue culture. Appreciation of the relationship between Streptococcal disease and glomerulonephritis has led to clinical regimens that prevent chronic renal failure and avoid the need for dialysis. Although diabetes mellitus is still a prevalent medical problem and is not completely understood, the increased knowledge of the basis for diabetic vascular complications has led to better management of patients and decreased serious complications, including the need for coronary artery bypass and renal dialysis. Finally, improvements in diet and drugs, especially anti-hypertensive agents, again based on fundamental understanding of biological processes, have led to a decreased incidence of coronary artery disease.

What is the ultimate solution to medical problems that are now treated by transfusion with blood components. It does not seem that we will ever be able to ask donors all the questions or test them for all possible pathogens. Let us consider the other possibilities:

- Completely effective infectious agent inactivation? I think all the words are important here. It must be *completely effective*, since the transmission rates are already extremely low and we are seeking zero transmission. We must speak of *infectious agents* since there may be categories of such entities that are yet to be discovered. Can all this be accomplished without damaging red cells or platelets? This will be a difficult challenge;
- Can cells be produced using in vitro culture systems? The scale production must be beyond anything that has been realised to date. The system must be genetically stable. There will be a possibility of infection of the system and testing or sterilisation will be needed. In a sense, the in vitro system does not have many advantages over the human donor;
- We have heard status reports on non-cellular red cell and platelet substitutes and seen that, in spite of considerable effort, the goal has not yet been achieved. The possibility that substitutes for specific and limited indications will be available in the foreseeable future seems good. Platelet substitutes are receiving increased attention in recent years. These pose especially difficult problems but, once again, for specific indications the problems seem to be approachable;
- Gene therapy and transplantation offer solutions to basic defects underlying some of the diseases requiring transfusion. The risk/benefit considerations are often daunting, e.g. how does one compute the potential benefit/risk of bone marrow transplantation for treatment of thalassemia major compared to the risk/benefit of transfusion therapy, with associated iron overload, for that disease. There are also technical hurdles posed by these approaches that remain to be solved. Again, basic information is needed.

We can ask similar questions about potential ultimate solutions for the disorders now treated with plasma derivatives. Viral inactivation has been quite successful in dealing with lipid-enveloped viruses. Non-enveloped viruses, such as parvovirus B19, tend to be more resistant to the methods used for enveloped viruses and different procedures, such as nanofiltration are used to remove such viruses. Applicability of such procedures are limited. The spongiform encephalopathies, exemplified by CJD, are caused by poorly understood agents and procedures to protect plasma derivatives from such diseases must await better understanding of the underlying processes.

The complexity of diseases like CJD and the potential that other unexpected diseases will appear has led some to conclude that, in the future, the products now obtained from plasma should be derived via recombinant technology. Such approaches are already in use for production of coagulation factors (Factor VIII and Factor IX), for which the appropriate genes have been inserted into cultured cell expression systems. The coagulation products are administered in relatively small doses and are used by a limited population. In these cases, cell culture systems appear adequate to meet the demand. For protein products used in larger quantities, different approaches will be needed. Albumin is a case in point. When administered as a plasma volume expander, hundreds of millilitres of 5% or 25% solution may be used. Albumin is also used as an excipient for many therapeutic agents, including cytokines and vaccines. To meet this demand, a transgenic expression system would be the logical choice and plant systems may provide a measure of actual and perceived safety that exceeds that possible from animal systems. Will such approaches truly provide safety that is beyond that achievable with human donors, or will it still be a matter of risk perception? Only the future will tell us.

The blood bank of the future

What, then, will be the blood bank of the future? How will the future transfusion medicine specialist be involved in the delivery of medical care? Will the transfusion medicine specialist be:

- A provider of medical services related to transfusion?
- A manufacturer of transfusion products, with a full understanding of quality systems?
- A molecular biologist, transplantation expert, geneticist?

Obviously, there is no way for us to know the answer. When we consider the pace of change in recent years, the possibility of predicting the future seems even less possible. Consider that the very word "recombinant" did not exist when many of us were in medical or graduate school. There are few things, however, of which we can be fairly certain:

- Success will require resourcefulness and innovation. This has been immutable truth over the ages;
- An obvious corollary of the need for innovation is that the environment and resources that permit innovation must be preserved. This refers not only to financial support, although that is critical, but to the environment, the working conditions provided for creative people.

A closing thought

This symposium has realistically addressed the questions associated with changing attitudes toward transfusion. In doing so, it has conformed with advice given by the physicist and author, Isaac Asimov,

> *"No sensible decision can be made any longer without taking into account not only the world as it is, but the world as it will be."*

DISCUSSION

J.C. Fratantoni, P.C. Das

A. Laupacis, Ottawa, C: I listened to dr. AuBuchon's superb talk. He indicated that a lot of economic evaluations of technologies in the transfusion area have shown that they are highly cost-ineffective compared to other interventions. Yet we seem to be ignoring this information in health policy. One reason might be that, in Canada at least, I think part of transfusion medicine has functioned more or less outside the conventional health care system. So, when blood is ordered by a clinician, the clinician tends not to think about the costs of blood since the hospital does not pay for it. I wonder whether more attention needs to be paid in these economic analyses to whom actually pays for the blood. The second issue is that because we understand how much we as a society pay for blood, people tend not to pay that much attention to the increased aggregate costs of blood transfusion.

J.P. AuBuchon, Lebanon, NH, USA: I appreciate your comments and I agree with them. I think your observations are entirely correct. There is something different about transfusion, but even more specifically I think there is something different about viral infection transmitted through transfusion. Maybe it is related to how HIV has been transmitted outside of transfusion. That makes it part of a "sexy" issue because the public is not concerned about patients dying from receiving the wrong unit of blood, that rarely makes the headlines and certainly never gets any congressional attention. All you have to do is but whisper the word AIDS and it sends everyone running to the laboratory to perform another test or pushes us back into the laboratory to do another test. I am not sure exactly why that situation is so different in aggregate. Dr. Fratantoni, you may have better numbers than I do, but I believe it has been estimated that the cost of providing blood transfusion in the United States for about 250 million people is around 2 billion dollars a year.

J.C. Fratantoni, Rockville, MD, USA: Somewhere in that neighbourhood, which sounds like a lot of money and it is a lot of money. But when we look at interventions it pales in comparison to how else the Federal Government or society spends its money. I am privileged to sit on a national committee that is charged with looking at blood safety and availability and charged with including issues of costs; we recently considered hepatitis C in the United States and questions were raised about its costs and when numbers in the several hundred million dollar range were put out all the blood bankers gasped, because several million dollars in their budget meant a lot of money represented from the Federal Government. They really woke up from a slumber. So, there is something different about transfusion. I am sorry to give you a rambling answer but I do not really have an answer to the situation.

I guess the difference between HIV and dying from an AB0 mismatch is just that one can pass on HIV to relatives which I think is an issue that often is not discussed as much as it might be.

J.P. AuBuchon: I happen to deal with decision analysis and is it indeed a rational question to ask whether we did not spend money on p24 antigen testing would June Osborne have additional money to spend on AIDS prevention? Unfortunately the answer is no. The congress in the United States rarely looks at issues like that closely, starting with a fixed budget and allocating to one direction or another. They do have some trade-offs when they are talking about buying a hundred new warplanes versus an entirely new welfare system and there are some trade-offs between those, but when they get down to the "small change" they are not going to be involved in the trade-offs. The FDA had demanded that the testing be done by the blood centres; the blood centres are passing the cost of testing onto the hospitals; the hospitals are not getting any more money. In the case of my institution we are paying about 75,000 dollars a year more for the privilege of getting p24 antigen tested blood. We are not getting any more money to support our patient care so we have to decide not to spend the 75,000 dollars somewhere else. To a congressman that is immaterial but to us it has forced some decisions.

A. Brand, Leiden, NL: Dr. Hébert, you presented a study in which you compared transfusion triggers between two levels; you also referred to rabbits in which fresh blood and old blood was compared and you are doing now a large study. I think within the population that you study you can ask a very simple question which may have large consequences for final outcome of patients for instance fresh versus stored blood; do you consider that for your critical ill patients' study?

P.C. Hébert, Ottawa, C: When we designed our clinical trial, the study was undertaken at 30 centres and when the age of blood question came up because in our laboratory and in our patients we were looking at that, the study had already been approved without the age of blood issue as part of the design. What we had decided to do in the first few months prior to allocation of patients was to measure age of blood. So when the results of the trial came out neither during the full publication nor within the full publication or thereafter will be reporting age of blood or age of blood effects. If we were to do this study again and had we decided to do this prior to getting a large medical research council grant the age of blood issue might have figured more prominently. I think we would have undertaken a factorial design looking at high and low transfusion thresholds and then also allocating by fresh or old blood. I am sorry to ramble again but the other difficulty we had was a pragmatic one, we were not assured of getting fresh blood upon request in patients randomised within the trial. So not only did we have the problem with the design of the study that was done before the age of blood issue came out, we also had very pragmatic issues whereby we could not implement the trial the way we wanted to. So the question is important.

A. Brand: It is more or less a question to the whole of the panel; I think we are missing opportunities talking about these risks of viruses and AB0 mistakes. We are transfusing everyday with indications of which we do not know whether they are true and we can make comparisons, enormous numbers of comparisons.

P.C. Hébert: Getting back to the whole blood I think dr. Winslow pointed this out. When we decided to store blood on the shelf for 30 days the criteria for storage was cell survival and had nothing to do with the efficacy of the product. That is an unfortunate sort of side-track but I guess it was done for various reasons I was not aware of at the time. But now the age of blood issue I think is going to become a very real one and it is becoming more one because of available alternatives, but certainly age of blood and at least the laboratory setting are showing that the transport of oxygen is not the same as the product changes over time.

C.Th. Smit Sibinga, Groningen, NL: I think the opportunity is now coming closer to get more precise information on the effectiveness as you called it of transfusion in various situations because all over the world, at least in the industrialised world the part of the total quality system in the transfusion chain named haemovigilance is coming up. I think by doing studies based on more accurate documentation of the effectiveness so the actual outcome of the transfusion (not only the wanted one but also the other effects) may give us better ideas of what actually is on and how the risks are. A comment in that respect is: HIV is usually the example because that is surrounded with all the negativity but also with all the assumptiveness around risk. At this point in time we all know that no longer HIV is the major threat, the major occurring infection in blood transfusion is HCV and it is also known from studies[1,2,3] that there is a substantial nosocomial infection risk outside the transfusion. However, surprisingly this issue of the nosocomial infection risk has never gained any attention and there are to my knowledge no real studies done to unravel what it is in the nosocomial factors and how you could prevent that.

---

1. Allander T, Gruber A, Naphavi M et al. Frequent patient-to-patient transmission of hepatitis C in a haematology ward. Lancet 1995;345:603-07.
2. Bronowichi JP, Venard V, Botté C et al. Patient-to-patient transmission of hepatitis C virus during colonoscopy. N Engl J Med 1997;337:237-40.
3. Keur I, Schneeberger PM, v.d. Graaf Y, Vos J, van Dijk WC, van Doorn LJ. Risk factors for HCV infection in two haemodialysis units in the Netherlands. Neth J Med 1997;50:97-101.

P.C. Hébert: Maybe I can highlight a few things from your comment. The first point I guess because of time I did not conclude actually, but I mean the point of my talk was that randomised trials are crucial. A single randomised trial will not give you the answer; we are dealing with multiple diseases. Not just in critical care but with transfusion medicine you are dealing with a whole spectrum of diseases and it is very likely that a number of studies will be required to answer some of the even very basic questions that we have not addressed yet; so that is point number one. Point number two is that when you look at randomised trials one study does not do it. In transfusion medicine there are a lot of small 30 to 50 patient trials, when you read the literature on various topics. Those types of studies are highly select and people take with them the "will it work" answer. The problem is there was only one level one trial that we were able to find going from 1960 to now with multiple search techniques, that was the Vichinsky trial in the N Engl J Med[4] which randomly allocated 604 patients to the question of conservative liberal and looking at prevention of sickle cell crises; that is the only study in the whole domain of trying to determine whether you should give more blood or less and that would apply to any new intervention we undertake in this system. So one of the pleas I would have is we need to do not simple little trials which are necessary but not sufficient, but to start undertaking the larger studies that need to be done with blood substitutes. Fortunately, they will be mandated by other management strategies or clinical practice guidelines.

B. McClelland, Edinburgh, UK: Thank you for your review of the issues. Having just been struggling for the last 18 months with setting up a randomised controlled trial of transfusion in the clinical situation I think all the points that dr. Hébert made are extremely practical and I think we have encountered every one of them. They are all difficult because it is an old-fashioned intervention that has been around for a long time and everybody "knows" how to do it. Two points from our pilot study the same findings although we are looking at different groups of patients. The first is there is a zone uncertainty where clinicians do not know what to do. This is between a haemoglobin of 8 grams and 10 grams in an elderly population following the repair of hip fracture. So it is interesting that the uncertainties are the same in the ITU group although the population is very different. Secondly having randomised to an 8 and a 10 gram haemoglobin postoperative management protocol the amount of red cell transfusion is halved in the low trigger, which I think is rather similar to what came out of your study. I suspect what we will see is that we will have to study large numbers of patients before we will be able to see an outcome other than this difference in blood utilisation and nothing very striking in terms of other outcomes that are important to the patient.

P.C. Hébert: I will briefly comment on the issue of polarisation. As many of you are aware, the concept that I have outlined has been elaborated in a New

4. Vichinsky EP, Haberkern CM, Meremayr L. A comparison of conservative and aggressive transfusion regimes in the perioperative management of sickle cell disease. N Engl J Med 1995;333:206-13.

England Journal of Medicine publication by a gentleman called Benjamin Freedman[5]. A perceived difficulty with randomised control trials was the loss of control by clinicians in the decision making process. Thus, the issue of individuality in making patient based decisions was considered a huge problem. This can be defined as the concept of individual uncertainty or individual equipoise. The major revelation by Freedman was to move the concept of uncertainty from individual clinicians to groups of expert clinicians. In considering a patient for randomised control trial, both therapies would be considered of equally uncertain benefit by the expert medical community at the time of randomisation of a patient. Once uncertainty is no longer present then that patient can no longer be randomised into a clinical trial. At the bedside the clinician needs to be uncertain at an individual level regarding the risks and benefits of therapy and accept the judgement of the expert medical community. If the patient's physician has excessively polarised views regarding a therapy, then perhaps individual uncertainty should supersede the expert medical community's opinion. However, individual clinicians usually do not randomise patients when they believe that a therapy is either beneficial or risky. So, I quite agree with you. It becomes quite a difficult issue in management type trials when both therapeutic options are known to the practitioner. In drug studies physicians must only agree to the concept of drug A and drug B. Given that this study is blinded, there is less concern regarding randomisation.

R.M. Winslow, San Diego, CA, USA: I applaud this discussion about clinical trials to test transfusion triggers. I think we are going to learn a lot from them, but we have to be prepared that the outcome from those trials may not be so clear cut because of the problems about blood volume, because haematocrit and haemoglobin are only measuring a part of the issue. Dr. Valeri, I first really want to agree with what you said about the blood volume. It is critically important but it has not gotten the attention because it is so difficult to measure. Why has not some clever person come up with a handy way to measure plasma volume? It seems to me that it should not be that difficult; why is it?

C.R. Valeri, Boston, MA, USA: This is a very important question because for years everyone assumed that albumin would be the ideal molecule to measure the plasma volume. All the studies that have been published show that in patients albumin rapidly distributes into the extravascular space. At the time we were studying these wounded servicemen returning from Vietnam at the Chelsea Naval Hospital, our only way to document the contracted plasma volume was to use the IgM cold agglutinin molecule with a molecular weight of 1 million which was iodinated to measure plasma volume. The plasma volume can be estimated from the red cell volume measured using chromium and/or technetium and the total body haematocrit. We are now using biotin-X-NHS, which is a non-radioactive label, to estimate the red cell volume. The best way to estimate plasma volume in patients is to measure the red cell volume with 51-chromium and/or 99mTc and then to estimate the plasma volume from the total

5. Freedman B. Equipoise and the ethics of clinical research. N Engl J Med 1987;317:141-45.

body haematocrit. Albumin cannot be used to measure the plasma volume in patients. A substance which will circulate only in the plasma volume is needed, like IgM with a molecular weight of 1 million.

P.C. Das, Groningen, NL: Dr. Valeri, you were suggesting aggressive transfusion therapy in a clinical trial but would that be cost-effective?

C.R. Valeri: It is well known that the preoperative red cell volume of patients subjected to cardiopulmonary bypass surgery predicts outcome. The red cell transfusion requirements in patients undergoing cardio-pulmonary by-pass surgery are dependent on 1) the preoperative haematocrit, 2) length of by-pass 3) age of the patient and 4) the sex of the patient. Non-surgical blood loss following cardiopulmonary bypass surgery can be measured accurately following neutralisation of the heparin with protamine. Maintenance of normothermia, a reduction in the degree of haemodilution will reduce non-surgical blood loss and the requirements for red cell transfusion. I agree with dr. Winslow that the haematocrit is a very poor indicator of the red cell volume. We have data to support that red cell transfusions reduce non-surgical bleeding in patients following cardiopulmonary bypass surgery. The aggressive use of red cell transfusions may reduce mortality and morbidity and this approach may prove to be cost-effective.

C.Th. Smit Sibinga: So, what would then be your suggestion for a more optimal algorithm.

C.R. Valeri: Data are needed to define an algorithm for transfusion of red cells. Studies are needed to evaluate the treatment of patients with non-surgical blood loss. Prospective randomised studies should be done to evaluate the transfusion of red cells alone and the transfusion of red cells, platelets, and fresh frozen plasma, on mortality and morbidity. A critical haematocrit at the bleeding time site is needed to prevent non-surgical blood loss. In 1983, dr. Shukri Khuri told me that consultations with haematologists and neurologists provided him with little useful assistance to treat patients following cardiopulmonary bypass surgery. In 1983 dr. Khuri reported[6] that when he had a patient who was severely haemodiluted and was bleeding diffusely without a surgical cause, the transfusion of red cells alone would restore haemostasis. Today, in 1997, I am convinced that red cells have a critical role in haemostasis.

C.Th. Smit Sibinga: That then means actually that you would advise dr. Hébert and others to give the clinical picture parameter a higher rank.

C.R. Valeri: Yes, when I was trained in medicine, I was impressed that orthopaedic surgeons would feel the temperature of the patient's big toe following an

---

6. Khuri SF, Wolfe JA, Josa MT et al. Hematologic changes during and after cardiopulmonary bypass and their relationship to the bleeding time and nonsurgical blood loss. J Thorac Cardiovasc Surg1992;104;94-107.

orthopaedic procedure and then tell the resident to transfuse the patient a unit of red cells and then the following day again feel the temperature of the big toe and would order another unit of red cells. Peripheral perfusion of the extremity can be assessed by measuring the temperature of the big toe and the orthopaedic surgeon used this clinical technique to determine the need for red cell transfusions. Red cell transfusions increase the peripheral blood volume and blood flow to the extremities and the gastrointestinal tract. Restoration of the peripheral blood volume, especially to the gastrointestinal tract, is needed to reduce morbidity and mortality of following resuscitation of hypovolaemic-hypotensive patients.

P.C. Hébert: Can I address a few of these questions. First, a number of my patients die warm with warm big toes, particularly patients with multi-organ failure where I cannot find a source of infection in after intensive investigation. This group of patients usually has a peripheral vascular defect which does not enable skin temperature to be an accurate reflection of forward flow. Thus, patients do die warm and poorly perfused. Second, though I agree peripheral perfusion is crucial, in contradiction to dr. Valeri, I do not believe that haematocrit alone determines peripheral perfusion. In fact, in most of my patients, a number of resuscitative measures including fluids, inotropes, mechanical ventilation, will all change perfusion status. Indeed, there are at least six randomised trials evaluating various means of augmenting oxygen delivery in critically ill patients. One of these studies was done in Italy by dr. Gattinoni[7]. In this study three goal directed resuscitation protocols were evaluated. The study demonstrated that augmenting oxygen delivery through fluids and pharmacologic means did not improve outcomes. Therefore, over resuscitation of patients may not be beneficial and in fact may be harmful.

I would like to address dr. Winslow's comment regarding the interaction between haemstocrit, blood volume and diagnosis. First, there were no differences in baseline characteristics amongst patients randomised to both groups. All variables either directly or indirectly associated with oxygen delivery were comparable at baseline. Second, we were unable to detect any statistically or clinically important differences in various patient subgroups including patients with cardiovascular disease. We searched up and down looking for such differences and were unable to find them. Perhaps we do not understand the physiologic basis for our results, but outcomes of this study were the outcomes of the study. I believe we must now search to explain the results of this trial by examining various hypotheses. Indeed, the study illustrates why clinical trials often better illucidate mechanisms of disease. The results of this study would seem to indicate that amongst the number of possible reasons for our results, some of them appear to be more important than others.

---

7. Gattioni L, Brazzi L, Pelosi L et al. A trial of goal oriented haemodynamic therapy in critically ill patients. N Engl J Med 1995;333:1025-32.

A. Lust, Aalst, B: Did I understand well dr. Valeri that you make us forget every perioperative dilution, and every preoperative autologous "predeposit donation" haemodilution and therefore risk of more bleeding for the patient.

C.R. Valeri: I miss the point are you saying that under haemodilution you observe more bleeding, have you made that observation?

A. Lust: It is something I understood.

C.R. Valeri: Severely haemodiluted patients have an increased tendency for non-surgical blood loss. Dr. Shukri Khuri reported[8] that haemodiluted patients with non-surgical blood loss stop bleeding following transfusion of red blood cells. Dr. Khuri[9] reported that red cells act like Elmer's glue to reduce non-surgical blood loss in patients that are haemodiluted.

---

8. Valeri CR, Khabbaz K, Khuri SF et al. Effect of skin temperature on platelet function in patients undergoing extracorporeal bypass. J Thorac Cardiovasc Surg 1992;104:108-16.
9. Khuri SF, Valeri CR, Loscalzo J et al. Heparin causes platelet dysfunction and induces fibrinolysis before cardiopulmonary bypass. Am Thorac Surg 1995;60:1008-14.

INDEX

DEVELOPMENTS IN HEMATOLOGY AND IMMUNOLOGY

1. H.R. Lijnen, D. Collen and M. Verstraete (eds.): *Synthetic Substrates in Clinical Blood Coagulation Assays*. 1980 ISBN 90-247-2409-0
2. C.Th. Smit Sibinga, P.C. Das and J.O. Forfar (eds.): *Paediatrics and Blood Transfusion*. Proceedings of the 5th Annual Symposium on Blood Transfusion, organized by the Red Cross Bloodbank Groningen-Drenthe, The Netherlands (1980). 1982 ISBN 90-247-2619-0
3. N. Fabris (ed.): *Immunology and Ageing*. 1982 ISBN 90-247-2640-9
4. G. Hornstra: *Dietary Fats, Prostanoids and Arterial Thrombosis*. With an Introductory Chapter by A. Bleakley Chandler. 1982 ISBN 90-247-2667-0
5. C.Th. Smit Sibinga, P.C. Das and J.J. van Loghem (eds.): *Blood Transfusion and Problems of Bleeding*. Proceedings of the 6th Annual Symposium on Blood Transfusion, organized by the Red Cross Bloodbank Groningen-Drenthe (1981). 1982 ISBN 90-247-3058-9
6. J. Dormandy (ed.): *Red Cell Deformability and Filterability*. 1983 ISBN 0-89838-578-4
7. C.Th. Smit Sibinga, P.C. Das and H.F. Taswell (eds.): *Quality Assurance in Blood Banking and Its Clinical Impact*. Proceedings of the 7th Annual Symposium on Blood Transfusion, organized by the Red Cross Bloodbank Groningen-Drenthe (1982). 1984 ISBN 0-89838-618-7
8. A.M.H.P. van den Besselaar, H.R. Gralnick and S.M. Lewis (eds.): *Thromboplastin Calibration and Oral Anticoagulant Control*. 1984 ISBN 0-89838-637-3
9. P. Fondu and O. Thijs (eds.): *Haemostatic Failure in Liver Disease*. 1984 ISBN 0-89838-640-3
10. C.Th. Smit Sibinga, P.C. Das and G. Opelz (eds.): *Transplantation and Blood Transfusion*. Proceedings of the 8th Annual Symposium on Blood Transfusion, organized by the Red Cross Bloodbank Groningen-Drenthe (1983). 1984 ISBN 0-89838-686-1
11. H. Schmid-Schönbein, L.J. Wurzinger and R.E. Zimmerman (eds.): *Enzyme Activation in Blood-perfused Artificial Organs*. 1985 ISBN 0-89838-704-3
12. J. Dormandy (ed.): *Blood Filtration and Blood Cell Deformability*. 1985 ISBN 0-89838-714-0
13. C.Th. Smit Sibinga, P.C. Das and E. Seidl (eds.): *Plasma Fractionation and Blood Transfusion*. Proceedings of the 9th Annual Symposium on Blood Transfusion, organized by the Red Cross Bloodbank Groningen-Drenthe (1984). 1985 ISBN 0-89838-761-2
14. S. Dawids and A. Bantjes (eds.): *Blood Compatible Materials and their Testing*. 1986 ISBN 0-89838-813-9
15. C.Th. Smit Sibinga, P.C. Das and T.J. Greenwalt (eds.): *Future Developments in Blood Banking*. Proceedings of the 10th Annual Symposium on Blood Transfusion, organized by the Red Cross Bloodbank Groningen-Drenthe (1985). 1986 ISBN 0-89838-824-4
16. A. Berlin, J. Dean, M.H. Draper, E.M.B. Smith and F. Spreafico (eds.): *Immunotoxicology*. Proceedings of the International Seminar on the Immunological System as a Target for Toxic Damage – Present Status, Open Problems and Future Perspectives, in collaboration with the UNEP-ILO-WHO IPCS and the Commission of the European Communities. 1987 ISBN 0-89838-843-0
17. T. Ottenhoff and R. de Vries: *Recognition of M. leprae Antigens*. 1987 ISBN 0-89838-887-2
18. J.-L. Touraine, R.P. Gale and V. Kochupillai (eds.): *Fetal Liver Transplantation*. 1987 ISBN 0-89838-975-5
19. C.Th. Smit Sibinga P.C. Das and C.P. Engelfriet (eds.): *White Cells and Platelets in Blood Transfusion*. Proceedings of the 11th Annual Symposium on Blood Transfusion, organized by the Red Cross Bloodbank Groningen-Drenthe (1986). 1987 ISBN 0-89838-976-3
20. C.F.M. Hendriksen: *Laboratory Animals in Vaccine Production and Control*. 1988 ISBN 0-89838-398-6

21. C.Th. Smit Sibinga, P.C. Das and L.R. Overby (eds.): *Biotechnology in Blood Transfusion.* Proceedings of the 12th Annual Symposium on Blood Transfusion, organized by the Red Cross Bloodbank Groningen-Drenthe (1987). 1988 ISBN 0-89838-404-4
22. C.Th. Smit Sibinga, P.C. Das and C.F. Högman (eds.): *Automation in Blood Transfusion.* Proceedings of the 13th Annual Symposium on Blood Transfusion, organized by the Red Cross Bloodbank Groningen-Drenthe (1988). 1989 ISBN 0-7923-0488-8
23. S. Dawids (ed.): *Polymers: Their Properties and Blood Compatibility.* 1989 ISBN 0-7923-0491-8
24. C.Th. Smit Sibinga, P.C. Das and H.T. Meryman (eds.): *Cryopreservation and Low Temperature Biology in Blood Transfusion.* Proceedings of the 14th Annual Symposium on Blood Transfusion, organized by the Red Cross Bloodbank Groningen-Drenthe (1989). 1990 ISBN 0-7923-0908-1
25. C.Th. Smit Sibinga and L. Kater (eds.): *Advances in Haemapheresis.* Proceedings of the 3rd International Congress of the World Apheresis Association (Amsterdam, The Netherlands, 1990). 1991 ISBN 0-7923-1312-7
26. C.Th. Smit Sibinga, P.C. Das and P.M. Mannucci (eds.): *Coagulation and Blood Transfusion.* Proceedings of the 15th Annual Symposium on Blood Transfusion, organized by the Red Cross Bloodbank Groningen-Drenthe (1990). 1991 ISBN 0-7923-1331-3
27. C.Th. Smit Sibinga, P.C. Das and J.D. Cash (eds.): *Transfusion Medicine: Fact and Fiction.* Proceedings of the 16th International Symposium on Blood Transfusion, organized by the Red Cross Bloodbank Groningen-Drenthe (1991). 1992 ISBN 0-7923-1732-7
28. C.Th. Smit Sibinga, P.C. Das and T.H. The (eds.): *Immunology and Blood Transfusion.* Proceedings of the 17th International Symposium on Blood Transfusion, organized by the Red Cross Bloodbank Groningen-Drenthe (1992). 1993 ISBN 0-7923-2380-7
29. C.Th. Smit Sibinga, P.C. Das and H.J. Heiniger (eds.): *Good Manufacturing Practice in Transfusion Medicine.* Proceedings of the 18th International Symposium on Blood Transfusion, organized by the Red Cross Blood Bank Groningen-Drenthe (1993). 1994 ISBN 0-7923-3009-9
30. C.Th. Smit Sibinga, P.C. Das and E. Briët (eds.): *Hereditary Diseases and Blood Transfusion.* Proceedings of the 19th International Symposium on Blood Transfusion, organized by the Red Cross Blood Bank Groningen-Drenthe (1994). 1995 ISBN 0-7923-3694-1
31. C.Th. Smit Sibinga, P.C. Das and E.L. Snyder (eds.): *Trigger Factors in Transfusion Medicine.* Proceedings of the 20th International Symposium on Blood Transfusion, organized by the Red Cross Blood Bank Noord-Nederland (1995). 1996 ISBN 0-7923-4225-0
32. C.Th. Smit Sibinga, P.C. Das and B. Löwenberg (eds.): *Cytokines and Growth Factors in Blood Transfusion.* Proceedings of the 21th International Symposium on Blood Transfusion, organized by the Red Cross Blood Bank Noord-Nederland (1996). 1997 ISBN 0-7923-4787-0
33. C.Th. Smit Sibinga, P.C. Das and J.C. Fratantoni (eds.): *Alternative Approaches to Human Blood Resources in Clinical Practice.* 1998 ISBN 0-7923-8305-2

KLUWER ACADEMIC PUBLISHERS – DORDRECHT / BOSTON / LONDON

MIX
Papier aus verantwortungsvollen Quellen
Paper from responsible sources
FSC® C105338

If you have any concerns about our products,
you can contact us on
ProductSafety@springernature.com

In case Publisher is established outside the EU,
the EU authorized representative is:
Springer Nature Customer Service Center GmbH
Europaplatz 3, 69115 Heidelberg, Germany

Printed by Libri Plureos GmbH
in Hamburg, Germany